THE WOMANLY ART OF
breastfeeding

THE WOMANLY ART OF
breastfeeding
Seventh Revised Edition

A PLUME BOOK

PLUME
Published by the Penguin Group
Penguin Group (USA) Inc., 375 Hudson Street, New York, New York 10014, U.S.A.
Penguin Books Ltd, 80 Strand, London WC2R 0RL, England
Penguin Books Australia Ltd, 250 Camberwell Road, Camberwell, Victoria 3124, Australia
Penguin Books Canada Ltd, 10 Alcorn Avenue, Toronto, Ontario, Canada M4V 3B2
Penguin Books India (P) Ltd, 11 Community Centre,
Panchsheel Park, New Delhi – 110 017, India
Penguin Books (NZ), cnr Airborne and Rosedale Roads,
Albany, Auckland 1310, New Zealand
Penguin Books (South Africa) (Pty) Ltd, 24 Sturdee Avenue,
Rosebank, Johannesburg 2196, South Africa

Penguin Books Ltd, Registered Offices: 80 Strand, London WC2R 0RL, England

Published by Plume, a member of Penguin Group (USA) Inc.

First Plume Printing (Seventh Edition), May 2004
10 9 8 7 6 5 4 3 2

Published by arrangement with La Leche League International.

REGISTERED TRADEMARK—MARCA REGISTRADA

CIP data is available.
ISBN 0-452-28580-1

Printed in the United States of America
Designed by Digital Concepts, L.L.C.
Seventh edition revised and edited by Judy Torgus and Gwen Gotsch

Photo credits are listed in the appendix.

DEDICATION

We dedicate this book with much love to the many caring parents who have helped make La Leche League what it is today, and to our patient, loving husbands and children, all of whom helped the seven of us learn the womanly art of breastfeeding.

This book could not have been written and the basic principles underlying the work of La Leche League would not have withstood the test of time, had it not been for the unfailing counsel of Doctors Herbert Ratner and Gregory White, both of whom recently passed away. These two physicians wholeheartedly supported us from the earliest days of La Leche League. For this, we are most grateful.

CONTENTS

FOREWORD

I would not be alive today if not for breastfeeding.

In 1941, when I was born, the little village at the foothill of the mountain range between Thailand and Malaysia was caught madly in the battles of the start of World War II. But I was fortunate. My mother nursed me with the goodness of her milk and the love and care that came with it.

The natural power of breastfeeding is one of the greatest wonders of the world. It is about real love. It is about caring and celebrating the wondrous joy of nurturing a new life. It is about enjoying being a woman.

In a world too often dominated by materialism and greed, every act of the natural power of breastfeeding reminds us that there is another way, the natural way, the breastfeeding way.

Breastfeeding is about the power of peace, the power of goodness, and the power of responsibility.

Today, all over the world, women demonstrate this power by choosing to breastfeed. They celebrate this power and joy by helping other mothers who wish to exercise this natural choice.

Today, all over the world, the people in La Leche League International (LLLI) make breastfeeding happen. Through the partnership that LLLI forges with the World Alliance for Breastfeeding Action (WABA), groups all over the world act in unison to protect, to promote, and to support breastfeeding worldwide. And from August 1 to 7, every year, thousands of groups and millions of people celebrate this great cause through World Breastfeeding Week.

The United Nations, particularly through the United Nations Children's Fund (UNICEF), and the World Health Organization (WHO) have provided a Code that serves as a global framework to ensure that the culture of breastfeeding is not undermined.

The greatest power of all in ensuring the maintenance of the culture of breastfeeding is going to be the living example of breastfeeding mothers everywhere, demonstrating and sharing their knowledge and their wisdom about this universal heritage. This is why LLLI is so important and why this book is so necessary.

Mother-to-mother support is the warm, family, and community way and this book helps to gather the great wisdom into useful information. Don't be without it and don't forget to give a copy to a friend. It is this kind of assertive action, this linking and multiplying, that will help more and more mothers, and children, to share in the joy and power of a breastfeeding culture. It's baby-friendly, it's mother-friendly, it's family-friendly, it's community-friendly, it's eco-friendly, and good economics, too.

Enjoy!

Anwar Fazal
Chairperson
World Alliance for Breastfeeding Action (WABA)
Recipient of the Right Livelihood Award,
popularly called the "Alternative Nobel Prize"
Penang, Malaysia, May 1997

INTRODUCTION

Breastfeeding a baby—what could be more natural? Just cradle that precious newborn in your arms and offer him your breast. It sounds easy enough.

Breastfeeding a baby is simple and natural—if you know how to do it and what to expect. But it takes information and encouragement and some motherly know-how to breastfeed a baby, as the seven of us who founded La Leche League quickly discovered with our first breastfeeding attempts. How often should you nurse? How long on each side? How do you know if baby is getting enough to eat? What other foods does he need? And what if he seems hungry again only an hour after he has been fed?

When the seven of us found each other in 1956 and formed La Leche League, answers to such questions were as scarce as mother's milk itself. But we had breastfed a combined total of twenty-four babies, and by then had a good idea of what did and didn't work, what was and wasn't helpful. The secret of success in breastfeeding a baby, we had discovered, was having the right information and having another breastfeeding mother to turn to for advice and reassurance.

In THE WOMANLY ART OF BREASTFEEDING we have attempted to put a philosophy about being a mother and nurturing an infant between covers. This book is our way of sharing the sense of satisfaction and fulfillment countless mothers have found through breastfeeding their babies, and the special joys that are awaiting as you embark on the great adventure of motherhood.

Our first two editions, published in 1958 and 1963, were based largely on our own personal experiences. The third edition, published in 1981, was enlarged and expanded to include the combined wisdom accumulated from thousands of breastfeeding mothers who had shared their stories and experiences with us. The fourth edition included new information, reflected current medical research, and continued the tradition of providing practical suggestions based on the experiences of breastfeeding mothers from all over the world.

The fifth edition commemorated the organization's thirty-fifth anniversary. While it was not a major revision, specific information was updated throughout the book and current research was reflected in the chapters on the benefits of breastfeeding.

The sixth revised edition, published in 1997, was considered a major revision. A great deal of new information was added, reflecting the broad range of research that had been done up to then on breast-feeding management and the benefits of human milk. That edition celebrated La Leche League International's 40th Anniversary and was designed to reach mothers who would breastfeed in the 21st century. In the sixth edition, references were included for the first time.

This seventh revised edition reflects a broader perspective of experiences and research as more information has become available from countries beyond the United States. New research from Australia has prompted us to change the way we explain certain aspects of milk production. The details of how to get the baby to latch onto the breast most effectively have been modified because closer observation of babies has taught us what works best. And, of course, continued research into the differences between human milk and artificial feed-ing products has reinforced our conviction that breastfeeding is the gold standard for infants.

In this edition, you will notice that we still write from the perspec-tive of a household consisting of husband, wife, and child or children. Some have pointed out to us that times have changed and this is no longer a realistic approach to family life. But we are convinced that breastfeeding and mothering progress more easily in such an environ-ment. From personal experience, we also know that this situation does not always hold true in real life. Sometimes the father is missing from the family, and mothering then becomes a solitary endeavor. It is not an easy situation for a woman to be in. Our hope is that any mother in that situation finds the support she needs in other ways. But no matter what else happens in her life, a mother can take great satisfaction in breastfeeding her baby and staying close to him. Her efforts in this regard bring a feeling of accomplishment that will increase in value as time goes by.

Our wish is that every mother anywhere in the world who wants to breastfeed her baby will have the information and support she needs to do so. Yes, breastfeeding is simple and natural—and an exquisitely beautiful way to nourish and nurture a new life.

We appreciate and applaud the fact that babies come in two gen-ders, but in this book, we refer to baby as "he," not with sexist intent, but simply for clarity's sake, since mother is unquestionably "she."

PART ONE

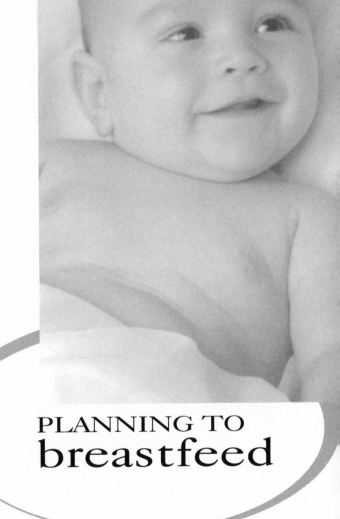

PLANNING TO
breastfeed

CHAPTER ONE

WHY CHOOSE
breastfeeding?

Breastfeeding is the most natural source of nourishment and security for your baby. For many mothers, breastfeeding is a fulfillment of what it means to be a woman. Pregnancy, childbirth, and breastfeeding comprise a special phase in your life—one that is bound up with an extraordinary array of emotions.

Expecting a baby brings with it a sudden realization that your life will never be the same. You recognize the need to learn more about being a mother, but you may feel doubt and uncertainty about being able to cope.

You may even share the feeling of this mother:

> When I was expecting my first baby, my husband and I didn't feel comfortable about becoming parents. We had no friends or relatives living near us who had babies. We were confused by what we read, what we were told, and what we felt.... After four years and two breastfed babies, we now feel better about being parents and we also know what to listen to—our hearts.

As you watch your body grow and change to accommodate the growing child within you, you can be reassured that your own capabilities to care for your baby after he is born will also adjust to meet your baby's needs. Breastfeeding offers a beautiful transition for mother and baby alike as they learn about each other in those first hours and days following birth.

A Special Journey

During early pregnancy, your baby's development is nothing short of remarkable. Eighteen days after he is conceived, his heart is beating. About the fourth month or so of your pregnancy, you feel the flutter, the unmistakable stirring that is like no other. It's the revelation of a new life. Your body changes to meet your baby's needs. There's the swelling readiness of your breasts, the expanding cradle of your womb. You are beautiful, as lovely as a tree that is heavy with fruit.

During the last trimester—the seventh, eighth, and ninth months—you may be impatient, eager to complete this stage and have the baby. Then, often when you least expect it, you feel a twinge. And another. The time is here. Mingled relief and anticipation can bring a catch in your throat. Today, sometime soon, your baby will be born!

The doctor or midwife is contacted, and the preliminary details are taken care of. You settle down to the work of giving birth. This day is like no other. Your mind and your whole body center on the process that is taking over inside of you.

The birth force rises, swells as a great wave, peaks, and recedes. You try to concentrate on relaxing, on willing your muscles to cooperate. In the welcome interim between contractions, there's time to rest.

The tempo quickens. Contractions are strong, they come quickly. You've probably never worked harder in your life. Labor is a fitting term! Just when you're most likely to feel exhausted and discouraged, you hear the reassurance of those who are with you—"Don't give up! We'll soon have a baby!"

And, at last, there is the moment you've been waiting for all those months, the bursting forth, the moment of blessed birth! As you catch your breath, you hear his cry. Was a sound ever before so priceless?

The umbilical cord is cut, marking the first separation. Who is to bridge this change of worlds for your newborn, who will soothe him and let him know he is again secure? Who better than his mother?

Again your body cradles him. You touch him, kiss his cheek, stroke his damp little head. Will he nurse? Perhaps. At some time within the

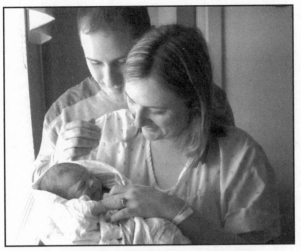

Parents lovingly cradle their newborn child
knowing their lives will never be the same.

first hour or so he will take the breast. You hold him close and he nuzzles your breast. His tiny mouth grasps your nipple. It seems no less than amazing! You and your baby can relax. After the enormous effort of giving birth, this is sweet reward.

Without thought or conscious effort on your part, your milk will come. You can look beyond to the many days together as a nursing couple. The security and warmth of your arms, the ready comfort of your milk, the familiar smell and pulse of your body are all precious food to fill out your baby's body and quicken his mind and spirit. Such accomplishments take time. But is there a more awe-inspiring task? This is the ageless beauty of mother and child—a time of grace and peace.

You'll hug him to you, intensely aware of his dependence upon you. Of course he will grow, reach out, and eventually leave you. But not for a while. Give yourself time together; let there be no regrets. Together you'll begin to weave a new cord to replace the one so recently severed. This one will be plaited simply and naturally by your continuing closeness through many unhurried days. Not to be cut, it will form the first link to all human love and understanding.

But perhaps, instead of the natural birth you prepared for, you have a cesarean delivery. Or the months of waiting are not long enough, and the baby arrives prematurely, to be whisked away for specialized care. For the moment there is little sense of rapport with the baby.

These things happen. They may slow down a mother and baby's start as a nursing couple, but they need not end it. Given the right support, mothers and babies have untold levels of strength and adaptability. Mothers through the ages have happily breastfed their babies, and you can do it, too.

The groundwork is laid before your baby is born. Nothing is more important in your advance planning than your preparation for breast-feeding. There is no better time to start than now.

Best for Baby—Best for You

When you breastfeed your baby, you're providing him with the best possible infant food. No product has ever been as time-tested as mother's milk. Human milk contains all the nutrients your newborn needs and is more easily digested and assimilated than any other infant food. As reassuring as this is, superior nutrition is only one of the many advantages you and your baby gain from breastfeeding.

Putting your newborn to the breast within minutes after delivery causes the uterus to contract and reduces the flow of blood. It also results in the uterus getting back in shape more quickly than it would if you were not breastfeeding.

With his small head pillowed against your breast and your milk warming his insides, your baby knows a special closeness to you. He is gaining a firm foundation in an important area of life—he is learning about love.

As his tiny mouth eagerly milks your breast, your baby is perform-ing an exercise that promotes the proper development of his jaw and facial structure. Breastfeeding also encourages a normal weight gain for your particular baby, which is good insurance against a future tendency toward obesity.

There is no better safeguard for your baby against the onset of allergies than breastfeeding. A diet of your milk alone for about the first six months of his life readies his body for other foods. Human milk protects your baby against infection as well as allergies. Living substances that are unique to your milk inhibit the growth of harmful bacteria and viruses in his still maturing system. With fewer health problems, you can look forward to having a happier baby. Many of these benefits are explained more thoroughly in later chapters.

Brain development is essential for the human infant and human milk contains all the right components to aid the development of baby's brain and nervous system. One study showed that premature infants who had been given human milk scored significantly higher on IQ tests at age 7 1/2 and 8 years of age than children who had not been fed human milk. Another study showed that higher IQs continued into adulthood.

For a woman, breastfeeding was meant to follow pregnancy and childbirth. The milk-producing breast represents a healthy progression in the natural sequence of reproduction that includes pregnancy, birth, and lactation. Nursing mothers find that breastfeeding is a naturally pleasurable experience.

The mother who is totally breastfeeding—not giving formula supplements or solid foods—will find that her menstrual periods will probably be delayed for six months or more after her baby's birth, especially if baby nurses often. During this time, a mother will have very little chance of becoming pregnant.

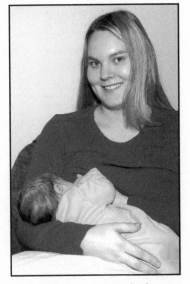

A newborn receives the best start in life at his mother's breast.

Breastfeeding uses up extra calories and a breastfeeding mother's metabolism changes, which enables most mothers to lose weight gradually without dieting.

Breastfeeding also protects a mother from certain health problems. Studies show that mothers who breastfeed for even a few months are less likely to develop breast cancer than women who have given birth but never breastfed. Breastfeeding also protects against ovarian cancer, urinary tract infections, and osteoporosis.

Breastfeeding results in an appreciable saving of time, effort, and money when compared to formula feeding. Minutes and hours of a mother's time are not diverted to the preparation of baby's milk. Feeding the baby is a time to relax. Day and night, automatically and accurately, milk is made and stored in the breasts. The temperature is always ideal; the supply is pure and practically unlimited.

Breastfeeding helps us appreciate the different yet complementary ways that men and women can participate in raising a child. If you have older children, breastfeeding the baby contributes toward their sex education. For a parent, it is an educational process itself, of a rank and value equal to a course of study at any prestigious institution of learning.

Breastfeeding is the best start in life for a baby. Unlike so much that is considered "best" and is often beyond even one's wildest dreams, in this instance the best is yours to give.

Solid backing

If you had been a new mother living in Rome in the year 180 AD, there is a good possibility that you would have heard the following advice from the physician Galen, who gave public lectures on anatomy and physiology.

> For if one places the nipple in the mouth of the newborn, they suck the milk and swallow it eagerly. And if they chance to be distressed or to cry, the best appeasement of their unhappiness is the mother's nipple put in their mouth.

Closer to our own time, the man who is usually referred to as the father of the modern natural-birth movement, Dr. Grantly Dick-Read, said:

> The newborn baby has only three demands. They are warmth in the arms of its mother, food from her breasts, and security in the knowledge of her presence. Breastfeeding satisfies all three.

Dr. Ashley Montagu, noted anthropologist and social biologist, wrote the following in his book, *Touching*:

> What is established in the breastfeeding relationship constitutes the foundation for the development of all human social relationships, and the communications the infant receives through the warmth of the mother's skin constitute the first of the socializing experiences of life.

In 1985, the late James P. Grant, who was then the Executive Director of UNICEF, wrote about the life-or-death consequences of the decision to breastfeed:

> Breastfeeding is a natural "safety net" against the worst effects of poverty. If the child survives the first month of life (the most dangerous period of childhood), ... exclusive breastfeeding goes a long way toward canceling out the health difference between being born into poverty and being born into affluence. Unless the mother is in extremely poor nutritional health, the breast milk of a mother in an African village is as good as the breast milk of a mother in a Manhattan apartment.... It is almost as if breastfeeding takes

the infant out of poverty for those first few vital months in order to give the child a fairer start in life and compensate for the injustice of the world into which it was born....

In many cities of the developing world, the incidence and duration of breastfeeding has begun to fall precipitously (in recent years)....The result can be a doubling or trebling of malnutrition, infection, and infant deaths.

In August 1990, participants from the World Health Organization (WHO), and UNICEF, an agency of the United Nations, met in Florence, Italy and adopted a sweeping statement in support of breast-feeding, known as the Innocenti Declaration. This declaration was signed by 32 governments and 10 United Nations agencies and has been the springboard for a variety of programs and initiatives to support breastfeeding.

In August 1994, a group of doctors representing specialties in family practice, obstetrics, pediatrics, and preventive medicine met to create a new medical society called the Academy of Breastfeeding Medicine. Their mission statement reads:

The Academy of Breastfeeding Medicine is a worldwide organization of physicians dedicated to the promotion, protection, and support of breastfeeding and human lactation. Its mission is to unite into one association members of the various medical specialties with this common purpose. The goals are: physician education; expansion of knowledge in both breastfeeding science and human lactation; facilitation of optimal breastfeeding practices; and encouragement of the exchange of information among organizations.

In 1997, the American Academy of Pediatrics published a statement declaring human milk to be the preferred food for all newborns and recommending exclusive breastfeeding with no supplements for the first six months. Their official statement reads:

The benefits of breastfeeding are so numerous that the Academy strongly encourages the practice during the first six to twelve months of life. Human milk is nutritionally superior to formulas for the content of fats, cholesterol, protein, and iron. In addition, there is evidence that human milk confers protection against infections and other diseases.

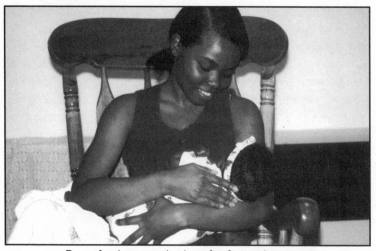

Breastfeeding provides benefits for mothers, too.

Exclusive breastfeeding is ideal nutrition and sufficient to support growth and development for approximately the first six months after birth. It is recommended that breastfeeding continue for at least twelve months, and thereafter for as long as mutually desired.

The American Academy of Family Physicians issued a policy statement in support of breastfeeding in 1989 which was reissued in 2001. It reads:

Breastfeeding is the physiological norm for both mothers and their children. The AAFP recommends that all babies, with rare exceptions, be breastfed and/or receive expressed human milk exclusively for about the first six months of life. Breastfeeding should continue with the addition of complementary foods throughout the second half of the first year. Breastfeeding beyond the first year offers considerable benefits to both mother and child, and should continue as long as mutually desired. Family physicians should have the knowledge to promote, protect, and support breastfeeding.

In 2001, the World Health Organization recommended exclusive breastfeeding for six months as the optimal way of feeding infants and formally declared:

As a global public health recommendation, infants should be exclusively breastfed for the first six months of life to achieve optimal growth, development, and health. Thereafter, to meet their evolving nutritional requirements, infants should receive nutritionally adequate and safe complementary foods while breastfeeding continues for up to two years of age or beyond.

In 2001, US Surgeon General David Satcher, MD wrote the following in an official report:

Breastfeeding is one of the most important contributors to infant health. Breastfeeding provides a range of benefits for the infant's growth, immunity, and development. In addition, breastfeeding improves maternal health and contributes economic benefits to the family, health care system, and workplace.

The Paediatric Society in New Zealand also recognizes that breastfeeding provides optimal nutritional, immunological, and psychosocial benefits for the baby and also provides benefits for the mother.

In Germany, the National Breastfeeding Commission states that:

Breastfeeding is much more than the best and most healthy way to feed your baby, it is also nourishment for the heart and maintains in a special way the close relationship a mother and her baby develop during pregnancy.

The Canadian Paediatric Society, the Dietitians of Canada, and Health Canada published a combined statement supporting breastfeeding in 1998:

Breastfeeding is the optimal method of feeding infants. Breastfeeding may continue for up to 2 years of age and beyond.

The National Health Service of Great Britain says:

Breastfeeding confers significant short and long-term health benefits for both the mother and her infant, which go beyond the period of breastfeeding itself.

> **The Government is fully committed to the promotion of breastfeeding, which is accepted as the best form of nutrition for infants to ensure a good start in life.**

In order to focus the efforts of the many worldwide organizations that promote and support breastfeeding, a group of them, including La Leche League International, joined together in 1991 to form a network called the World Alliance for Breastfeeding Action (WABA). To commemorate the Innocenti Declaration, WABA has established World Breastfeeding Week held the first week in August every year.

Breastfeeding is more than just another lifestyle choice. It's an important health choice for mothers and babies, and that's why agencies that care about health support breastfeeding. The US Department of Health and Human Services, in cooperation with the Ad Council and La Leche League International, initiated an ad campaign to promote breastfeeding that began in 2003. The slogan for the ad campaign is—Babies were born to breastfeed.

The Key to Good Mothering

Even though your milk is important to your baby as a food and as a source of elements that protect him against infection, breastfeeding is more than a method of feeding your baby. Breastfeeding is the most natural and effective way of understanding and satisfying the needs of the baby. An experienced mother made the following observation, "Nursing the baby is a do-it-yourself kit for learning good mothering."

One explanation of breastfeeding's effect on mothering lies in the fact that a breastfeeding mother is physically different than a mother who is not breastfeeding. She is in a different hormonal state. Because she is breastfeeding, she has a high level of prolactin—the "mothering" hormone.

We all know that motherhood can be very demanding, and breastfeeding helps balance the give-and-take of caring for a young child. It serves as a bridge from mother to child, child to mother. Lucy Waletzky, MD, a psychiatrist who breastfed her children, explains:

> **The more intimate bodily communication inherent to the breastfeeding situation leads to a feeling of psychological oneness with the child, which allows the mother to satisfy her own dependency needs (needs to be cared for and loved) at the same time she meets the baby's dependency needs. A mother's dependency needs may be accentuated postpartum**

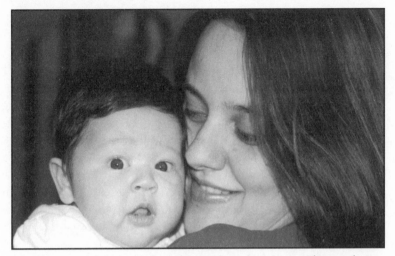

Getting to know your baby helps you learn how to meet his needs.

by pain, fatigue, and the psychological stress of adjusting to new motherhood. When her dependency needs are thus met, her resentment of the child's dependency (often a very difficult problem) is alleviated, and the positive maternal feelings can flourish unencumbered.

What is mothering?

Mothering is caring for your baby, communicating with him and encouraging him to communicate back. It encompasses all of the many things that you will do to keep your baby healthy and comfortable, to help him grow in body and spirit. Breastfeeding is an unequalled form of communication between mother and baby. All of the senses are brought into play. Your baby tastes your milk. He knows you through the smell of your skin and your milk. He experiences a sense of closeness to you by feeling your skin next to his. In the nursing position, he can easily look into your eyes. He hears your voice. The many times that you nurse your baby tell him, "Yes, you are loved. You are safe. You are doing all right!" and he, of course, communicates back to you that he feels loved and is reassured. It is a learning and comforting experience for both of you.

From time immemorial, mothers have comforted their babies at the breast. They know that a few minutes of nursing can soothe an upset child's feelings of fear or anger. Nothing is more reassuring to a small one than being close to mother and tasting her warm milk.

In explaining how breastfeeding improves the interaction between a mother and her baby, Dr. William Sears, pediatrician and author, writes:

Breastfeeding mothers respond to their babies more intu-
itively and with less restraint. The baby's signals of hunger or
distress trigger a biological response within the mother
(a milk let-down) and she feels the urge to pick up the baby
and nurse him. This responsiveness rewards both mother and
baby with good feelings. If a mother is not breastfeeding, her
response to her baby's hunger or distress cues is quite different. She must initially divert her attention away from the
baby to an object, the bottle, and take time to find and prepare it. ... In my practice, I have noticed that breastfeeding
mothers tend to show a high degree of sensitivity to their
babies, and I believe this is a result of the biological changes
that occur in a mother in response to the signals of her baby.

Good mothering means babying the baby, accepting that his wants
and needs are the same. It includes holding him when he is too full to
nurse, but he is not yet ready to sleep. Mothering is changing a diaper
or playing peek-a-boo. It means recognizing that each child has an inex-
haustible need to be loved for what he is—a person with his own individuality. As he grows, his needs will change. A toddler needs freedom
and guidance, with an ever-watchful eye. The manner in which these
early needs are met, or not met, has a great deal to do with a child's
response to people and situations in later life. The way the child is
mothered is important not only to mother and child, but to society as
well. Marian Tompson, one of La Leche League's co-Founders,
observes, "No matter how far our world advances technologically, the
decisions of how to use that technology still have to be made by people.
And so the kind of people we produce is crucial to the direction our
world takes. Raising a loving, caring child is the most important contribution any of us can make to the progress of the world."

Getting to know your baby

Mothering is not something you can learn from a book. We can tell
you, for instance, that most young babies like the secure feeling of
being snugly wrapped up and cuddled. We can tell you that at about
three months, most babies like company. They like to be propped up
in the midst of the family. Instead of wanting to be fed or cuddled,
what they often want is just to be sociable. These may be perfectly
true observations for many babies—but your newborn may prefer to
have his arms and legs free, or your three-month-old may be overstim-
ulated by too much activity and end up feeling miserable. You have to
be sensitive to the individual needs of your baby.

The sensitivity that helps you do the right thing at the right time comes from knowing your baby. It develops as you spend time with him, but it develops more quickly, and to a greater degree, if you are nursing your baby. The very closeness and intimacy of breastfeeding give you a quicker and surer perception of the feelings and needs of this tiny person, and help you to know how to meet them.

Ann Van Norman, a mother from Ontario, Canada, tells how breastfeeding helped her learn about her baby's needs:

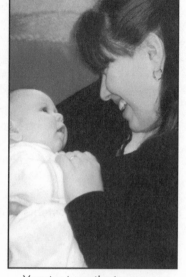

Your joy in mothering grows as you get to know your baby as a person.

I thought I had prepared myself for mothering before Sarah's birth. I learned about diapering, bathing, and breastfeeding, but there was no way to prepare for "mothering." I found out that mothering is only learned by doing. Learning to respond flexibly to baby's needs for love, care, and stimulation, putting our own desires on temporary hold, and accepting the constancy and intensity of baby's needs are lessons only learned by living them.

I believe nursing has helped make my learning relatively painless, mainly through the positive reinforcement I have received from Sarah. She showed me how much I was needed and loved. Nursing her meant that I had to take time to respond, relax, and reflect. I am a different person now. Sarah has changed me from a compulsive time-and-task oriented tiger to a go-with-the-flow housecat.

Your joy in mothering grows as you experience the quick, strong feeling of affection so natural between a nursing mother and her baby; as you develop an understanding of your baby's needs and gain confidence in your own ability to satisfy them; and as you see the happy dividends from the good relationship as the baby grows. As one nursing mother, Shirl Butts, from Louisiana, expressed her feelings:

Those who have never nursed a child might find it hard to understand just how special a nursing relationship can be.

Now as I nurse my second child, I can appreciate what I missed with my toddler, whom I did not nurse.

My favorite moments are just before bedtime, nursing my four-month-old daughter. We snuggle together in our rocking chair, her tiny mouth eagerly searching for the warmth of my milk, until at last she latches on and drifts into peaceful sleep. Her chubby little hand is outstretched on my arm, her cheek nestled against my breast. I continue to rock, lovingly studying every crease and fold of her soft body. Times like this make me look forward to the next night and the next. Sometimes she stops nursing to look up at me and give a big smile as if to say, "Thanks, Mom!" and then resumes nursing again. Those moments make me wish time would stand still.

Breastfeeding is not a guarantee of good mothering, and formula feeding does not rule it out. The most important thing is the love you give your baby and the fact that you are doing your best to be a good mother. Mary White, another of LLL's co-Founders, reminds us:

We're all learning, all the time. We're all still reaching up to the top of the ladder, and we've all got a long way to go. But for each and every one of us, the person from whom we can learn the most is our own baby; listen to him. Give to him; in the giving we are growing, as mothers and as women. As we watch him grow and thrive, we are watching an achievement that can really make us proud.

PLANS ARE
underway

Planning for a new baby is one of the most exciting adventures in the life of a couple. You will dream the dreams that belong exclusively to parents. Your family's future is full of hope.

Planning usually begins with making practical arrangements. You'll select a doctor, look into childbirth education classes, and attend La Leche League meetings. Then your attention will turn to the need for rearranging the priorities in your life. Babies take time, and adjustments will have to be made. How can you change a routine here or eliminate an activity there in order to fit the new family member into your already busy life?

From long experience, we have learned that whenever a routine comes into conflict with the needs of one of the family members, it's the routine that has to give. "People before things" is a handy slogan to remember.

It should be said, too, that this change of emphasis is not a temporary interlude, with life reverting to its former style once the baby is older. Having a baby, loving a child, is forever. New experiences, endless opportunities, and depths of feelings that you can know in no other way lie ahead of you.

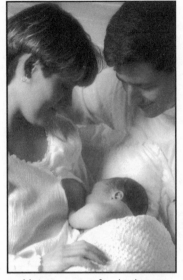

Nursing soon after birth gets breastfeeding off to a good start.

True, the investment in a new baby is enormous. As you are probably well aware, the financial output is a definite concern for many couples. But money is seldom the most critical or the rarest commodity that parents must provide. The coin that has greater value and is more difficult to part with is that which represents the continuous giving of one's self, emotionally and physically. Babies have no way of knowing how much it costs their parents to tend to them, worry about them, and love them day and night. They can't know, of course, until they themselves become parents someday. Then the gift is recognized and passed on as lovingly as it was given.

Plans for the Baby's Birth

We learned early in La Leche League's existence that a woman's experience in giving birth affects the beginning of breastfeeding and many of her attitudes about being a mother. Alert and active participation by the mother in childbirth is a help in getting breastfeeding off to a good start.

Childbirth can be a rich, joyful, and maturing experience. Those of us who have given birth without drugs or medical intervention know that helping a baby to be born and hearing his first cry can be a crowning moment of achievement in the life of a woman. After doing a survey of women's long-term memories of their birth experiences, childbirth educator Penny Simkin reports that the women who felt the most satisfaction about their childbirth experiences "described feelings of accomplishment, control, increased self-esteem, and/or confirmation of worth. Most of those with low satisfaction expressed disappointment or anger that they were not in control." And she concludes, "a sense of maternal fulfillment and personal self-worth are hallmarks of a healthy outcome" of the birth experience.

Having a baby is a natural, normal function for which a woman's body is superbly designed. The healthiest birth situation for both mother and baby is one that is completely drug-free. Almost all mothers are physically able to deliver their babies without medical intervention. You do need a doctor or trained midwife attending the birth of your baby but this is similar to having a lifeguard on duty in case there are complications. In the natural, normal birth, it is not the doctor who delivers the baby; it is the mother.

Ten tips for a normal birth

Today's woman is inundated with mixed messages about birth; obstetric care practices once reserved for complicated labor and birth are often used routinely and can hinder a woman's effort to give birth normally. To combat this alarming trend, Lamaze International has developed a set of ten tips promoting normal birth which are adapted here with permission:

Choose a place that supports normal birth, a place where you'll be comfortable. This may be at home, in a birth center, or in a hospital.

Choose a health care provider who supports the practices that promote normal birth. Many women have found that the care provided by midwives includes more labor support and less intervention.

Don't request or agree to induction of labor unless there's a medical indication for doing so. Allowing your body to go into labor on its own is usually the best sign that your baby is ready to be born. Allow your labor to find its own pace and rhythm.

Plan to move around freely during labor. You'll be more comfortable, your labor will progress quickly, and your baby will move through the birth canal easily if you stay upright and respond to the pain of your labor by changing positions.

Consider hiring a doula or other professional labor support person to give you, your partner, and any other support person continuous emotional and physical support.

Ask that your baby's heartbeat be monitored intermittently instead of all the time so that belts, cords, or wires do not tie you to a machine or specific place.

Eat and drink as your body tells you. Drinking plenty of fluids during labor will give you energy and keep you from getting dehydrated.

Use nonpharmacologic pain management strategies. For many women, warm baths and showers give powerful pain relief. Practice using birth balls, massage, hot and cold packs, aromatherapy, focused breathing, and other comfort measures learned in childbirth classes.

Don't give birth on your back! Upright positions (sitting, squatting, or standing), on all fours, or on your side are more comfortable, increase the effectiveness of your contractions and enable you to work with gravity. Push when your body tells you to, and ask that support persons give only quiet encouragement. Simply work with your body's own cues and rhythm.

Keep your baby with you after birth. Skin-to-skin contact keeps your baby warm and helps to regulate your baby's heartbeat and breathing. Staying in the same room helps you to get to know each other, and it lets you respond to early feeding cues and get breastfeeding off to a good start.

See the Appendix for more information about Lamaze International as well as other organizations working to support women in achieving a normal and satisfying birth experience.

Effects of medications

Research has shown that pain relievers and anesthesia used during labor or delivery may contribute to breastfeeding problems. In one study, babies whose mothers had received an epidural were less alert, less able to orient themselves, and had less organized movements than babies whose mothers had given birth without medication. Furthermore, these differences in behavior were measurable during the entire first month. Other medications commonly used during labor have also been found to affect baby's sucking behavior after birth.

Learning about childbirth

Advance preparation can pay off for you and your baby by resulting in a safer, happier birth experience. You and your husband can begin to prepare for this event by learning as much as you can beforehand. Many of the fears, doubts, and misconceptions you may have about childbirth will disappear as you become better informed and more confident. Attending childbirth classes will help you learn about the process of giving birth as well as how to participate and cooperate in the event. In addition, childbirth options are explained in many books that are listed in the Appendix.

With concentration and practice, you can learn relaxation techniques that are invaluable in the first stage of labor. Then in the second stage of labor, by pushing with contractions, you move your baby out of the womb and into the world, perhaps even into his father's hands. The experience of seeing and holding his newborn bonds a father to his child and to the mother of his child in a special way. When you are all together—mother, father, and baby—you "claim" each other for your own.

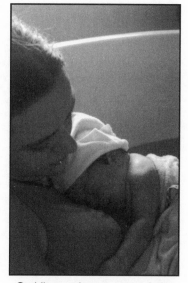

Cuddling and nursing your baby right after birth is soothing and comforting for both of you.

If all goes well, you'll be able to hold your baby immediately after birth and put him to your breast. The outflow of love and warmth to your child at this time is a spontaneous continuation of the comfort and security he has known for so long before his birth. This early contact can be very soothing and satisfying for both of you. Nursing the baby soon after birth encourages your milk to come in and starts you on your way as a breastfeeding mother.

Studies have shown that if mother and baby are separated after birth and the first nursing is delayed, even by as little as twenty minutes, the baby may have difficulty latching on well. So it is definitely worthwhile to discuss this with your doctor or midwife ahead of time and be assured that you and your baby can be together soon after birth.

Childbirth options

Nowadays, mothers are approaching the birth of their baby as the natural, normal event it really is, instead of a medical situation. They are looking into alternatives to the traditional hospital birth. Home birth and freestanding birth centers are becoming popular choices in some areas. Hospitals have responded to this by offering birthing rooms and family-centered care to replace traditional labor and delivery rooms. Many of these changes have been in response to the patients' demands.

Judy Unruh, from California, gave birth to her two daughters in the hospital. When she was expecting her third child she planned to return to the same hospital. But at her doctor's suggestion she visited the new birthing center. The positive atmosphere and the enthusiasm of the staff made her decide she wanted to have her baby there. She writes:

> When we arrived at the birthing center to have the baby, we were told to go right to the room we had chosen ahead of time. There weren't any strong hospital odors, no people rushing around, no papers for Gary to fill out while I was wheeled off down a long hall without him. We just walked together to our room.
>
> There is always some amount of anxiety in starting labor, but the atmosphere at the birthing center was so relaxing that it had a calming effect on me. The thing that meant the most to my husband was his feeling that he belonged there. No one made him feel that he was in the way.
>
> I can remember how great it felt to be able to get up and shower to relieve my back labor and to take a walk out in the hall when I felt the need to walk. I wasn't confined to bed; I was in control.
>
> Several hours later, our third daughter was born. She never left us to go to the nursery with harsh lights and lots of crying babies. She remained in our quiet room with us. We could hold her when she wanted to be held and feed her when she wanted to be fed. Gary and I both were there when the pediatrician checked her.
>
> Even though it was my most difficult labor and delivery, it was our happiest. My husband and I look back on our daughter's birth with good memories and love for all the wonderful people who have worked so hard to make having a baby an enriching experience for the entire family.

You'll want to find out as much as possible about the choices available as you plan for your baby's birth. Books and organizations listed in the Appendix will be helpful.

The cesarean question

The cesarean birth rate in the USA was 5.5 percent in 1970 and increased to 24.4 percent of all births in 1987, according to the National Center for Health Statistics. In 2002, the figure was reported to be 26.1 percent, the highest level ever reported in the United States. This means one-fourth of all births in the USA are done by cesarean, an alarming fact that many health professionals consider to be an epidemic.

The decision to perform a cesarean is a serious one, often made at a critical point in labor when parents are not likely to question their doctor's decision. Parents will want to thoroughly discuss their doctor's views on the need for a cesarean birth early in the pregnancy. A few doctors have come to believe that cesareans are always necessary for twins, babies who are breech, and so-called "prolonged" labor. Other doctors view cesarean deliveries as only a last resort and find that in many such cases all that is needed is a little more time and patience. With proper medical support and care, most babies, even the big ones, can be successfully delivered vaginally with greater safety for both mother and baby.

The incidence of prematurity, respiratory distress syndrome, and other complications is far higher with cesarean deliveries, and the likelihood that the baby and mother will be separated from each other, often for some time, is much greater. Morbidity and mortality rates are higher for mothers who have cesarean births. The mother is more likely to experience infection, pain, and discomfort, as well as psychological effects such as depression after a cesarean birth.

If your doctor thinks it may be necessary to plan on a cesarean birth for your baby, don't hesitate to consult another doctor before making this decision.

If you have already had a previous cesarean birth you should know, too, that most mothers are able to have vaginal deliveries for subsequent babies. Having future babies by cesarean is not inevitable. Frequently the reason for the first cesarean delivery does not apply to subsequent births. Organizations listed in the Appendix can offer further information about this.

Dottie Leach, from Oklahoma tells of her experience:

Two months ago I gave birth to Daniel, my second child. I had a vaginal birth after a cesarean (VBAC). At six months into my pregnancy, I changed obstetricians, choosing one whom I felt had a positive attitude about natural delivery and who had demonstrated success with VBACs. I prepared a birth plan stating my intentions, explaining that I wanted an unmedicated, intervention-free birth.

Probably the most important factor in having a VBAC was my labor support. My husband was there as well as a woman who was familiar with childbirth and acted as my labor assistant. They supported me through every contraction for nine hours, talking to me and praising and comforting me. Everyone was very positive and loving. I felt most comfort-

able standing and walking, and this was supported by the hospital staff. The last two hours of transition were intense and exhausting. I was ready to give up by the time I was ready to push, but my coaches were so incredibly positive and encouraging, they somehow gave me the energy to continue. After about forty-five minutes of pushing, my son was born weighing ten pounds and nine ounces.

     My feeling about natural childbirth is that it can help build self-esteem and self-awareness that carries over to every other part of life. It has shown me how strong I really am, and that I can be courageous in other parts of my life, too. It felt right to me.

A growing number of doctors and hospitals permit fathers to be present for a cesarean birth. Mothers appreciate the comfort and support, and fathers are glad to be able to participate in the birth of their babies. Discuss these options with your doctor.

Health Professionals Who Care

There's no doubt about it—your choice of health care providers makes a difference. The doctor or trained midwife who attends you in childbirth will greatly influence how your infant is delivered, and the health care provider you choose for your baby afterward can affect the course of breastfeeding. Even the doctor who prescribes medication should you become ill must take both you and your nursing baby into consideration. A doctor who has little opportunity to learn about breastfeeding may be readily inclined to take the baby off the breast when treating either you or your baby. Such a move is rarely necessary.

    Many young couples are devoting a considerable amount of time and care to finding health care professionals whose priorities are similar to their own. If you are in a situation where the choice of health care providers is limited, then it becomes even more important to have a dialogue with the doctor.

    Attendance at La Leche League meetings and childbirth education classes is a good way to learn about other parents' experiences. As you become better informed, through reading and talking to others, you'll know the questions to ask in order to learn more about a doctor's or a hospital's practices.

    Your first step will probably be to select the doctor or trained midwife who will attend the birth of your baby. Seek out a doctor who does not routinely use epidurals, other medications, or IVs during labor, who does not routinely induce labor or use fetal monitors, who does not routinely give anesthesia or do episiotomies. Be sure to ask about the cesarean rate among the doctor's patients and what situations would be considered as indications of a need for a cesarean birth. Discuss whether routine procedures might interfere with breastfeeding your baby soon after birth. Ask about rooming-in policies at the hospital or other facility where your baby will be born.

You may want to meet and talk with several health care professionals before selecting one. Before the interview, write out a list of the points you want to discuss. When you make this appointment, ask what the fee will be for a consultation visit. Tell the receptionist you do not want a complete examination at this visit.

Find out, too, if the doctor or midwife is in a group practice with other doctors or midwives. You'll be interested in knowing if an associate, rather than the person you have selected, might attend the birth of your baby. Be sure to find out if the associates are also willing to respect your wishes.

After discussing your concerns with your doctor or midwife, it's a good idea to put in writing what is acceptable to all of you and ask the doctor or midwife to indicate his or her agreement by signing your list. (Of course, a health care provider must reserve the right to change procedures in any emergency.) Take this with you to the hospital. Mothers say that producing their signed list was often all the authority needed to stop someone who was ready to administer a routine procedure or medication in childbirth or give the baby a routine bottle of formula or water in the nursery.

The baby's doctor

In the United States, parents are usually able to choose the doctor or health care provider they want for their baby. You'll want to find someone who is knowledgeable about breastfeeding and has a positive attitude toward it. A family doctor may be caring for both you and your baby and you can discuss breastfeeding at your prenatal visits. Otherwise you may select a pediatrician or family doctor to care for the baby after birth. Make an appointment to talk to the doctor before the baby is born and let him or her know that you plan to breastfeed your baby. Ask questions. Are most of the doctor's patients breastfed? How does he or she deal with situations such as slow weight gain? A doctor who has not dealt with many breastfed babies may want to give supplementary formula or recommend that you start solid foods too early. If you are not satisfied with the answers you receive, shop around for another doctor. If this is not an option in your situation, discuss your concerns with the doctor and explain why breastfeeding is so important to you.

A need for dialogue

When dealing with health professionals, you may have to take the initiative in letting them know what you want. A simple, direct statement can begin a dialogue between the two of you. "Doctor, I need to discuss this with you. It's important to me." When there's a need for medication or hospitalization for the baby, you need a doctor who will treat him yet not interrupt breastfeeding—or do so as little as possible. Staying close to your baby at a time of illness, nursing him when possible, is always best.

If the doctor who is treating you or caring for your baby is not willing to discuss the options you prefer, you may want to seek another medical opinion.

Preparing to Breastfeed

As you talk to other mothers about your plans to breastfeed your baby, you will probably hear stories about sore nipples. At one time, nipple soreness was a common reason for mothers to give up breastfeeding, so a great deal of emphasis was put on the need to "prepare your nipples" before your baby was born. In recent years, it has been found that the major cause of nipple soreness is incorrect positioning of the baby at the breast and/or improper latching on and sucking techniques. Nipple preparation is no longer considered necessary as you prepare to breastfeed.

Kittie Frantz, RN, CPNP, who is a La Leche League Leader and also the Director of the Breastfeeding Infant Clinic at the University of Southern California Medical Center, was one of the people who first emphasized the importance of correct positioning for comfortable and effective breastfeeding. In evaluating 300 breastfeeding mothers, she found that 57 percent reported nipple soreness and 43 percent said they were not sore. Kittie reports on her findings:

> We observed a difference in the two groups—in the way mother held the baby and the way the baby accepted the breast into his mouth. When we taught the mothers with sore nipples the technique we observed the mothers without sore nipples to be using, they almost all exclaimed that the pain significantly lessened or, in most cases, vanished.

More information on correct latch-on and positioning of the baby at the breast can be found in the chapter called "Your Baby Arrives."

What you can do

Some women apply a lubricant to their nipples and breasts to moisturize their skin during pregnancy. Many mothers use Lansinoh Brand Lanolin for Breastfeeding Mothers®, the purest form of USP modified lanolin available. It can be used during pregnancy to moisturize the nipples. Some mothers with very dry skin who experienced nipple soreness when they breastfed a previous baby report that they were able to nurse comfortably after using Lansinoh Brand Lanolin for Breastfeeding Mothers® to moisturize their nipples during pregnancy.

Soap can be very drying so it should be avoided entirely in the nipple area. Rinsing with plain water when you bathe will keep the nipple area clean. When your baby is nursing, the Montgomery glands that surround the nipple secrete a substance that lubricates the skin and discourages the growth of bacteria. There is no need to use alcohol or other antiseptics on your nipples.

For some couples, a normal part of their lovemaking includes caressing the breasts and sucking the nipples. This can be a natural way of preparing the wife's breasts for the coming work of nourishing their child.

Breast massage

Gentle breast massage will help you feel more comfortable handling your breasts and can be useful later on if you need to express your milk. Support one breast with both hands, your thumbs above and fingers underneath. Press your fingers and thumbs together gently as you slide your fingers forward from the chest wall out toward your nipple; circle the breast with this gentle massaging motion. Then switch to the other breast.

Another type of breast massage involves using your fingers to press gently on one area of your breast and moving your fingers in a circular motion on one spot. After a few seconds, move your fingers to another spot. Start at the top of your breast and spiral around the breast toward the nipple using this massage.

Check for flat nipples

In order for the baby to suck effectively, he will need to draw your nipple far back into his mouth. If you have flat nipples, the baby may have a problem latching on correctly.

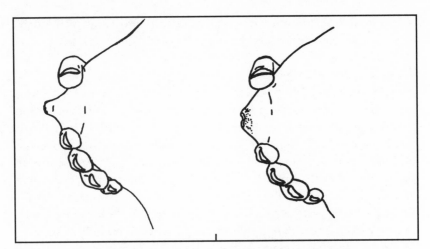

A normal nipple protrudes when the areola is pinched;
an inverted nipple retracts.

To bring the nipple out, place a thumb and forefinger near the base of the nipple and gently press together. You'll be able to feel where the larger mass of the breast tissue ends and the nipple begins. Then, holding the nipple, slowly pull it out, and gently turn it up and then down. Some authorities believe doing this exercise several times a day with each nipple will increase the elasticity of your nipples and help baby grasp them more easily. Others believe it is not necessary.

If you try these nipple pulls and find that your nipples do not come out far enough for you to grasp them easily, you may have flat or inverted nipples. Squeezing or pinching gently about an inch behind the base of the nipple should cause the nipple to project away from the breast.

One method for encouraging the flat nipple to be more outgoing was developed by Dr. J. Brooks Hoffman of Connecticut. Place a thumb on each side of the nipple. Your thumbs should be directly at the base of the nipple, not at the edge of the areola (the darker area of skin surrounding the nipple). Press in firmly against the breast tissue and at the same time pull the thumbs away from each other. Some believe this will stretch out the nipple and loosen the tightness at the base, which can help the nipple move up and outward. If you feel comfortable doing this exercise, repeat this stretch five times first thing in the morning, moving your thumbs around the base of the nipple.

Inverted nipples

If you find your nipples do not come out at all when you do these exercises, then you may have inverted nipples. An inverted nipple shrinks back into the breast when the areola is squeezed. Some inverted nipples appear as though they're pushed in all the time. One mother who had this type called it "the folding model of the nipple world." A full-size nipple is there, ready and able to do the job for which it was intended, but left on its own, it folds back into the breast instead of coming out when the baby tries to nurse.

Inverted nipples may or may not require treatment. Some breast-feeding experts believe that a baby who is latched on well can draw an inverted nipple far back into his mouth to nurse. Others suggest using breast shields or shells that are designed specifically to draw the nipple out. Breast shells can be comfortable to wear, lightweight, and inconspicuous under your bra. If you want to try using them, you can begin wearing them during pregnancy for a few hours a day and gradually increase the time. There are two sections to each shell, the bottom part, which has an opening for the nipple and fits directly over the breast, and the top part, which holds the bra away from the emerging nipple.

When flat or inverted nipples are discovered after the baby is born and the baby is not able to latch on properly, breast shells can be worn between feedings to draw the nipple out. Other methods can also be used to draw out a flat or inverted nipple. If your newborn is not latching on well, be sure to discuss the situation with someone who is knowledgeable about breastfeeding—a La Leche League Leader or board certified lactation consultant (IBCLC).

Expressing colostrum

During pregnancy, your breasts begin producing colostrum to prepare for the task of feeding your baby. You may notice a few drops leaking from your nipples during the last few weeks of pregnancy, or some may leak out if you massage your breasts.

At one time, experts recommended squeezing a few drops of colostrum from your breasts every day during pregnancy, but this has not been proven to be helpful in preventing engorgement or sore nipples.

What to Wear—Nursing Fashions

You'll probably be glad to shed your maternity garb after your baby is born and your figure changes to the smaller tummy and the temporarily fuller breasts of a nursing mother. Actually, you can make almost any clothes work for nursing, but a few special items can make life easier.

During pregnancy, and when the milk first comes in, the breasts often enlarge, and the support of a well-fitted bra can be most welcome. Let comfort be your guide. If you usually go braless, you may not need to wear one while breastfeeding.

You will probably find that you are more comfortable with a bra designed for nursing mothers. The traditional nursing bra has a flap on the cup that is opened for feedings. We suggest that you start with two to three bras and try them for fit and ease of use before purchasing more. Bras purchased during the last weeks of pregnancy should have extra room both in the cup and around the rib cage. The breasts will enlarge after the baby is born and the milk comes in, and nursing bras must be fitted with this in mind. A bra that is too tight, either around the ribs or in the cup, can cause a plugged milk duct or breast infection, and you don't want that to happen.

When trying on nursing bras in the store, be sure to note how the flap is attached in front. You'll want a fastener that you can manage with one hand so that you don't have to put the baby down every time you open or close the cup. You can also purchase washable or disposable nursing pads which fit inside your bra and absorb the milk that may leak from the nipples between feedings.

If you often wear skirts or dresses, half-slips are probably the handiest while nursing, but you can adapt full slips to your needs by replacing the adjustment clip with a small piece of a Velcro-type fastener. For outer apparel, two-piece outfits—skirts, jeans, slacks, or shorts with a loose top or sweater are ideal. With your top, blouse, or sweater lifted from the waist for nursing, the baby covers any bare midriff. When wearing a blouse that buttons down the front, you can unbutton from the bottom up. If you wear a three-piece outfit, with a jacket or shawl, you will be able to nurse so unobtrusively that the person sitting next to you won't know that your baby is having lunch.

La Leche League publications often carry ads for nursing bras and clothing designed especially for nursing mothers. Today's breastfeeding mother has her choice of many fashionable and comfortable styles of clothing designed with special openings for discreet breastfeeding. Maternity shops and specialty catalogues often carry nursing fashions. Companies who specialize in designing clothing for breastfeeding mothers often advertise in La Leche League publications and may be listed on the LLLI Web site at www.lalecheleague.org/.

Nursing discreetly

This brings us to a concern you may have about breastfeeding. You may worry about feeding the baby while you're away from home or when other people are around. As the American Academy of Pediatrics noted, "It is a curious commentary on our society that we tolerate all degrees of explicitness in our literature and mass media as regards sex and violence, but the normal act of breastfeeding is taboo."

Embarrassment is a reason mothers sometimes give for not breastfeeding or for weaning within the early weeks. Interestingly, studies of breastfeeding mothers show that the mothers who stop early seldom know another nursing mother and have no one to help them in their new undertaking. Experienced breastfeeding mothers know how to nurse a baby so discreetly that only the mother and the baby are the wiser. Breastfeeding can be as private as a mother wishes it to be, yet it need not unduly confine her and her baby.

There may be occasions when someone is extremely sensitive to the prospect of the baby being put to mother's breast when others are present. Breastfeeding mothers note that,

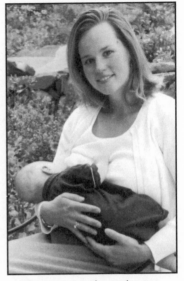

Mothers soon learn they can breastfeed discreetly in public.

at such times, discretion can be the better part of valor. Some mothers find it easiest to leave the room for a few moments just to get the baby started on the breast. Then, with baby nursing contentedly, a shawl or lightweight blanket can be draped over your shoulder to cover the baby and you can return comfortably to your group of friends.

A mother from California, Sue Ellen Jennings Austin, tells how attending La Leche League meetings helped her learn how to nurse discreetly:

> I have managed to feed my baby in just about every place imaginable, from teenage brother's basketball games to a large holiday party. This came about gradually of course—after practicing in front of the mirror and becoming brave in desperate situations, but most importantly after observing other mothers nursing discreetly at LLL functions and being able to share my concerns with them.

Don't let a concern about feeding your baby in public keep you from enjoying the advantages and convenience of breastfeeding. In later chapters, we offer more tips on trips and outings with your breastfed baby.

CHAPTER THREE

YOUR NETWORK OF
support

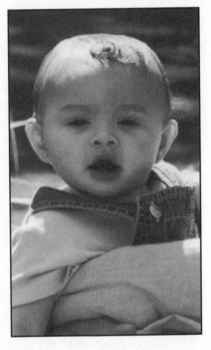

How can we adequately convey to you the tremendous value of being in touch with other nursing mothers? No book about breastfeeding can equal talking to an experienced nursing mother and seeing her happy baby. When you know a woman who enjoys being a nursing mother, you have access to a continuing source of information and inspiration. It is our hope that you can join with other mothers and together find the same reinforcement and satisfaction that we have known.

The best place we know of to receive this mother-to-mother support is your local La Leche League Group. Attending LLL meetings during your pregnancy is the ideal preparation for breastfeeding and a good way to learn what being a mother is all about. Betty McLellan, a La Leche League member from Ontario, Canada, puts it this way:

> I have a background in psychology, but it was attendance at LLL meetings and the example of a wonderful Leader that showed me alternatives to many of the typical ways of handling children in our culture. The "psychology of mothering" is learned best from other mothers and comes through loud and clear at La Leche League meetings.

La Leche League Meetings

"Doesn't breastfeeding just come naturally? My great-grandmother never went to a La Leche League meeting, and she nursed all her babies." "Why should breastfeeding women need a worldwide organization for support?" Many who are unfamiliar with La Leche League ask these questions. More and more mothers today are choosing to breast-feed their babies, but they may not understand just how much a support group like La Leche League can help them enjoy the experience.

When La Leche League began nearly fifty years ago, breastfeeding had become a lost art. Mothers had begun seeking advice from medical professionals about caring for their babies instead of learning from the wisdom of other mothers.

Today, La Leche League gatherings are held monthly in all parts of the world. The information is divided into topics for a four-meeting series. As no two series of meetings are exactly alike, many mothers continue to attend for many months beyond the first series and even for many years.

LLL meetings are sometimes held in the home of a La Leche League member or in a convenient public meeting place. Mothers are encouraged to bring along their nursing babies. The meetings are conducted by an experienced breastfeeding mother who has been accredited to represent La Leche League. She presents a specific outline of information at each meeting, but these meetings are not classes; they are open, informative discussions. At the LLL Group meetings in your area, you will learn about much more than the basics of breastfeeding.

The first meeting of the series is usually about the advantages of breastfeeding. You will discover benefits of breastfeeding that may have never occurred to you—results of research on the value of human milk and mothers' own stories of breastfeeding advantages. Many mothers have remarked after this meeting, "I knew that breastfeeding was good for my baby and good for me, but I didn't know how good it was. This information makes me more confident than ever in my decision to nurse, and it makes me feel proud to know that I am doing something so wonderful for my baby."

At the next meeting, the discussion usually centers on the family and the breastfed baby. Mothers share tips on how to get off to a good start in the hospital and at home with the new baby. Knowing what to expect in the way of procedures and routines at local area hospitals or birthing centers can be helpful to a pregnant mother. Easing the emotional adjustment of all family members, lightening the workload, establishing a good milk supply, and preventing problems from ever beginning are all topics of discussion.

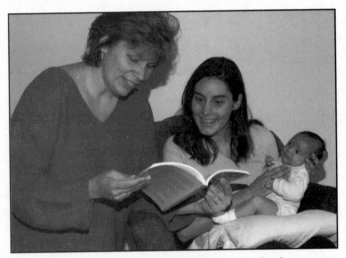

Mother-to-mother support helps a new mother learn
about breastfeeding.

Another meeting covers basic breastfeeding techniques and problem-solving. You can receive specific advice from the best breastfeeding experts in the world: experienced nursing mothers. The overall message is that no matter what problem may arise, there is almost always a solution that does not require weaning the baby.

At another meeting, the proper diet for lactating and pregnant women is discussed, as well as starting the baby on solid foods and when and how to wean the baby. Often discipline of toddlers is also explored at this meeting.

Almost all La Leche League Groups have an extensive lending library available to their members. Current titles on breastfeeding, childbirth, parenting, and nutrition that may not be widely available can be found at LLL meetings. Most Groups also have books, booklets, and breastfeeding-related products that LLL members can purchase.

All mothers are welcome

All women who have an interest in breastfeeding are invited to attend La Leche League meetings. All mothers are accepted with open arms at La Leche League: mothers of all races and religions, single mothers, working mothers, and mothers whose philosophy on various aspects of infant care and childrearing may differ from La Leche League's. Each mother is encouraged to take from La Leche League's philosophy what seems sensible and helpful to her. The ideal time to begin attending is during pregnancy, because the information received in advance may prove to be vital to a mother when her baby arrives.

After her first La Leche League meeting one pregnant mother commented, "I had read all the books, and didn't think there was anything else I needed to know. I learned so much more tonight than I expected to." Another mother, Heather Karlheim from Ohio, had a similar response after attending La Leche League meetings:

> As a pharmacist and avid reader, I spent the months of my first pregnancy reading everything I could find on topics related to birth, breastfeeding, and childrearing. I anticipated my child's birth with confidence.
>
> Since I have a close friend who is a La Leche League Leader, I knew a little about LLL, but I was not convinced that I "needed" such an organization.
>
> In my fifth month of pregnancy, I was persuaded by a co-worker, who was also expecting a baby, to accompany her to a La Leche League meeting. This meeting was a real turning point for me, providing specific suggestions and lots of reassurance from other mothers.
>
> As the months passed and my daughter and I became a happy nursing couple, I continued to benefit from La Leche League meetings and friendships made there.
>
> As I look back now I can't believe how naive I was, thinking that I could "learn it all" from books. La Leche League has been, for me, a safe island in the tumultuous sea of first-time motherhood, and you can bet I'm not about to jump back into the water alone!

Why Do You Need Support?

Though the majority of mothers in the USA start out breastfeeding, within a few months, weeks, or even days, most of them switch to formula. Why? Insufficient milk supply, breast infections, sore nipples, embarrassment, criticism from relatives, and general confusion about newborn behavior are some of the reasons. These problems can be avoided for the most part or resolved quickly with the correct information and support. If a breastfeeding mother has questions or concerns, she can contact a La Leche League Leader for help at any time. Sometimes just being able to dial the phone number of a sympathetic, informed mother who has had breastfeeding experience is the key to the resumption of a successful breastfeeding relationship. Mothers can also receive help from a La Leche League Leader on our Web site at www.lalecheleague.org/.

Ruth A. Lawrence, MD, a physician who breastfed her own children and the author of *Breastfeeding: A Guide for the Medical Profession*, emphasizes that mothers need information and support as they learn about breastfeeding:

> Breastfeeding is not a reflex; it is a learned process. In our present culture, many women have never witnessed an infant at the breast. When a woman is called upon to nurse her own infant, much of her success depends on a learning process. Successful lactation depends on proper information.

Mothers who attend LLL meetings soon find there is more involved than basic breastfeeding information. There is something very special about the sharing and companionship of other mothers. Cynthia Webb, from Montana, found this out:

> When I was seven months pregnant and wondering if I could survive pregnancy and parenthood, I found a place that celebrates motherhood in a quiet, sustaining fashion: my first La Leche League meeting.
>
> I believe motherhood touches the soul of a woman in a way that nothing else can. After being infertile for ten years, motherhood came as quite a surprise to me. Without LLL, I'd probably still be in shock. La Leche League members have helped me cope with many situations. Problem-solving and support are important, but so is having a place to share the special joys of each day's experience. An LLL meeting is a haven for all of these things.

And another LLL member, who wrote to us anonymously, told how La Leche League helped her overcome memories of her own unhappy childhood:

> The reason I am so grateful to La Leche League is that it has helped me understand what "mothering" means and has given me confidence with my own children. My own upbringing was scary and chaotic. I was terribly afraid of becoming a mother. By having a stable nursing relationship I was able to tune in physically and emotionally to the needs of my baby.
>
> At meetings I saw other mothers at peace with their infants and toddlers, learning like me and still available to be learned from. I became friends with several of these mothers

and that, too, has enriched my life and my children's lives. And of course, those things that enrich us are of benefit to my husband as well.

I read your bimonthly magazine, NEW BEGINNINGS, including all the back copies in the Group's library. I am grateful I received adequate doses of support in favor of nursing to counterbalance the negative input I had received.

Sally Olson, from Nebraska, already breastfed two babies when she attended her first La Leche League meeting. Her third son was just a month old. She explains:

I really went to the meeting to meet some other mothers, as we had just moved to a new town and I did not know a soul. I found what I went for—friendship with other nursing mothers—but I also found much more. The mothers in my Group and the LLL pamphlets and books found in the LLL Group Library helped me to put into words and actions what I felt in my heart.

How Do I Find La Leche League?

There are several ways for you to find out the name of your local La Leche League Leader. You may find La Leche League listed in the white pages of your telephone directory, however many LLL Groups are not able to afford such a listing. You might check at your local library to see if they have information about a nearby LLL Group. If you are attending childbirth classes, your instructor may know of an LLL Group in the area. A local newspaper may have LLL meeting notices from time to time so they may know the local Leader's phone number.

You can also write or call LLLI's central office for the name and number of your local Leader. Our business hours are from 9 AM to 5 PM (Central Time in the USA); the phone number is 847-519-7730. By following the directions on the menu, you can put in your zip code (in the USA) and be directed to a Leader near you. You can also use our toll-free number to find the name of a local Leader. Call 1-800-LA LECHE. The address is: P.O. Box 4079, Schaumburg IL 60168-4079 USA. In Canada, the toll-free number is 800-665-4324 and the office for LLL Canada is located at 18C Industrial Drive, Box 29, Chesterville, Ontario K0C 1H0. The phone number in Canada is 613-448-1842.

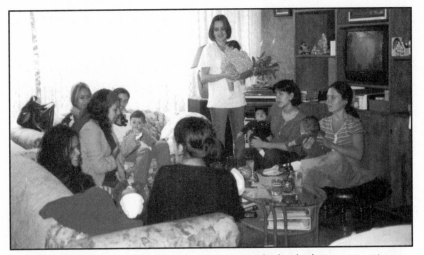

Mothers find information and encouragement at La Leche League meetings.

Local Group meetings that are held all over the world are listed on the Internet at www.lalecheleague.org along with a wealth of breast-feeding information in many languages.

When you join LLL, you participate in an international mother-to-mother helping network, a valuable resource for parenting help and support. Paying your annual dues brings you six bimonthly issues of NEW BEGINNINGS, a magazine filled with stories, hints, and inspiration from other breastfeeding families. Members in the USA receive our LLLI Catalogues by mail and they are entitled to a 10% discount on most purchases from LLLI's wide variety of outstanding books and publications on breastfeeding, childbirth, nutrition, and parenting. Your membership dues also support La Leche League activities all over the world. Additional benefits of LLL membership may also be available; they will be explained by your local Leader or in current LLL publications. Membership fees and benefits may vary in countries outside the USA.

Even mothers who cannot attend LLL Group meetings find the support they need through LLL membership. Elizabeth Hunsaker was living in Belgium, far from her family and friends, when her first baby was born. She writes:

I had always wanted to breastfeed because I had read it was best for the baby and that it helped to create a special bond between mother and child. I bought many books on caring for a baby, and I joined La Leche League. Our baby boy is now ten months old and is still nursing. It has been an experience

I will always treasure. But it hasn't always been easy; and at times I felt very frustrated and discouraged.

Receiving NEW BEGINNINGS helped me through a lot of trying times and made my nursing experience a happier one. Reading letters from other mothers who had the same experiences and the same attitudes about nursing made me feel as if I weren't alone and that it was worth the effort.

And another mother, Elena Hannah from Newfoundland, Canada, found a friend's collection of back issues helped her get through some difficult times:

When I was almost overwhelmed with problems I was having with my first baby, a friend sent me her two-year collection of back issues of NEW BEGINNINGS. As soon as I starting reading them I felt I had found what I needed. Reading others' stories, many of them with problems more serious than mine, put everything back in perspective for me, and the main message seemed to be: "You can do it! You can overcome the difficulties!" By the time I finished devouring the collection I felt calmer and more confident. So today I want to say: Thank you to all the mothers who shared their stories with me and thank you, La Leche League, for having such a wonderful publication.

Soon thereafter, Elena paid her membership dues and started receiving her own copies of NEW BEGINNINGS on a regular basis.

Is La Leche League just for brand new mothers? The answer is "no." Experienced mothers provide the backbone of LLL Groups because they can offer the advice and encouragement that help a new breastfeeding mother cope. But mothers of older babies and toddlers find advantages, too, from their continued association with La Leche League. Elizabeth Hormann, who is an experienced mother and La Leche League Leader, writes:

Why would anyone want to continue with LLL once their children are weaned? It is not always easy to explain, but support is a large part of the reason. LLL addresses more than breastfeeding; there is a philosophy of mothering that grows from our experience as nursing mothers and that philosophy is not widely shared outside La Leche League circles. We need each other, especially as our children get beyond infancy and develop more facets to their personalities.

Mothers of toddlers are particularly likely to need the kind of support LLL provides. Shifting gears to care for toddlers is not easy.

Above and beyond information, La Leche League offers a special advantage to mothers summed up this way by one La Leche League Leader: "LLL gives me an opportunity to surround myself with the kind of people that I want in my life: caring, intelligent, family-oriented women who look on their children as assets, and who enjoy being mothers."

Beyond the basics

In addition to the basic meetings offered by LLL Groups all over the world, special meetings are often scheduled in response to the interest of the mothers in the Group. Toddler Meetings are held routinely for mothers who want to discuss meeting the needs of their older babies and toddlers. Employed Mothers' Meetings may be scheduled when mothers in the Group want to discuss routines that are specifically directed to combining working and breastfeeding. Couples' Meetings or Fathers' Nights give men the opportunity to share their experiences with one another.

In addition, La Leche League periodically sponsors International and Area Conferences. These are one, two, or three day events providing information on breastfeeding and parenting that goes beyond the topics of regular LLL meetings. Doctors, health professionals, educators, and experienced parents lend their expertise to a variety of sessions throughout the day. Often luncheons are scheduled featuring a special guest speaker or allowing time for open discussion. Mothers, fathers, and babies enjoy the opportunity to spend the day together at an LLL Conference.

At International Conferences, which are usually held every other year, thousands of parents and professionals from all over the world meet to share their experiences and expertise. La Leche League International also sponsors annual Physicians' Seminars on Breastfeeding. Currently, these seminars are cosponsored by the American Academy of Pediatrics and the American College of Obstetricians and Gynecologists, The American Academy of Family Physicians participates as a cooperating organization. These seminars are also accredited by other major medical associations. Lactation Specialist Workshops are also scheduled in various locations and offer continuing education credits for board certified lactation consultants and registered nurses.

La Leche League International offers training opportunities for Breastfeeding Peer Counselors who work in local communities to support and encourage breastfeeding mothers.

The LLL Alumnae Association continues to link Leaders and members together as they explore the application of LLL philosophy in new stages of their lives. It is open to all current and retired Leaders and members.

La Leche League has been a source of inspiration and encouragement for breastfeeding mothers for almost fifty years. If there is an LLL Group in your community, we urge you to become a part of this mother-to-mother network.

PART TWO

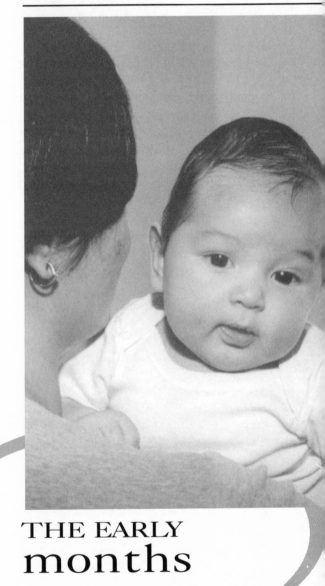

THE EARLY
months

CHAPTER FOUR

YOUR BABY
arrives

The newborn child is a rare and incredible sight. He seems so tiny and helpless, yet he does have certain survival skills. Held up close, a newborn baby can see his mother's face clearly, and in fact has a preference for the human face. He can also hear quite well. For a period during the first hour of life, most newborns are quietly alert and receptive. A lively and intricate exchange of messages passes between the mother and baby who are together at this time. The hours and days immediately after birth also seem to be an especially sensitive period for a mother to form an attachment to her newly arrived baby.

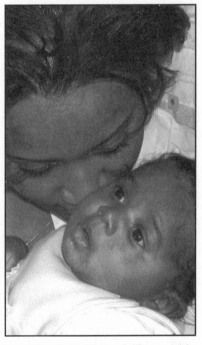

In their book, *Your Amazing Newborn*, Marshall Klaus, MD, and his wife, Phyllis, tell about a newborn's capability:

> Right after birth, within the first hour of life, normal infants have a prolonged period of quiet alertness, averaging forty minutes, during which they look directly at their mother's and father's face and eyes and can respond to voices. It is as though newborns have rehearsed the perfect approach to the first meeting with their parents.

45

Baby's First Feeding

The sooner you put your baby to the breast, the better. Most babies are ready and even eager to breastfeed at some time within the first hour. Amazingly, a healthy full-term newborn who is placed on his mother's abdomen soon after birth is able to find his way to her breast and latch on without assistance, provided he is not drowsy from drugs or anesthesia used during labor and delivery. The sucking reflex of a full-term healthy newborn is usually at a peak about twenty to thirty minutes after he is born. If this prime time to begin nursing is missed, the baby's sucking reflex may be less strong for about a day and a half.

Early breastfeeding is mutually beneficial to mother and baby. Aside from getting breastfeeding off to a good start, your newborn's immediate nursing hastens the delivery of the placenta. You will have less blood loss because the baby's sucking causes the uterus to contract. For the baby, being so close to his mother is comforting, and the first milk, the colostrum, is priceless as a source of protective immunities against disease.

When mothers are able to greet their newborns by cuddling and nursing, and infants remain with their mothers to nurse at will, breastfeeding usually progresses with few problems. Mother and baby need to be together early and often to establish a satisfying relationship and an adequate milk supply.

Your first attempt to breastfeed your baby is a learning experience, a get-acquainted effort for both of you. There are many variations in babies' responses. He may only nuzzle at your nipple or lick it a few times. You will be very emotional from the excitement of giving birth and you may feel awkward trying to position your baby at the breast. It will be hard for you to relax if there is a lot of activity going on around you.

The important thing is to hold your baby close, talk to him, and comfort him. Cup your breast in your hand (as described in the sections that follow) and tickle your baby's lips with your nipple. If he opens his mouth wide, pull him in close to you so he can easily grasp the nipple and a large portion of the areola, the darker skin area that surrounds your nipple. He may take a few sucks and fall asleep. Or he may let go and prefer to look around at his new surroundings. Don't worry if he doesn't latch on right away. He will soon. This first opportunity to nurse sets the stage for the hours and days ahead when you and your baby will be getting to know each other.

If medical complications prevent you from breastfeeding immediately after your baby is born, all is not lost. You and your baby can make up for lost time once you are able to be together and begin breastfeeding. In later chapters of this book, we discuss breastfeeding in certain medical situations or unusual circumstances. If you are in the hospital, there may be a board certified lactation consultant on staff who can help you. You'll also want to be in touch with your local La Leche League Leader if difficulties or special problems arise.

Getting started

Getting your baby started at the breast smoothly and easily will soon be second nature to you. Breastfeeding a baby is actually much less involved than any description of the process.

One benefit of attending La Leche League meetings during your pregnancy is seeing other mothers breastfeeding their babies. This can help you more than photos or written explanations because you can observe a variety of mothers with babies of different ages and sizes who have adopted comfortable ways to breastfeed. They will probably be using pillows, cushions, footstools, and armrests to help them position their babies for nursing. Of course, no two mothers and babies are alike and as a baby gets older and nurses well, correct positioning becomes less of a concern.

Breastfeeding in Slow Motion

The following steps explain the correct way to position your baby at the breast in order to ensure that baby sucks well and gets plenty of milk. Correct positioning and latch-on of the baby at the breast will also prevent nipple soreness and pain.

1. *Position yourself properly.* It's easiest to get started breastfeeding the first few times if you are sitting up. Sit up in bed, in a comfortable armchair, or in a rocking chair. Pillows are a must. Use them behind your back, under your elbow, and on your lap to support the baby. Use a footstool to bring your knees up or use pillows under your knees if you are sitting up in bed. You should be relaxed with none of your muscles straining.

2. *Position your baby properly.* Baby should be lying on his side with his whole body facing you and his knees pulled in close to your body. In the cradle hold, his head should rest on your forearm. His back should be supported by your forearm and you can hold his bottom or his upper thigh with your hand. Baby's ear, shoulder, and hip should be in a straight line. His head should be in line with his body, so he does not need to turn sideways to reach your nipple.

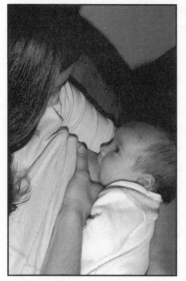

When baby is latched on well, it does not hurt to breastfeed.

3. *Hold the baby at the level of your nipple,* so you are not leaning forward to reach him and he is not straining to latch on. Using a pillow on your lap will help.

4. *Offer your breast to the baby.* Your thumb and index finger should form a "C" or "U." Be sure your fingers are well behind the areola. Support the breast as close to its natural height as possible while the baby latches on and throughout the feeding, with your thumb in line with the baby's nose and four fingers on the other side of the breast. Keep fingers and thumb well back from the nipple so they don't get in the way as the baby latches on.

5. *Encourage baby to latch on properly.* If baby turns his head away, gently stroke his cheek on the side nearest you. The rooting reflex will make him turn his head toward you. Encourage the baby to open his mouth wide by moving him toward and away from the breast, touching his lips lightly and repeating until baby opens wide. Baby's mouth should be open really wide, like a yawn, as he latches on. Talk to him and encourage him to open his mouth. When the baby opens his mouth wide, pull him onto the breast chin first, so that his lower jaw (which does all the work during feedings) is as far back on the breast as possible.

6. *Move baby onto the breast quickly and firmly,* so that he takes the breast deeply into his mouth. Once he is latched onto the breast, keep him pulled in very close, so his chin is pressed into the breast. If his nose seems blocked by the breast, pull his hips and legs in closer to you to angle out his nose. If the baby is latched on well, it should not hurt to breastfeed.

7. *Encourage baby to suck effectively.* In order to suck effectively, the baby must take a large portion of your areola into his mouth along with the nipple. The milk sinuses that must be compressed in order to release the milk are located under the areola. Baby's gums

should completely bypass the nipple and cover all or most of the areola behind the nipple. Be sure your nipple is above his tongue. Baby should be pulled in so close that his chin is pressed into your breast. If baby's nose seems blocked by your breast, try lifting up your breast or pulling baby's body in closer to you rather than pressing down on the top of your breast.

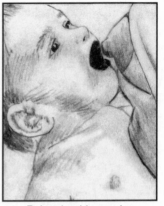

Baby should open his mouth wide.

8. *Avoid nipple soreness or pain.* If your baby is latching on and sucking correctly you should not feel any painful pressure on your nipple. If baby seems to be sucking incorrectly or you feel pain as he nurses, you will need to remove the baby from your breast and start over again. Break the suction by putting your finger in the side of baby's mouth and either pressing on your breast or gently pulling on baby's cheek. Don't let your baby continue to suck incorrectly because it can lead to nipple soreness; poor sucking patterns can be hard to correct later on. Perhaps the baby's mouth needs to be open wider, you need to adjust the angle so that his lower jaw is farther back on your breast, or he needs to be pulled in closer to you.

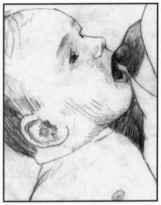

Baby goes onto the breast chin first.

Some babies catch on quickly, while others need more time. For some babies, it may take many tries at each feeding before breastfeeding feels comfortable. You need to coordinate your actions with baby's reactions so that all goes smoothly. If baby gets frustrated, you may have to stop and soothe him a bit before starting again.

Getting a good latch-on during the early weeks is well worth the

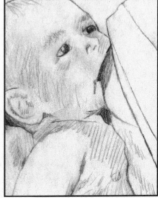

This baby is latched on well.

effort. Not only does it prevent sore nipples, but it also makes sure the baby gets the most milk for his efforts and stimulates a healthy milk supply. Within a short time, it will become quick and automatic, and you will not need to follow these steps. But in the meantime, plan to spend some time at each feeding helping your baby learn to do it right.

If you continue to feel discomfort, check into these possible causes of nipple pain:

- Do not let baby slide onto the nipple, stopping short of the correct sucking position. Be sure he opens his mouth very wide so your nipple goes far back into his mouth.

- If baby persistently clamps down too hard as he starts to suck, depress his lower jaw with your finger by pulling down on his chin as you tell him to "open" in a clear, commanding tone of voice. Open your mouth wide and baby may imitate you.

- If nipple pain continues, have a helper gently pull baby's lower lip down while he is nursing and check to see if his tongue is visible between his lower lip and the breast. If his tongue is not visible, baby may be sucking it along with your nipple. Take baby off the breast and restart him, being sure his mouth is open very wide and his tongue is below the nipple and forward in his mouth when he latches on

- If baby's chin is not touching the breast, he is probably not sucking effectively. Take him off the breast and start again. Be sure his mouth is open very wide and pull him onto the breast chin first.

9. *Watch for effective sucking patterns.* Many babies know exactly how to suck correctly from the moment they are born. Others take a few days to learn and need specific guidance as outlined above with lots of comfort and patience. But once baby is sucking properly you will take great satisfaction in watching him. As baby sucks vigorously, the muscles in his face work so hard that even his ears wiggle. You can see the strong action of his jaw muscles and hear him swallowing. Then once his initial hunger is satisfied, he becomes relaxed, sucking less vigorously, with fewer swallows, as he enjoys the closeness and comfort of being at his mother's breast.

10. *Let the baby finish at one breast and then offer the other breast.*
In the early days of breastfeeding, it is a good idea to offer both breasts at each feeding. If the baby is latched on and positioned well, there is no reason to limit a feeding. Once baby is nursing actively, let him nurse from the first breast until he comes off on his own, either by letting go or by falling asleep, and then offer the second breast. Sometimes he will take the other breast, and sometimes he will not, which is fine. If a baby falls asleep or stops nursing actively within a few minutes, he may need to be latched on again and encouraged to continue.

Supporting your breast

You will sometimes see photos of mothers using just two fingers to position their breast for the baby to latch on. At one time, this technique was recommended and some mothers do find it effective. But more recently it has been found that positioning the thumb and fingers to form a "C" or "U" allows the mother to support her breast and avoid pressing on the areola or squeezing too hard. It is suggested that the way you hold your breast should be adjusted so that the widest part of the breast lines up with the widest part of baby's mouth. In other words, use the "C" hold when baby is facing you and the "U" hold when baby is coming toward the breast with his head sideways.

Other Breastfeeding Positions

It can be useful to know how to breastfeed your baby in different positions so you can find the ones that are most comfortable for you.

Lying down to nurse

Learning how to comfortably breastfeed your baby while lying down can be very helpful.

Breastfeeding your baby in the side-lying position will allow you to get more rest in the early weeks. You will need to use pillows to support yourself and the baby. At first, you may need some help getting the baby positioned properly so he can latch on correctly. Lie on your side with a pillow under your head. Have baby lying on his side facing you with his mouth in line with your nipple and his knees pulled in close to your body. You may be comfortable with the baby lying directly on the bed or you may want to place your arm under him. Lean back into the pillows that are behind your back. Offer your breast to the baby by supporting it with your fingers underneath and your thumb above, well behind the areola. Encourage the baby to latch on properly

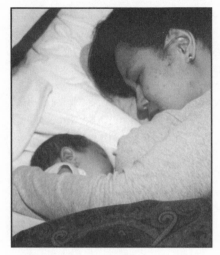

Nursing lying down.

as described above. Wait until he opens his mouth wide. Then quickly pull him in close to you so he can latch on well and suck effectively.

After you get baby started, you may want to place a pillow behind his back to hold him close and tuck your arm under the pillow supporting your head if that's more comfortable for you. Some mothers also place a pillow between their knees. To change sides, sit baby up and pat his back to see if he needs to bring up a burp, then hold him flat against your chest and roll over on your back. Lie on your other side and position baby at your other breast. This is especially good for mothers who have had a cesarean birth; while still in the hospital you can use the side rails on the bed to help you roll over.

The football hold

Another useful position for you and your baby to learn is the football or "clutch" hold. Seated in a wide chair or on a sofa, position baby at your side with his legs under your arm and his head near your breast. Support his head by placing your fingers on his neck and shoulders. Use pillows to bring baby up to the level of your nipple. When you pull baby in close to latch on, be sure his legs are not pushing against the back of the chair or sofa. If this seems to be happening, bend his legs upward, behind you. This position is helpful for babies who are having trouble latching on as it gives the mother good visibility of what's going on and good control of baby's position as he latches on.

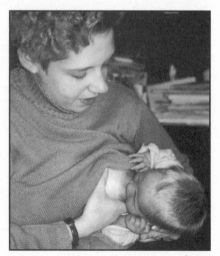

The football hold.

Crossover, cross cradle, or transition hold

This position is similar to the cradle hold described above, but you are holding the baby with the opposite arm. To feed the baby with the left breast, support the breast with your left hand and hold the baby with your right arm. This position gives you a good view of baby's latch-on and may be a good choice at first for a premature baby or a baby who is having trouble latching on. Support

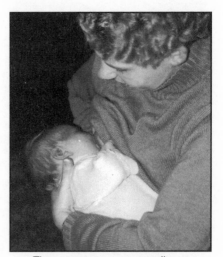

The crossover, cross cradle, or transition hold.

your baby's head by resting his neck on the palm of your hand, with your thumb and fingers at the base of his head. Don't hold onto the back of baby's head as this will cause some babies to pull away from the breast. Some mothers use pillows under the baby's body to support his weight and bring him up to the level of the breast. By using the "U" hold, your elbow is at your side. Support your breast with the hand on the same side as the breast you are offering.

Follow these procedures carefully at first

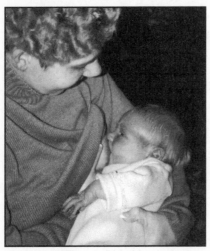

The cradle hold.

Since it is important that the young baby learn to suck effectively, we recommend that you use these techniques step-by-step when you and your baby are learning. After a while, when both of you are breastfeeding experts, you can use whatever positions and procedures are comfortable for you. You may find yourself breastfeeding in different positions at different feedings. This is just fine. Breastfeeding should be a comfortable and relaxing time for you and your baby.

The milk-ejection reflex (the let-down)

After the baby has been sucking vigorously for several minutes, many mothers feel a tingling sensation and notice a strong surge of milk. This is known as the milk-ejection reflex or the let-down. It occurs several times during a feeding, and mothers sometimes notice that milk drips from the other breast when a let-down occurs. Baby usually responds to the let-down with more frequent swallowing. Even if you don't feel a tingling in your breast, you'll know a let-down has occurred by watching baby's pattern of sucking and swallowing. Sometimes, hearing your baby cry will initiate a let-down even before he starts to nurse.

Occasionally a baby will be caught off-guard by mother's strong let-down and he will choke and sputter a bit. It's a good idea to keep a towel or clean diaper handy to mop up the drips as you sit baby up and let him catch his breath.

Some mothers do not feel the milk-ejection reflex at all, but it is still occurring if their babies are nursing well. For other mothers, the tingling sensation may be very strong, especially in the early weeks. One mother, Jo Ellen Carson from Georgia, had the following thoughts about the let-down:

> One quiet evening as I nursed my daughter to sleep, I reflected on the term "let-down" and I began to wonder how this term came to be used in regard to breastfeeding. It usually means disappointment and hurt. The total opposite is what occurs when I nurse my infant daughter.
>
> The breastfeeding let-down was by then a very familiar feeling to me, yet it can't really be described. My daughter sucked and wriggled and sucked more to coax the milk out. After a few brief moments, I felt the fullness—almost an ache—my breasts seemed hard and ready to overflow. And then the change in her breathing as she began drinking in with long, slow gulps, eyes closed, in utter peace and abandonment.
>
> I looked down at this small being who was cradled against my body. As I stroked her soft, sweet skin, I felt the overwhelming release of love which, to me, is what the let-down truly is.

Engorgement—
When the Milk "Comes In"

Your milk will become more plentiful, or "come in," at some time between the second to the sixth day after delivery. Before that time, your baby will get colostrum, which will provide him with all the nourishment he needs, plus important elements to protect him against infections. It takes about two weeks for the colostrum to gradually change into mature milk.

A combination of factors influences when a mother's milk becomes more plentiful. Nursing the baby soon and often after birth encourages milk production. An unmedicated delivery and having your baby with you make an important difference. It also helps if you are reasonably at ease. For most mothers, being in the familiar surroundings of home, with the freedom that gives you to cuddle and nurse your baby frequently, is all that is needed to bring in the milk.

When the milk becomes plentiful, your breasts may seem fairly bursting. You feel as though you could satisfy twins—or triplets! This fullness comes about because additional blood has rushed to the breasts in order to assure that there will be adequate nourishment for the new baby. It is like the marshaling of the grand army—all the forces come to the fore to get things in good working order. The extra blood, along with some swelling of tissues, produces the fullness. Some mothers notice only moderate or little fullness, while other mothers become engorged with each of their babies.

In the usual course of events, this feeling of fullness subsides in a matter of days. It is especially important to continue to nurse the baby frequently, at least every two hours, since removing milk from the breasts relieves the congestion. A comfortably warm shower, followed by a nursing, often reduces any discomfort. For some women, the normal feeling of fullness develops into engorgement with the breasts becoming hard and painful. The mother may even develop a low-grade fever. Some mothers find applying warm moist compresses and expressing some milk before feedings help to relieve engorgement. Ice packs can be used between feedings to reduce swelling.

A gentle breast massage may also help to relieve engorgement. Sometimes the engorged area is mainly in one part of the breast, perhaps high up toward the arm. With the palm of your hand, gently stroke the breast downward toward the nipple. This is most effective when done under the shower or while leaning over a bowl of warm water and sloshing the water over the breasts.

An effective home remedy to relieve engorgement is the use of cabbage leaves. They can be refrigerated or room temperature. Rinse the cabbage leaves, remove the hard vein, and cut a hole for the nipple. Apply directly to your breasts, inside your bra. In two to four hours, the cabbage leaves will become soft and wilted. Reapply, between feedings, for up to eight hours or until your breasts feel comfortable. Cabbage leaves should not be used for longer than that because they can affect your milk supply.

Cynthia Webb, from Montana, tells how her La Leche League Leader helped her to overcome the problem of engorgement and get off to a good start breastfeeding her daughter:

> The day after we got home from the hospital was the day my breasts became engorged. With the baby crying in the background and the sample bottle of formula from the hospital looking temptingly easy, my LLL Leader gave me advice and solutions that had us back on the right track in half an hour.
>
> It took Kelli and me a little longer to really get the hang of nursing. Then one day everything seemed to fall into place. The reward for perseverance has been tremendous. Kelli has shown me the gentle joys and subtle pleasures of motherhood. More than the baby at the breast, it's the first smile of recognition, little arms around my neck, a sleepy head on my shoulder, or snuggling under the covers during an early morning feeding.

Engorgement can present a problem if the fullness causes the nipples to flatten making it difficult for the baby to latch on properly. It may be helpful to massage your breasts and pump or hand-express some milk first to relieve the fullness. Some mothers worry that expressing even a small amount of milk will increase their milk supply and make their breasts even more engorged. This is not the case. Enabling the baby to latch on effectively will help to soften the breasts and eventually eliminate the problem. Sometimes briefly holding a cold washcloth or ice pack on your nipple will help to bring it out.

Breast shells, made of hard plastic, can sometimes help to draw out flat nipples if they are worn for thirty minutes before feedings. Some suggest using a breast pump for a few minutes to draw out flat nipples and relieve engorgement.

Nipple shields, made of soft silicone, can be worn over a mother's nipples during feedings. If engorgement is making it difficult for a baby to grasp the nipple, using a nipple shield on the breast for a few feedings may be helpful.

How Long to Nurse?

At one time new mothers were often told to limit nursings in the first few days to three to five minutes on each side at each feeding. Such advice was meant to help avoid sore nipples. However, nursing frequently—every two hours or so from the beginning of one feeding to the beginning of the next—is easier on the nipples and at the same time stimulates the production of milk and helps to prevent exaggerated levels of jaundice in your newborn.

We now know that correct positioning of the baby at the breast and effective latch-on techniques are the best protection against nipple soreness, so limiting baby's time at the breast is not necessary to prevent sore nipples.

The length of a breastfeeding session should be determined by the baby's interest and response. He will usually suck eagerly, swallowing often, for the first ten to twenty minutes. Then the flow of milk decreases and he begins to doze or lose interest. That's the time to switch him over to the other breast. You may want to stop at this point to burp him or change his diaper, and then get him started on the other side. As long as he is sucking effectively, you can let him nurse as long as he wants on the second side.

Taking baby off the breast

If you must end a nursing session while baby still has a firm grip on your nipple, you can comfortably remove your baby either by gently pressing the breast away from the corner of his mouth or by pulling back on his cheek near the corner of his mouth. Pulling your baby off the breast without releasing the suction may be painful, and it can also be damaging to your nipples.

One side or both?

Most mothers find it best to offer both breasts to the baby at each feeding in the early days. The baby's sucking stimulates milk production and offering both breasts at each feeding will help keep the breasts from becoming overfull.

At each feeding, alternate starting sides. For instance, if at one feeding you start nursing on the right and then switch to the left, reverse the order for the next feeding. You'll be using the last-used side first and the first, last. To help remember the starting order, mothers have come up with all kinds of ideas from fastening a small safety pin on the bra on the side used last to transferring a small ring or bracelet from hand to hand.

If you do forget, your baby and your own full breast will probably soon let you know you've offered the "wrong" side. No harm is done if this happens from time to time; there's no need for you to worry about it.

"Emptying the breast"

In normal situations, when a baby is nursing effectively and frequently, a mother does not need to worry about "emptying" her breasts. If, however, you have a baby who does not suck well at first, you may need to pump after each feeding in order to provide sufficient stimulation to keep up your milk supply and to provide your own milk for your baby.

New research on milk production shows that emptying the breasts does help to stimulate milk production more effectively. In other words, if a large amount of milk is left in the breasts after a feeding, the breasts will begin to produce less milk for subsequent feedings. This allows a baby who is breastfeeding effectively to regulate his mother's milk supply to meet his needs. However, a decrease in a mother's milk supply can occur if a baby consistently falls asleep before he takes in enough milk, if he is not latched on well to the breast, or if a baby had a birth trauma or a physical injury that causes poor feeding. In these circumstances, you would want to be in touch with someone who is knowledgeable about difficult breastfeeding situations in order to keep up your milk supply and provide your baby with your milk until he is ready to breastfeed effectively.

Keeping your nipples clean

There is no need for special cleansing techniques for your nipples either before or after nursing. The Montgomery glands that surround the nipple secrete a substance that lubricates the skin and discourages the growth of bacteria. When you bathe or shower, use only plain water on the breasts and nipples as soap can be drying. It is important to wash your hands before a nursing session, especially while you are in the hospital.

Burping the baby

During a feeding a baby sometimes swallows air that needs to be expelled or burped if the little one is to be comfortable. Your experience with your own baby will be your best guide as to when and if he needs burping. Some breastfed babies never seem to need burping, while others will swallow air when mother's breast is very full and the milk comes quickly. The baby who by nature is a "gulper" is always a likely candidate for burping. Burping is one of the things to try whenever the baby is fussy.

There are any number of ways to burp a baby. You can try placing your baby on your shoulder and gently patting his back. A clean cloth diaper, small towel, or blanket tossed over the shoulder will absorb any milk that comes up. Just holding your baby in a more or less upright position will bring up most air bubbles in an easy and relaxed way. Another tried and true method is to sit baby in your lap and slowly lean him forward, bending at the hips, while patting or rubbing his back. When he is very small, take care to support his head and back, and hold him in this position for only a few seconds. Some mothers rest the baby, tummy down, across their knees and

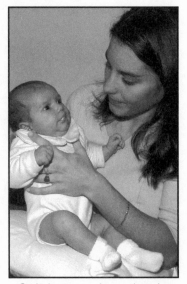

Sit baby in your lap and pat his back to bring up a burp.

rub or pat his back. Try burping the baby when you switch from one breast to the other during a feeding and again when your baby is finished nursing. If there is no burp after a few moments, you can forget the idea—unless, of course, he is fussy. Then you'll want to try again.

Anytime your baby burps especially heartily, see if he wants a little more milk. The big bubble may have made him feel full when he really wasn't. But if baby falls asleep at the breast while nursing, you don't need to disturb him with the burping routine.

Hiccups

We'd also like to mention hiccups here. Little babies seem to be prone to them, often hiccupping after every feeding. Don't worry about them; they're perfectly normal and more upsetting to the parents than the baby. If you like, you can let the baby nurse for a few more minutes. This may stop the hiccups.

Hospital Routines

Hospitals want what is best for the patients, but often their size and bureaucracy come between their good intentions and the kind of care you need. Be prepared to speak up for what you want. Often, getting what you want is simply a matter of persistence. One mother said that whenever she was told "I'm sorry, we can't do that" in answer to a request, she would say that she did not want anyone to go against hospital policy, but that she would like to talk to someone who had the authority to alter the policy. Carrying her appeal up the line did at times result in a happy resolution of the problem.

You may also need help

Assertiveness takes energy, of course, and may be an effort that you aren't up to at the time. Your husband can be your partner in helping to bend or bypass routines that hamper your breastfeeding efforts. You concentrate on caring for the baby, and he can take the position of running interference against red tape and regulations that get in your way. After all, this is your baby, a fact that is sometimes obscured in the delicate balance between institutional and parental authority.

Susan and Larry Kaseman of Virginia tell of their experience when their son Peter was born:

> As my husband, Larry, and I planned for the birth of our second child, one major concern was that our family be together as much as possible. When a cesarean became necessary, we quickly changed plans, but not priorities. With a combination of diplomacy and determination, Larry communicated our wishes and began a dialogue with the hospital staff. They would state hospital policy, we would offer an alternative, and they would consider and sometimes cooperate.
>
> "May I please have my baby?" became my theme throughout my hospital stay. I had been reluctant to refer to our first child as "my baby" for fear of being thought an overpossessive mother. I have since decided it is an effective way of emphasizing to myself and the staff exactly who has the primary responsibility.
>
> Again and again I found that exceptions could be made to many of the rules. Peter was brought to us in the recovery room, two hours old and sleepy, but eager and able to nurse. What a tremendous help that contact was! When a nurse said an injection of painkiller might make me too woozy to be trusted with Peter, I declined the injection and she found a milder, oral drug that worked well enough.
>
> Throughout my hospital stay, I had to keep asking for Peter. If one person refused to bring him, I'd ask someone else. Staff members were generally cooperative in responding, but seldom offered to bring him. I felt like a minority of one because of my "unusual" ideas, and was grateful for the reassurance of those who agreed with me.

My initial concern had been that Peter be with me so I could meet his needs, but I was continually amazed at the strength of my need for him—how much better I felt, physically and emotionally, when he was in my arms, and how difficult it was for me to relax when he was in the nursery.

No supplements—frequent nursing

In the hospital your constant refrain should be that you do not want your baby to be given any artificial nipples, especially bottles of water or formula, and you do want to be able to breastfeed him often. This is very important because artificial nipples and supplementary formula are the greatest deterrents to establishing a good milk supply. Frequent nursing will also help to limit jaundice in your newborn. Your milk is regulated by what your baby takes, and the more he nurses, the more milk your breasts produce. If your baby is given formula, he will take less from the breast. Also, your baby will be confused if he is given an artificial nipple before he learns how to suck properly at the breast. A baby uses his tongue, jaws, and mouth differently when sucking on an artificial nipple. If he is given bottles or other artificial nipples at this point, it may be a long hard struggle before he learns to breastfeed effectively.

If you do not have rooming-in, be sure to let everyone know that you want your baby brought to you as often as he wants to be fed. This should be at least every two hours during the day and whenever he wakes at night. Babies need to be fed at night and if your newborn is not brought to you, he may be receiving a bottle of water or formula in the nursery.

Rooming-in

Problems caused by hospital routines can often be avoided if it is possible for you to room-in with your baby. Rooming-in allows you to have your baby in your room for all or most of the time. You care for the baby, and others care for you. Connie Horenhamp of Illinois tells of her experience:

My first two children were totally breastfed, but they were forced to live those first precious days behind the glass wall of the hospital nursery. I spent many hours standing at the window making sure everything was all right. When Marissa was born, hospital policy was more relaxed and I was more determined; we roomed-in together. We nursed frequently, napped together, and just cuddled. The first day she slept very

**little as she adjusted to her new life, but I was able to phone a
Leader for the reassurance I needed. Now I keep remembering (three months later) how Marissa slept in my arms and in
the arms of my husband. Those first days were ours in which
to grow together. I went home confidently knowing my baby.**

Sleeping or screaming?

If you are able to have rooming-in or at least nurse your baby on
demand, you won't be bothered with problems that can be caused by
hospital feeding schedules. Still, there may be times when baby is not
waking up to be fed as often as he should. A newborn needs to nurse at
least eight to twelve times in twenty-four hours.

If your baby has been sleeping for more than two or three hours,
try gently to awaken him. Rough handling is very disturbing to a newborn, but you can jiggle him a bit, rub his head, talk to him, stroke his
cheek with your nipple; try rubbing his feet or blowing on them.

One suggestion is to sit baby on your lap with his chin in your
hand and bend him forward at the hips. Usually he awakens in just a
few seconds. If not, try walking your fingers up and down his spine. Or
gently bring him from a horizontal to a vertical position, one hand supporting his head, the other holding his bottom.

You can also try undressing him or changing his diaper. If nothing
works to awaken him, you may have to give it another half hour or so
and then try again. If the nurse comes to take him back to the nursery,
be sure to let her know the baby did not wake up to nurse, and should
be brought back for a feeding as soon as he wakes up. Make it clear
that you do not want your baby to be given a bottle in the nursery.

If for some reason your baby is crying very hard before you get a
chance to start feeding him, a little patience may be needed to calm
him down before he's ready to nurse. Try rocking him or putting him
over your shoulder and patting his back. Sing a soothing melody—baby
will be calmed by hearing your familiar voice. Then try offering him
your breast and see if he calms down and starts to suck. If he's not
ready yet, try a few more minutes of calm mothering to help him relax.

With either the sleeping or screaming baby, squeeze a few drops of
your milk onto his lips to give him a taste of what he's missing. We do
not advise putting anything else, such as honey, on the nipple to entice
the baby to take it. Anything other than your milk can cause a reaction
in a sensitive baby. Also, these products may have impurities in them
which could cause problems for baby—a certain type of botulism
spores, for example, has been found in honey and can be very dangerous. Honey should not be given to babies under one year old.

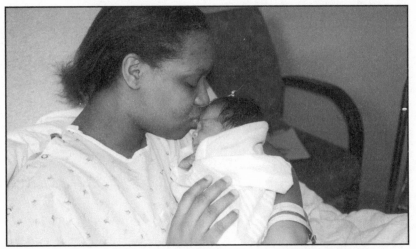

Sometimes baby sleeps right through a "scheduled" feeding time.

Breastfeeding Products

Experience has taught us that breastfeeding proceeds most smoothly when kept as simple and natural as possible. But there are some circumstances when a product designed to aid breastfeeding can be helpful. Breast pumps and other breastfeeding products may be available from your local LLL Leader or a board certified lactation consultant in your area. Some are also sold through the La Leche League International Catalogue and on the LLLI Web site at www.lalecheleague.org. See the Appendix for details.

Breast pumps

Not every breastfeeding mother will need a breast pump. If a mother needs to remove milk from her breasts on a short-term basis, she can usually learn to use the techniques explained for hand-expression in a later chapter and in the Appendix. But there are situations when a breast pump is useful, for example, when a mother is saving her milk for a premature or sick baby, when a mother plans to return to work, or when a mother and baby must be separated for other reasons. More information on breast pumps can also be found in Chapter 7.

In the hospital, you may be advised to use a breast pump to relieve engorgement. If used for this purpose, be sure to pump only enough to soften the breast for baby to grasp the nipple. You will probably not need to do this for more than one or two feedings.

Breast shells or breast shields

These two-piece hard plastic shells are sometimes recommended for use during pregnancy to correct flat or inverted nipples. They can be used for thirty minutes or so before feedings to draw out flat or inverted nipples. One type of breast shell has large holes that allow air to circulate around the nipples. Milk often collects in these breast shells but it should not be saved or fed to the baby. It should be discarded.

Nipple shields

A nipple shield is made of soft silicone and is worn over the mother's own nipple during a feeding. A nipple shield can be a useful tool in helping some babies learn how to breastfeed effectively. When used under the guidance of someone who is knowledgeable about difficult breastfeeding situations, a nipple shield can help some mothers and babies establish a satisfying breastfeeding relationship.

It was once thought that the use of a nipple shield affected a mother's milk supply, but the newer silicone nipple shields do not seem to cause a decrease in milk supply. When a baby is having trouble learning to breastfeed, the use of a nipple shield can keep him at the breast instead of requiring him to adjust to other feeding methods. Some babies need to use a nipple shield for just a few feedings before their sucking ability improves. Others may need to use a nipple shield for weeks or months. Follow baby's cues about discontinuing the use of the nipple shield. Babies are usually willing to nurse without the nipple shield once the initial problem that led to its use has been resolved.

Your LLL Leader or a board-certified lactation consultant will be able to answer any questions you have about the use of a nipple shield or she may be able to offer specific suggestions that will help your baby learn to suck effectively without the use of a nipple shield.

Leaving the Hospital

Nowadays, there is a lot of controversy in the United States about how long new mothers should stay in the hospital after giving birth. Some mothers have been forced to leave sooner than they were ready. Some believe the mother needs to stay in the hospital for two or three days to get breastfeeding well established. Others believe nothing can duplicate the relaxed atmosphere at home that allows you to get to know your baby.

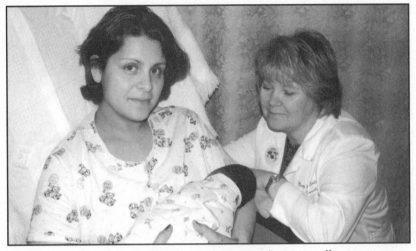

Some hospitals have a lactation consultant on staff to
assist breastfeeding mothers.

The mother who leaves the hospital in twelve to twenty-four hours needs to realize she is not fully recovered from the birth. She needs help at home so she can rest and breastfeed her baby. Also, she should be in touch with a La Leche League Leader or other breast-feeding specialist if she has questions or problems. It is recommended that the baby be checked by a health care provider within the first two weeks to be sure he is gaining weight and breastfeeding well.

Karen Stange of Nebraska went home from the hospital twelve hours after her baby's birth. Karen explains how it worked out:

> The doctor said the baby should be observed for twelve hours, but after that we were allowed to go home. Thus began three of the best days in eleven years of marriage. All of us got to know each other better than ever, and Clay seemed to thrive on the added love of five-year-old Sean and three-year-old Eric. The evening of Clay's birth all five of us sat in our home and, I'm sure, glowed with the love we felt.
>
> Larry took three days off and we did nothing but be a family. We had few visitors as no one realized we were home. I was free to rest as I chose, and needless to add, breastfeed-ing went very well. For us it was a time that will be remembered fondly all our lives.

You can do yourself and your baby a favor by not taking any formula home from the hospital. You won't need it, and if it isn't in the house, you won't be tempted to use it at one of those moments of doubt that

most mothers have. The take-home packs of formula are simply advertising, a promotion for artificial infant feeding. Research has shown
that these formula gift-packs interfere with a mother's determination
to breastfeed.

Hospitals have become much more consumer-conscious in recent
years and want to know what patients like or dislike about their hospital stay. By taking a few minutes to write a personal letter or fill out a
patient questionnaire stating your preferences, you can support the
practices you found helpful and point out the ones you'd like to see
changed. Your suggestions could make it easier for the next breastfeeding mother giving birth in that hospital and, who knows?—you may
find a delightfully improved atmosphere during your next visit.

If for some reason your breastfeeding experience in the hospital
has not been the best or if you could not relax, don't fret. The hospital
stay is now in the past. When you are at home with your baby, you will
be able to breastfeed him. Thousands of mothers have done so and you
can, too.

CHAPTER FIVE

AT HOME WITH
your baby

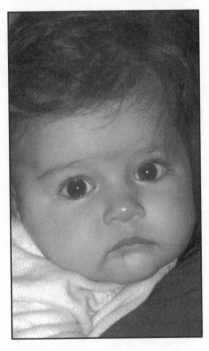

There is a sense of joy and satisfaction on everyone's part when your newborn is settled at home, in the heart of the family. Things are as they should be—you are all together. But don't be surprised if you feel unsure of yourself and even a bit panicky at times. Taking care of this tiny baby is your responsibility day and night, and the realization can seem overwhelming at times. You can be confident that your mothering skills will improve every day as you get to know your baby.

Many of us can say that we've been there; we know the feeling. One of La Leche League's co-Founders thinks back with amazement at her own ineptness when she and her husband brought their firstborn home:

The picture is vivid in my mind. My baby was lying in her basket, which was beautifully done up with a frilly, ruffled liner that I had made before she was born. She was crying her heart out, oblivious to this finery. She had been fed and changed and was supposed to sleep. I remember thinking, "If only she were old enough to talk. She could tell me what is bothering her." Unfortunately, I was not yet aware of a far

more basic form of communication with a little baby—a caring touch. How much more effective than speech! How simple if only I had picked her up! Instead I was feeling somewhat put out at the turn of events, disappointed in myself and my baby.

Think of the baby's first four to six weeks as an adjustment period for both of you, a time of getting to know each other. Your baby is mastering the skill of nursing to bring in milk, and your body is fine-tuning the system for producing it. It's not unusual for a new mother to feel as though her breasts are "bursting" with milk one day, and then be frantic a few days later because she thinks "there's nothing there."

Is the baby getting enough? Why is he crying? Haven't we all asked ourselves these questions and more? A good many of us announced firmly at some point in those early weeks that breastfeeding was "impossible." But at the urging of a supportive husband or with the help of another nursing mother, we decided to keep going for just a few more days.

Nowadays, new mothers have the advantage of being able to call an LLL Leader when questions or problems arise. She can give you reassuring answers and mother-to-mother encouragement. Diane McAleer, a mother from Florida, is still enjoying her breastfeeding relationship with her one-year-old daughter. But she recalls the early weeks:

> **The first six weeks were rough but well worth it. It took a while for me to recover from my daughter's long, difficult birth. We made it through together—Tiffany receiving the best through my milk and her nursing helping me to get back into shape. Six weeks, I had been told, was the magic number. I was told not to give up the idea of nursing until after that period, as both mother and child need time to adjust to one another. We had problems in the beginning, but nothing that a phone call to one of my LLL Leaders could not resolve.**

Babies Are to Love

Through doubts and anxious moments, remember—babies are to love. The task of caring for your new baby will not seem nearly so awesome if you keep this thought in mind, "Tender loving care" is what the very best authorities recognize as the prime need of babies. Look to your own baby. Is he happiest when snuggled close to you, nursing very often, perhaps even every hour? Or does he respond best when laid down after a nursing and patted to sleep? Your baby's well being, comfort, and security are your guides.

James Kenny, a clinical psychologist, who together with his wife, Mary, has authored many books and articles about childrearing, writes about baby's needs:

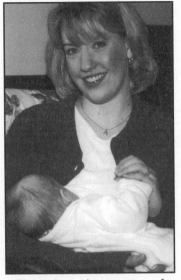

The needs of the infant are urgent. They are necessary for survival. When adults meet these needs day after day and week after week with reasonable consistency and promptness, the infant gradually develops a sense of trust.

The early weeks are a time of learning for you and your baby.

There is a beautiful simplicity about the care of the young baby that does not apply at any other stage of childrearing. With sureness we can say that a baby's wants are a baby's needs. The wants of a two- or three-year-old, however, may not always be what he needs. Parents will not respond any less lovingly then, but their approach will adjust to the changing world of the mobile child.

Mary Ann Cahill, one of La Leche League's co-Founders, talks about the needs of a newborn:

From living in the womb with the umbilical cord supplying all his needs, he has progressed to a position outside of, but near, mother's body. He is meant to be within close proximity of her warm breast and the sound of her voice. It is nature's careful way of providing a transition from the infant's old world to his new one. The little newcomer has the freedom needed to grow, yet is assured of continuous, loving support. The all-important mother-child bond replaces the umbilical cord.

Don't be afraid to "give in" to your newborn. "Giving in" to him is good parenting. Feed him according to his own time schedule. Comfort him when he is upset. But, you may ask, won't such permissiveness spoil the baby? This question is asked by many parents who are sincerely concerned about their children and want to do what is best.

A mother, grandmother, and La Leche League Leader, Marion Blackshear, had this to say on the matter of spoiling and babies:

> When you think of a piece of fruit as spoiled, you think of it as bruised, left on the shelf to rot, handled roughly, neglected. But meeting needs, giving lots of loving care, handling gently, is not spoiling. I could carry this one step further and say that a piece of fruit is at its best when left to ripen on the tree, its source of nourishment—and a baby is at his best when held close to his source of physical and emotional nourishment—his mother.

And others agree. Dr. William Sears, pediatrician and author of numerous child care books says, "Spoiling is a word that should be forever stricken from parenting books.... Babies do not get spoiled by being held. Babies 'spoil' when they are not held."

And in his classic book, *How to Really Love Your Child*, Dr. Ross Campbell explains:

> We cannot start too early in giving a child continuous, warm, consistent affection. He simply must have this unconditional love to cope most effectively in today's world.

How Many Times Do I Feed the Baby?

Throughout this book, we refer repeatedly to feedings "every two or three hours" since it is a common time span for babies' appetites. And it is a fact that when baby's tummy is filled often enough, and mother's breasts are emptied regularly enough, most breastfeeding problems are avoided. But no timetable can tell you how often you should nurse your baby. Some babies, some of the time, will nurse more often than every two hours. Others will nurse less often, or perhaps go for one longer stretch at night or in the early morning hours.

Some people are more comfortable with the explanation that a newborn usually breastfeeds eight to twelve times in twenty-four hours. This way, a mother is not watching the clock to see if two hours have passed since baby's last feeding.

Mothers who live in a world that is not as mechanized and scheduled as ours would be aghast at the thought of regulating the comfort their babies receive at their breasts. In a study of New Guinea tribeswomen, it was found that infants nursed about once every twenty-four minutes. The babies were carried close to their mother's body all the time and an average feeding lasted about three minutes.

In the *Journal of Tropical Pediatrics and Environmental Child Health*, guest editor Babette Francis wrote:

> **Successful lactation is an expression of a woman's femininity and she doesn't need to count how often she feeds the baby any more than she counts how often she kisses the baby.**

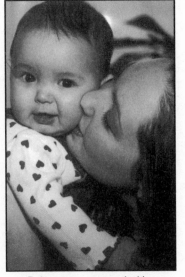

Babies are not spoiled by too much love.

Spitting up

While almost all babies bring up a little milk occasionally after a feeding, some babies spit up regularly after feedings and in-between time.

Some babies spit up because they're getting too much milk too quickly. If your baby gulps and gasps just after you have a let-down, try taking him off the breast for a moment or two as the milk rushes down. Have a diaper handy to catch the overflow. Let baby start nursing again as the milk flow slows to a rate he can handle. Some babies may even let the overflow trickle out of their mouths, which is a nice way of alleviating the problem. Your main response should be very gentle handling, with no sudden movements. Too vigorous burping can bring up milk that would otherwise stay in the baby's stomach. Gentle handling after a feeding will help your baby keep down his lunch. It may help to raise the pad or mattress in baby's bed by a few inches at the head end as laying baby flat is sometimes what triggers the spitting up.

Occasionally a baby will finish nursing as usual and promptly bring up what seems to be the entire feeding, perhaps even with jet-like force. If the baby does not show any signs of illness—no fever or unusual crying—it is probably just one of those things. After things calm down a bit and you've cleaned up the mess, go ahead and nurse the baby again. Of course, you'd want to check with your doctor if this happens often. (For more information on frequent spitting-up or vomiting, see Chapter 17.)

A handy supply of cloth diapers or small towels is a help in protecting your clothing with a spitter in the family. And along with diapers, take extra changes of clothing for baby (and maybe for yourself!)

when going out. As the late Dr. Gregory White often observed, "In a healthy baby, spitting-up is a laundry problem, not a medical problem."

Getting bigger is a sure cure for this tendency in a baby. While spitting-up is a nuisance at the time, there is less odor and staining with human milk than there would be if baby were formula-fed. And really, what's a little milk between a mother and her bosom buddy?

About the pacifier

Be forewarned that the pacifier can create more problems than it solves, often because it works too well. Pop it into a crying baby's mouth, and the room is suddenly blanketed with silence. What could be handier? But therein lies trouble. The use of a pacifier has a way of sneaking up on you by making it so simple to take the easy way out. While a pacifier can sometimes substitute for mother's breast, it is never a substitute for mother.

Used judiciously, however, for a short period of time and in a limited number of circumstances, a pacifier can be a help to the breastfeeding mother. Sucking can be very soothing to a baby, and a pacifier may be convenient when you find yourself in a situation where you absolutely can't nurse him. A pacifier may satisfy him briefly until you can. Sometimes a baby with colic will find it soothing to suck on a pacifier between feedings. If you want to give your baby a pacifier, don't introduce it until the baby is nursing effectively and gaining well.

A problem can develop when a pacifier is used routinely, for instance, as a way to put the baby to sleep. Ordinarily, if your baby likes to fall asleep sucking, let it be at the breast. You have the best pacifier in the world from baby's point of view. And more nursing at the breast means more milk for the baby.

If your baby sucks on a pacifier regularly every day, your milk supply could be adversely affected and the baby may not gain well. One study showed that mothers who gave their babies pacifiers regularly tended to wean sooner than those who did not.

Is Baby Getting Enough?

How will you know if your baby is getting enough milk? He is probably getting enough to eat if he nurses every two or three hours. Is he "filling out" and putting on weight? Growing in length? Active and alert? A "yes" to these questions is an indication that your baby is thriving.

A quick, easy way to reassure yourself that your infant is getting enough milk is to check the number of wet diapers. If he has six or more really wet diapers a day, you can be sure he is getting plenty of milk. (You can learn how to identify the "feel" of a really wet disposable diaper by pouring two to four tablespoons of water into a dry disposable diaper.) Frequent bowel movements are also a sign that baby is getting enough to eat. For the first six weeks or so, a breastfed baby will usually have at least three bowel movements a day.

From time to time, your doctor will weigh the baby as a way of measuring his physical progress. Some babies never lose an ounce from the day they're born, and put on weight with the greatest of ease. Most babies lose some weight during the first week but get back to birth weight by two weeks of age. After that, one and one-half pounds a month (680 grams), at least six ounces (170 grams) a week, is considered an average weight gain, although some babies occasionally gain less in some weeks and others gain as much as a pound a week in the early months. Family characteristics and the baby's individual makeup need to be considered. Remember—healthy, happy babies come in all shapes and sizes. Rapid weight gain in the early months is not a reason for concern as long as the baby's food is human milk and nursings are according to his needs. If baby is gaining less than the average of six ounces a week, you may want to evaluate his nursing patterns to be sure he is nursing effectively and frequently. Slow weight gain is discussed later in "Increasing Your Milk Supply" (in Chapter 7) and "Slow Weight Gain" (in Chapter 17).

With regard to baby's size and appetite, Malinda Sawyer of Missouri observes, "Mothers who give birth to large babies and mothers who give birth to small babies have at least one thing in common: They can expect to have their ability to totally breastfeed the baby questioned."

Marian Tompson, one of La Leche League's co-Founders, remembers when two of her nieces had identical weights of seventeen pounds—but one baby was six months old and the other was one and one-half years old. Yet the doctor for each was satisfied that the baby was healthy.

Leaking

A common occurrence while you are breastfeeding is for milk to drip from one breast when baby starts to nurse on the other. If your breasts are very full or engorged, there is good reason to let the milk come out rather than hold it back. It's a great way to relieve that full feeling. To catch the overflow and keep yourself dry, hold a diaper or something equally absorbent under your breast.

Sometimes a breastfeeding mother will find her milk is leaking at inopportune moments. This is most likely to occur during the first weeks of nursing. Suddenly, to your dismay, you realize that milk is leaking from your breasts. Often, it is nearly time for a feeding and the sight, sound, or even the thought of your baby triggers the let-down reflex.

Nursing mothers have learned that pressure applied directly against the nipples will keep the milk from dripping out. If you notice the tingly, stinging sensation of the let-down—or if you feel milk starting to leak—fold your arms across your chest and apply pressure with the heels of your hands directly on your nipples. Another unobtrusive way to stop leaking is to rest your chin on your hands and press against your breasts with your forearms.

Nursing pads that are designed to absorb leakage are available in drug stores, discount stores, and maternity shops. They are also sold through the LLLI Catalogue and on the LLLI Web site at www.lalecheleague.org. Some are disposable; others can be washed and used over and over again. You'll want to avoid pads that have a plastic liner as they can keep air from getting at your nipples. Some mothers make their own pads by stitching together circular pieces cut from old diapers or other absorbent material. The pads can be washed along with baby's other things and reused. A folded cotton or linen handkerchief works well, too, but avoid the no-iron variety as they are less absorbent.

The possibility of your milk leaking when you least expect it can lead to a certain amount of embarrassment, as Sue Ellen Jennings Austin, from California, recalls:

> I remember an early outing with our first nursing baby. I had carefully planned to be out between his every-two-hour nursings and was even armed with a water bottle in case (heaven forbid!) he should want to nurse in public. We were strolling down the aisle of a grocery store when a woman approached me and whispered, "Excuse me, Miss, your milk is leaking."
>
> Glancing down at the floor, I was horrified to see a trail of milk all around me and my shopping cart. Panicked, I clasped both arms across my chest. It was only then I realized that the milk had not come from me but from a milk carton in my shopping cart that had overturned.

But where has all the milk gone?

When the milk comes in and your breasts feel quite full, you are overjoyed and supremely confident that you will have plenty of milk for your baby. Then the fullness goes away, and you may find yourself thinking that the milk must be gone, too. At this point you may feel discouraged. You begin to wonder, "Have I lost my milk?"

You haven't, we can assure you. The absence of that full feeling and dripping is no indication that the amount of milk you have for your baby has been diminished. The making of milk is an almost continuous process. As the baby takes some out, more comes in. Just keep nursing, and your eager eater will be rewarded with milk, even though you do not feel "full."

The more often your baby takes milk, the more milk you will have. When a mother has twins, there is twice the stimulation to the breasts to produce milk, and so she has enough for two babies. When your baby nurses less often or with less vigor, the amount of milk you produce decreases accordingly. If it drops too low to suit his needs, he will want to nurse more often. With added nursings, your breasts will respond by making more milk.

As you will see, breastfeeding is an excellent example of the law of supply and demand in operation. Problems arise when rigid feeding schedules, bottles of water, or supplementary feedings hamper the natural balance. It takes a little while to establish a good balance between baby's appetite and your milk supply, so be patient. The first six weeks are usually the most challenging. This is the time when you'll really want to be in touch with other breastfeeding mothers, especially your La Leche League Group.

Breastfeeding becomes easier as it continues. As your baby's personality emerges, the fun increases. There are smiles and love pats. The time you spend with baby at your breast helps you get to know each other in a very special way. The concerns of the early weeks will soon give way to the enjoyment awaiting you in the months ahead.

Baby's bowel movements

For the first few days after birth, baby's stool will be very dark—greenish-black—and sticky. It may be a nuisance to wipe off his little bottom, but it's a reassuring sign that all is well with baby's digestive system. This first stool is called meconium. Nursing the baby soon after birth and often in the first few days assures that your baby will get the colostrum he needs to help get rid of the meconium.

Once the meconium is cleared out, the stool of the baby who is receiving only mother's milk differs a good deal from that of the formula-fed infant. The stool of the breastfed baby is usually quite loose and unformed, often of a pea-soup consistency, and may be yellow to yellow-green to tan in color. The odor, unlike that of the formula-fed baby's stool, is mild and not unpleasant.

Frequency of bowel movements varies from baby to baby and even from week to week with the same baby. In the early weeks, a breastfed baby should have at least three bowel movements per day and the amount should be about the size of a US quarter (2.5 cm). Some babies may have even more frequent bowel movements that are little more than a stain on the diaper. At first, your baby may have a bowel movement with every nursing. This is definitely not diarrhea in the breastfed baby. It is a sign that he is getting plenty of milk. As he gets older, past six weeks or so, he may have only two to three large bowel movements a week, sometimes only one a week; even less often is normal for some babies. As his bowel movements decrease in frequency, they will increase in volume. There is room for considerable variation among perfectly normal breastfed babies. Even an occasional green, watery stool is not a cause for worry in the otherwise healthy baby. Bowel movements can also change in color after exposure to the air.

Happily enough, because human milk contains enough water for his needs, your breastfed baby does not get constipated. Constipation (hard, dry stools) has nothing to do with the time interval between bowel movements. Some older breastfed babies go five to seven or more days between bowel movements and have perfectly normal, though very profuse, stools.

Babies sometimes fuss just before or at the time they have a bowel movement, and a change of position may help them. Some can get down to business more easily when in a semi-reclining position, either in your lap or in an infant seat. Others want to brace their feet against something. If you hold the baby against your shoulder, hold one hand under his feet. If your baby is one who seems to have a difficult time with this, you might try helping him by sponging the rectal area gently with warm water. If that doesn't help, some doctors suggest inserting a small glycerin suppository. This is seldom necessary, and there's no need to bother unless your baby has a real struggle and seems very uncomfortable. Be assured that your baby will outgrow this problem.

Caring for Your Baby

As a very new little person, your baby continues to need many of the same conditions that helped him to grow in the womb. He needs to be close to you most of the time, whether awake or sleeping. Being close to you is very reassuring to your new-born. The rhythms of your breathing and heartbeat are familiar to him. In addition, he has been hearing your voice since about five months before he was born, so talking to him in soft, loving tones is especially soothing. For the time being, you are his world.

As the late Herbert Ratner, MD, philosopher and long time friend and advisor to La Leche League, often said, "It is a wise and providential nature that gives each newborn his or her private caretaker and tutor—the mother."

Selma Fraiberg, professor of child psychoanalysis at the University of Michigan Medical School and author of many books and articles on child development, talks about baby's needs:

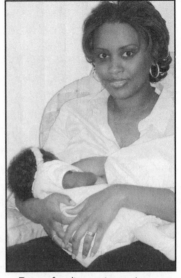

Breastfeeding gets easier as mother and baby get to know each other.

> In the biological program of mother and baby there are built-in guarantees for the satisfaction of the baby's needs that ensure the formation of human bonds in the first eighteen months of life. The mother is the primary "need satisfier," and that need satisfaction should lead the infant through a series of stages in the first year in which the mother is loved more than any other person in his small world.

Viola Lennon, one of La Leche League's co-Founders, tells a story of a young mother who had what seemed to her a hundred and one problems. Vi recalls: "I invited her over for a visit. As she sat down in the living room with me, she immediately began asking questions. Soon I noticed she was not listening to my answers but was watching me handle my baby, Marty, who was rather fussy that day. I nursed him, walked him, bounced him, rocked him, and carried him with me to the kitchen while I made a pot of tea. Finally, she blurted out, 'Does he often act this way?' When I said yes, she smiled and said, 'I don't think I have any real problems. I just didn't know that babies needed all that attention.'"

Keep your baby close

Along with whatever else you are doing during the day, you will want to have your baby close to you as a matter of course. You don't have to have him in your arms every minute, although you will be holding him often, both when you are nursing and between times whenever he needs this contact. But you will just want to be there because what your baby needs most of all is you. No one else can take your place. To him, there is nobody quite like his mother.

In many cultures it is the custom for mothers to be practically inseparable from their babies during their first years, with the baby either strapped to his mother's body or sleeping cuddled next to her. In these cultures, it is unusual to hear a baby cry.

So it is not surprising that a recent study found that more human contact makes for a happier baby. Those babies who spent more time being held or carried either in mother's arms or in a baby carrier—even while contented or asleep—cried less. The younger the baby, the more dramatic were the results. Three extra hours of carrying a day reduced the amount of crying in a four-week-old infant by forty-five percent.

These findings confirm what our mothering instincts tell us—that plenty of loving contact does not "spoil" a baby or make him more demanding, but instead helps him feel more comfortable and happy in his new world.

For many mothers, owning some type of a sling or baby carrier is essential. Helen Nichols of Massachusetts can't say enough "in praise of the baby carrier." She writes: "As with breastfeeding itself, the benefits of the baby carrier are not entirely for the baby. In fact, as I discovered, mother receives a generous portion of them. I could cook, clean house, wash dishes, care for the older children, even sew while Benjamin slept blissfully in his cozy nest. It was, purely and simply, the very easiest thing to do."

When you are considering what kinds of equipment you'll need for your new baby, you might want to put a sling or baby carrier at the top of your list. Remember that very little specialized baby equipment is really necessary; more important to the baby are mother's sweet milk and loving arms. Lee Stewart of Missouri sums up the subject well:

Children's natural values are very human and simple. They want to be held and loved. They want to be with those who care for them. They want to be comfortable. Given a choice between the warmth of human values and material values, babies will almost always choose the human.

A mother from New York, Michele Acerra, gives credit to La Leche League for helping her learn about her baby's needs:

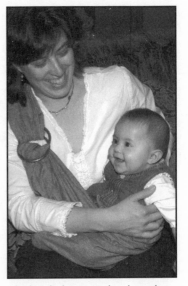

A sling helps a mother keep her baby close and happy.

I want to thank La Leche League, not only for the breastfeeding information, but for their outlook on babies and mothering. There are many baby gadgets and gimmicks around these days to substitute for mother's time and closeness. I don't think our society is really comfortable with babies and their simple needs: security in mother's presence and the best possible food, mother's milk.

Taking Care of Mother

As a brand new mother, you may find yourself concentrating so completely on your baby that you forget about taking care of yourself, so a quick review of the basics of "mother care" is worthwhile here. Mother care isn't elaborate or demanding; it involves mostly common sense things that are important to any new mother, breastfeeding or not.

Good food, plenty of fluids, and adequate rest come quickly to mind. We also include in our list the need for plenty of loving exchanges—if only a hug or a quick squeeze of a hand—between the new baby's parents. Such shared moments will help keep you going during this demanding time in your life.

Choose between-meal snacks carefully. A nursing mother gets hungry almost as often as her baby, and there's the temptation to nibble on sweets. Choose instead nutritious snacks such as fresh fruit, raw vegetables, whole wheat crackers, or cheese. Getting enough to drink can be taken care of by keeping unsweetened juice or water handy at all times.

Sufficient rest is right up there with the most important recommendations for a new mother. In the days immediately following your baby's birth you will want to spend a good part of your day relaxing. A certain amount of being up and about provides needed exercise, but this is the time to enjoy being pampered. "Mothering the mother" is an integral part of the care of a new mother and baby in many cultures.

A handy rule of thumb for a new mother is to sleep, or at least rest, whenever baby dozes. Even the baby who "never sleeps" catnaps more often than parents may realize. True, the times when the baby sleeps are probably not when you are accustomed to sleeping, and it will take some discipline on your part to put aside what interests you at the moment, close your eyes, and think "sleep." When baby's eyes close at the breast, settle back in your chair with your feet up, your little bundle still in your arms, and try to drop off to sleep. And even if you can't sleep, just closing your eyes, forgetting work that needs to be done, and relaxing can be refreshing.

Other times, mothers find that lying down, closing their eyes, and listening to soft music for ten minutes or so is refreshing. Try it! Think of tension draining away as water drains from a basin. Or snuggle with baby and a book. The important part is to forget about those things which "must be done." Remember, "people before things," and that includes you!

Every so often take a moment to think through the ways to make the most of this time in your life. Use your own good judgment as to what is or is not important. Your baby and the rest of the family, too, need and appreciate a mother who is relaxed and feels good about herself.

A nursing corner

Many breastfeeding mothers find it convenient to set up a comfortable spot for their nursing sessions. Since you'll be spending a lot of time there in the early weeks you'll want everything as handy as possible to save time and effort.

You'll probably start with a comfortable armchair or rocker. We'd go so far as to say that a rocking chair is one of the most essential items you'll need for your new baby. A footstool is another handy item as it helps to lift your knees when positioning your baby for breastfeeding. There's nothing like putting up your feet to help you relax!

Lots of cushions or pillows are another essential aspect of your nursing corner. You need these to properly support yourself and your baby for comfortable feedings.

A good reading lamp should be nearby, as there will be occasions when you'll want to lean back and enjoy reading a book or magazine as baby nurses the time away. Some mothers want the phone and the TV remote handy, too. A small table allows you to keep a large glass of water or juice within easy reach—something you should bring along every time you sit down to nurse the baby.

You might want to keep a stack of diapers, a wastebasket or diaper container, and other baby items (wipes, undershirts, and a few small blankets) close at hand. With these essential supplies always nearby, you can feed and change baby with a minimum of effort.

Visitors—A help or hindrance?

Friends or relatives may offer to help out when you have a new baby. While an extra pair of hands is always welcome, some well wishers may bring advice and comments that are not at all helpful. Be specific about the kind of help you would appreciate—a nice hearty casserole or a nutritious dessert perhaps. Don't be afraid to ask your mother or mother-in-law to stop at the grocery store if you need supplies—or to throw a load of laundry in the washer when she stops by to see the baby.

It may seem unusual for you to sit back and be waited on by your guests—but that's very much the way it should be for a new mother. If you enjoy visiting with friends, then welcome them but let them know you won't be up to the role of "perfect hostess" for a few weeks. One way to reinforce this message is what one mother calls "robe play." Slip into your robe when the company knocks on the door, even if you have been wearing daytime clothes. Without saying a word, the message is conveyed that you are not yet up to entertaining as usual.

In general, a new mother can be as active as she wants to be, provided that she stops whatever she is doing the instant she begins to feel tired. You will find that this little reminder covers a multitude of new-mother indiscretions. By taking care of yourself in the early weeks, you will feel better in the months ahead.

When relaxing isn't enough

If your baby happens to be one of those fussy, active babies who is always looking for mother's attention and who thrives on change, you may find it hard to follow our advice to relax and take it easy. If this is the case, you have our sympathy, because we've had this kind of baby too, and we know how trying it can be. The very busy, alert baby is almost always more contented as he gets older and can do more for himself. He can't wait to conquer the world on his own!

If you find that you just can't relax, ask yourself if you are trying to pack too much into your day. We hope you have taken to heart our remarks about the baby being more important than housework or other commitments. But if you do find yourself tense and jittery and you know the baby will want to nurse again soon, take a breather for a minute or two. An exercise break can do wonders. The activity will loosen tight muscles and perk up the blood circulation. There are books and video-tapes available that explain exercise routines that include your baby.

Weather permitting, look forward to a walk outdoors each day. Take baby with you, of course, in his carriage, sling, or baby carrier. The fresh air, sunshine, and change of scenery will do both of you a world of good.

It may be that, when you begin to feel on edge, you could be hungry. How long has it been since your last good meal? Why not eat a piece of fresh fruit or nibble on a tasty piece of cheese?   A hard-cooked egg, ready in the refrigerator, will furnish you with the staying power of protein. A slice of whole-grain bread with peanut butter is also quick and good. Or brew a fragrant cup of hot tea to enjoy as baby nurses.

The end of the day is often a troublesome time for mothers and babies. Clare Vetter of Kentucky tells of one particularly trying evening that worked out well in the end:

> After a very busy day, my son, Isaac, was too "wired-up" to nurse. Of course, I was worn out also and perhaps a bit low on milk supply. Each time Isaac would start to nurse, he would stop suddenly, sit up, and fuss loudly.
>
> My husband, Tom, came in and put on some lovely, relaxing music. It seemed to be just what our family needed. I stood up with Isaac in one arm and the three of us began a lively yet soothing waltz. Our dance was spontaneous and improvised, and our aching muscles seemed to work out their pains. Gazing into Tom's eyes I remembered our first dance at a college waltz party ten years ago. There is so much more to our lives now than then!
>
> The music ended too soon. Bathtime, storytime, then bed and lights out. Isaac and I lay nursing and the melody played itself again inside me, and there was plenty of milk. Sometimes a little romance helps.

New baby blues

Occasionally, a woman feels down or depressed for no particular reason following the birth of her baby. "There I was, holding my beautiful new daughter in my arms, knowing that I had everything to be thankful for, yet I was dissolved in tears," one mother remembers. Another mother described the feeling as "combat fatigue following delivery." Dr. James Good, a wise family doctor, once pointed out the similarities between the depression a mother may feel following the delivery of her baby and that which often sets in the day after a special occasion. The anticipation and planning that filled the months before have come to an end. A high point of participation is over, and a period of adjustment follows.

This emotional seesaw may also arise as a result of the change of hormones in your body from a pregnant to a nonpregnant state. It is usually short-lived, but if the feeling persists, you will want to check with your doctor. Breastfeeding and having your baby close to you will help you to deal with this transition. The hormonal changes are more gradual when you breastfeed. The old standbys, eating well and getting enough rest, are important in helping you feel well, both physiologically and emotionally. Sometimes a new mother just needs to be in touch with someone who can understand how she feels. That's when a call to your local La Leche League Leader can help.

Marlane Edelman of New Jersey stresses the benefits of being in touch with La Leche League:

At our last La Leche League meeting our Leader asked all of the mothers to share with us what they liked most about breastfeeding. One mother said that she considered La Leche League meetings to be one of the advantages of breastfeeding. Her answer caused me to look back on the influence La Leche League has had in my life.

I became pregnant shortly after we moved to a new state. During my pregnancy I had no friends in our new hometown and I was very lonely.

I attended my first LLL meeting because after three months of breastfeeding I was still having considerable difficulty with sore nipples and breast infections. I was looking for information and consolation that things would get better. I went home from that first meeting with some helpful information and returned for the next three meetings.

It hadn't occurred to me to continue past those first meetings, but the Leader called to invite me, so I went. Now, sixteen months later, I am still attending LLL meetings. I have found they are more than just a place to learn about breastfeeding. I've learned about the nutritional, emotional, and physical needs of growing babies and ways of coping with people who ask, "Are you still nursing?" I've found a place where people understand why my career is my family. And, I've finally found friends. Friends who have joined together with their children to form a playgroup. Friends who understand how frustrating it is to be housebound on a long winter day.

LLL has meant so very much to me. I hope someday to
be able to give other mothers what I have found there—a
warm accepting environment where I'm encouraged to love
and nurture my child in the way I feel is best, beginning with
breastfeeding.

Going Out? Take Baby Along

You don't have to stay at home just because you have a breastfed baby.
Baby can go right along with you almost everywhere you want to go. In
the early weeks, it's a good idea to pace yourself—take things easy—
for your own sake. A brief shopping trip or a visit to see proud grandparents would be good to start with and can be a refreshing break in
the everyday routine. When you're ready to go, baby and a diaper bag
are easy bundles to take along.

Feeding your baby or comforting him at the breast is not a problem, since it is possible to nurse inconspicuously almost anywhere. In
most parts of the world no one gives a second thought to the sight of a
nursing mother. But if you feel more comfortable nursing your baby
without drawing attention to the fact, this can be easily accomplished.

Two-piece outfits are probably the most convenient for nursing
away from home. A loose-fitting sweater or overblouse can be lifted
from the waist for easy nursing. You remain covered on top, and a diaper or small blanket can be a casual cover-up. The never-out-of-fashion
shawl also lends itself to discreet nursing. Maternity shops and specialty catalogues feature special tops and dresses for nursing mothers
with concealed openings for breastfeeding Many La Leche League
publications carry advertising from companies which specialize in fashionable clothing designed for discreet nursing.

It's a simple matter to conceal the fact that you are breastfeeding.
You will need only a minute or so of privacy to get baby started at the
breast. Once he's nursing, your baby could be sleeping in your arms for
all anyone knows. Many large stores, airports, train stations, and shopping malls have rooms set aside for mothers and small babies. Another
possibility when shopping in a large store or shopping center is a visit
to the women's clothing department. If it isn't too crowded, you can
relax in a fitting room while you nurse the baby. If you sew or just
enjoy looking at fashions, take a nursing break in the fabric department—one with comfortable stools at the pattern-book counter.

You will soon be able to devise a way to nurse inconspicuously to
suit any occasion. At the beach, a large beach towel thrown casually
over your shoulders and arms can serve as a kind of private tent for
your nursing baby.

As a new breastfeeding mother, you may feel more at ease about nursing in different situations if you practice inconspicuous nursing at home first, with your husband or a good friend as critic. Mothers find that it doesn't take long to smooth out their performance. A Nevada mother, Charlene Brown, recalls:

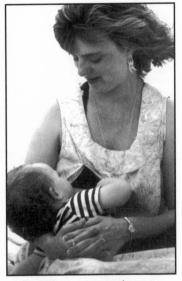

Today's nursing mother can find clothes designed for nursing discreetly.

> After the birth of our daughter, Dawn Michelle, Fred and I were invited to speak about our experience at a childbirth class. Toward the end, Dawn decided that she wanted to nurse. I continued answering questions as I put her blanket over her head and my shoulder, and she took the breast. One of the expectant mothers commented that I certainly had a unique way of quieting my baby—throwing a blanket over her head! I explained that the baby was nursing. Fred later said that I was getting to be such a pro, I didn't even pause in mid-sentence.

Breastfed babies go everywhere

A little advance planning or innovative thinking will often keep a young one and his mother together and happy. When Mary White, one of LLL's co-Founders, was the matron of honor at her sister's wedding, she brought a babysitter along for the sole purpose of holding her three-month-old baby during the ceremony. Between the ceremony and the reception, Mary slipped off, nursed the baby, and was back in the receiving line in time to shake a few hundred hands.

The women in the La Leche League Group in Hull, England, drew up a list of places they had gone with their nursing babies. In many of the situations, they felt it would be difficult to feed or comfort a bottle-fed baby. Lynne Emerson wrote the following account:

> Bridget said that she's nursed in restaurants, doctors' and dentists' offices, and in church. Christina took the minimum of equipment on a canalling holiday in contrast to another bottle-feeding mum on another boat. She has also nursed

baby Sarah in the changing room at the local sports centre. Lynne said she had nursed at a wedding reception, in a blizzard, while stuck in her car when her ten-minute car trip turned to all day after the car broke down, while football spectating, and on the beach.

I nursed Lucy, when only three months old, at a one-day yoga seminar. The yoga teacher was skeptical at first, but I assured her Lucy wouldn't distract the class. Our last excursion (to see the local pantomime) was really exciting. The whole family went, and there were a few raised eyebrows when we walked in, but afterward people remarked how good the baby had been. We hope this will help dispel the myth that breastfeeding the baby is confining.

Travel plans

On longer excursions, babies make good travelers if some thought is given ahead of time to their special needs. Breastfed babies have logged a phenomenal number of hours in the air. Judy Sanders of Washington flew halfway around the world to New Zealand with her daughter, Maria. Judy reports that it was easy to travel with Maria because she was breastfed. Wearing a caftan-type dress with hidden zippers was comfortable and convenient for discreet nursing.

You'll want to check with your specific air carrier for their regulations before planning a trip by plane. They may provide special infant safety seats or suggest you bring your own. Reserving a bulkhead seat will give you some extra room. Pack your tote bag with baby's diapers, soft toys, and a change of outfits—just in case your luggage does not land at the same time or place that you do. Nursing your baby at takeoff and landing will lessen the pressure on his ears, but this may not be possible if baby is restrained in a seat belt. This may be a time when a pacifier would be useful.

Kay McFerrin of Texas tells of her family vacation:

Last summer we traveled to Acapulco, Mexico, with our infant daughter, Monica. Thanks to breastfeeding, our little girl was a delightful travel companion. Monica was six months old then, and still on just mother's milk. All she needed for the trip was her mother, some diapers, and a bathing suit. We all had such a marvelous time. I had no worries such as what to do if the room doesn't have a refrigerator, or what if I don't take enough formula, or how will I warm the bottles, or how to take formula and feed baby away from the hotel, or any other problems a bottle-fed baby and mother might face. No matter where we were—beach, sightseeing, poolside, or plane—wherever Monica got hungry, she just did what came naturally.

At night we never had to bother with baby beds, we just tucked our baby in with us as we do at home. She didn't care where she was—no insecurity for her! She was happy just being with her mother and daddy. It never even occurred to us to leave her out of this adventure.

Lisa Gehring from Ohio tells about bicycling with her daughter. She and her husband ride a tandem bike, and they fastened the baby's car seat to a special trailer that attached behind their bike. She writes:

My husband and I, being avid bicyclists, decided that we did not want to give up our favorite hobby just because we had a baby—we would take her along!

Since Heidi is totally breastfed, going bicycling with her couldn't be any easier. We just put her in the trailer with her diaper bag, and off we go. It's great not having to pack bottles and formula.

When Heidi was four months old, we participated in a two-day tour along the south shore of Lake Erie. Whenever Heidi would get hungry, we would take a break. She had her lunch at a park on the shore of Lake Erie. We did attract quite a bit of attention, and at rest stops Rich would answer questions regarding our tandem and trailer. Meanwhile Heidi would nurse inconspicuously, oblivious to the crowd gathered around our bike.

I believe that a happy family is one that enjoys going places and doing things together. Taking Heidi with us is so easy that we would never dream of leaving her with a sitter. We're planning a cross-country ski vacation this winter, and guess who's going with us? That's right, have baby—will travel!

If you must leave your baby

If you must leave your tiny baby for a short time—and the shorter the time the better—leave him with someone he is happy with when you are around. Be sure to leave the baby well fed and contented. Don't rush—babies can sense when mother is in a hurry to get away. When he is happy and settled, then go off. For some time you won't leave him longer than an hour or two, and then only occasionally. Since you don't want your little one to miss you or go hungry, you'll want to be back soon.

Some mothers like to have the added security of leaving a container of their own expressed milk stored in the freezer in case it's needed while they're gone. (Information on expressing and storing human milk is found in Chapter 7.)

Mothers often ask about leaving a bottle of formula when they're gone. We cannot recommend that you do that. Leaving your own milk assures that your baby will continue to receive his favorite food. Even one bottle of formula can be a problem for some babies because of the risk of allergy. Animal studies have also shown that introducing formula may upset the balance of enzymes and nutrients in the digestive system and interfere with the protective qualities your milk provides.

Alone is lonely

You won't want to leave your baby any more than you have to because babies need their mothers. It's a need that is as basic and intense as his need for food. "That's all well and good," you may be thinking, "but what about me? I have needs, too."

Of course a mother has needs, and sometimes other responsibilities and obligations cause a mother to be away from her baby more than she wants to be. But you may be surprised to find how strong the bond is that develops between you and your baby. A mother often finds that when she does leave her baby for that long awaited "night out," she worries so much about how the baby is getting along that she doesn't really enjoy the occasion!

Dr. William Sears, pediatrician and author, explains how this can happen:

> When mother and baby are separated, both of them miss out on the full benefits of a continuous mother-infant attachment. When mother and baby spend most of their time with each other, responding positively to each other's cues, they get in harmony with each other...not only does the mother help the baby develop, but the baby also helps the mother develop.

Mothers do grow along with their children. Judy Kahrl from Ohio, tells of her experience in gaining an understanding of her baby's need for her:

> One thing that helped me when I wanted to leave the baby was to remember that a baby has no sense of time. When he

is left, he thinks it is forever. He can't understand that his mother will be back later tonight or whenever. Also, what seems like a short time to parents, for instance a weekend, is proportionately speaking, a long time in the baby's life. It has helped me to try to look at this from the baby's perspective, his sense of time, his understanding of the world. Of course, we mothers have needs, too, but because of our maturity, we are better equipped to cope with ours, to postpone them for a bit. A baby's needs are immediate.

CHAPTER SIX

A TIME TO
learn

The early weeks of caring for your new baby are a time of adjustment for both of you. Mothering is a learned skill and your baby is the best teacher you could have. As you learn to respond to your baby's needs, your baby learns to trust that his needs will be met.

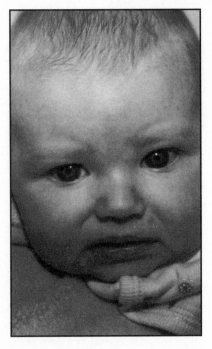

Why Is My Baby Crying?

The sound of a baby crying is not easy to ignore. It is not intended to be. Your baby's cry is meant to be disturbing, for it is his most important means of communication. Only by crying can he let you know that he needs you to help him—to come to his rescue. Something is bothering him or frightening him. It may be that he is hungry, or he may be lonesome for you. He only knows the security of your presence when his body is next to yours; as far as your baby is concerned, you might as well be on another planet as on the other side of the house. Vi Lennon, one of LLL's co-Founders, recalls that she once asked an older child to pick up the crying baby and hold him while she finished frying chicken. Her daughter responded, "I already tried that, but it's no use. He's having an attack of loneliness for you."

In THE FUSSY BABY, Dr. William Sears explains:

> Parents are led to believe that if they pick up their baby every
> time he cries, he will not learn to settle himself and will
> become more demanding as time goes on. This is not true.
> A baby whose cries have been promptly responded to early
> on learns to trust and to anticipate that a response will be
> forthcoming.

Responding to your crying baby

When a baby cries, a nursing mother's immediate instinctive response
is to offer her breast. Whether it's been ten minutes or two hours since
baby was fed, a few minutes of sucking may be all he needs to settle
down. A newborn needs to breastfeed often and his appetite can vary
from day to day, so he may really be crying because he's hungry. Or perhaps he just wants the comfort of being close to you. Either way, nursing him is often the best answer.

But what if that's not what he wants after all? Then you need to
check into other possible causes. Perhaps he's too warm, or maybe he's
too cold. Perhaps something he is wearing is causing the problem. Try
removing all of his clothes. Look for a pin or rough label, or something
binding around his leg or arm—sometimes a hair from a mother's head
can wrap tightly around baby's toe. Look him over carefully from top
to bottom, just to be sure that nothing is hurting or irritating his tender skin.

If he seems too warm, try leaving him in just a shirt and diaper. If
the room is chilly, try wrapping him in a soft blanket. Some babies feel
more secure if they are wrapped up snugly, or swaddled. To swaddle a
baby, place him in the center of a lightweight blanket or square towel
with his arms at his sides. His head and feet should point toward the
corners. Then fold the bottom corner up over his legs, and the other
two corners toward the center, wrapping him snugly. Pick him up with
the top corner folded lightly over his head. Rocking him back and forth
in this little cocoon can help him feel very secure and will often stop
his crying.

Once he is calm, offer him the breast again. This time, he just may
drift off to sleep. But sometimes the baby doesn't want to nurse, or has
downed so much milk he repeatedly spits it up, and still he cries. What
then? Try holding him against your shoulder and with a background of
soft music or your own lullaby, glide through the house doing the
"baby waltz." Some mothers put the baby in a baby carrier or sling and
vacuum. The droning noise of the vacuum cleaner and the accompany-

ing body movements often lull the baby to sleep. How about a drive in the car? Or a stroll outdoors? A warm bath may soothe and relax both of you—try taking baby into the tub with you.

A time-honored way of soothing a crying baby is time spent in a trusty rocking chair together. A steady rocking rhythm, some gentle patting on his back, and perhaps a soothing lullaby can work their magic on the fussiest of little ones. In fact, Becky Conley from Illinois swears by her "magic rocker":

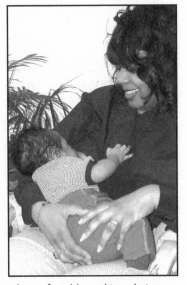

A comfortable rocking chair can help soothe a fussy baby.

No matter how hectic the day or how frantic the world may seem, we can retreat to the arms of our rocker, and be suddenly oblivious to it all. Peace descends on us; tensions float away; and love surrounds us like a cloud. We can go anywhere we please in our rocker. Over the years since Eli was born, we've been to desert islands, mountain ranges, endless beaches, and on a few, very special occasions, to what surely must have been heaven.

Some babies cry because they are overtired, but they aren't happy being held as they fall asleep. Try laying your baby in his cradle or on a blanket on the floor and talk or sing to him softly as you pat him gently. He may continue to fuss for a few minutes, then close his eyes and drift off to sleep. You'll soon know if he is truly tired and ready to sleep or not. If he becomes increasingly more anxious (even five minutes is a long time for a baby to cry), pick him up again.

Babies are sometimes fretful for reasons that no one, not even a mother, can understand. If you can't calm your baby right away, try not to let it upset you. "Don't take it as a personal rejection of you," a mother who has gone through the experience advises. Your baby will always benefit from a calm, loving mother. In handling any tiny baby, you have to move slowly and gently. Fast, jerky motions and loud noises may startle him. If he is already upset for some reason, accept the fact and work from there—slow and easy.

Should baby cry it out?

While holding and carrying the baby may comfort him, it may also elicit some stern advice from friends and relatives. The notion still persists that the baby who cries when put down, but is soothed when held, should be laid down gently but firmly to "cry it out."

Sometimes a mother wonders if it really makes a difference if the baby cries in her arms or in a crib. It makes a considerable difference. Jan Wojcik of Florida puts the matter in a different light by asking how any of us would feel if we were the ones who were upset. "If we were crying, wouldn't we feel better if someone were around to reassure us? To care that we were upset? Wouldn't we wives feel rejected if our husbands were to say, 'Go into the bedroom. I don't want to be around you until you regain control of yourself.' Don't we want to be loved in times of stress as well as in times of happiness?"

Our suggestion to the mother of a fussy baby is: Don't let your baby cry alone. The comfort and security extended by your loving arms is never wasted. Love begets love. Then, too, the next thing you try may be just the right thing to ease baby's discomfort and restore peace and serenity to the house.

Baby the baby

You can't spoil a baby; his wants are his needs. His need to be lovingly held when he is upset is as strong and important as his need to be fed and kept warm and dry. So, if your infant stops his crying when you pick him up and hold him, just keep on holding him and be happy that you are there to satisfy this important emotional need. By all means, "baby" the baby.

The late Dr. Lee Salk, who was a pediatric psychologist, wrote "The baby whose cries are answered now will later be the child confident enough to show his independence and curiosity. But the baby who is left to cry it out may develop a sense of isolation and distrust, and may turn inward by tuning out the world that will not answer its cry. And later on in life, this child may continue to cope with stress by trying to shut out reality." As for crying being good exercise for baby's lungs, according to Dr. Salk, "If crying is good for the lungs, then bleeding is good for the veins!"

A fussy time of day

Some babies have a regular fussy period, often late in the afternoon, that occurs predictably day after day. At other times, the baby is good-natured, and there doesn't seem to be any particular cause for these fussy spells. The baby is not uncomfortable, as with colic, but is not

happy either. Folklore refers to this
time as the "Granny Hour," meaning
that a loving grandmother is needed
who has nothing more urgent to do
than rock and cuddle the baby.

You may not always have someone
else around at baby's fussy time but it
can be a great comfort if your baby's
father or another family member can
take over for a spell. The change of
loving arms and voice often relaxes an
upset child. While dad and baby watch
the fish swimming in the fish tank or
the cars passing by, you may want to
take a refreshing shower—it can really
help wash the tension away.

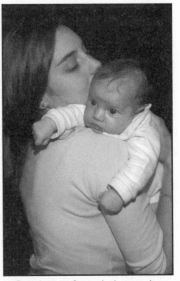

Soothing a fussy baby can be
exhausting for a mother.

Babies Who Are Colicky

When a tiny baby has long periods of hard crying and seems to be in
some sort of physical discomfort for which there is no apparent reason
that you or your doctor can discover, he is often said to be colicky.

"Colic" is a catchall word meaning essentially "loud, persistent
screaming for undetermined reasons." As many causes of colic are put
forth as there are doctors who have studied it. As far back as the turn
of the last century, colic was referred to in one widely used pediatric
text as "a scientifically inaccurate and unsatisfactory term which serves
such a useful purpose in practice and covers so well a multitude of
abdominal pains that it maintains its place in our medical books." The
same loose definition could apply today; doctors still seem to know little or nothing about the true cause of this kind of crying.

In his book, THE FUSSY BABY, Dr. William Sears has this to say
about colic:

> I suspect that colic is the result of many causes, tempera-
> mental, physiological, and environmental, that overwhelm a
> baby's immature coping skills.... In light of present knowledge
> about colic, the best anyone can do is to comfort the baby
> and minimize the factors that may contribute to the baby's
> fussiness.

So what can a mother do about colic? Calm, gentle handling is essential. Many doctors feel that frequent, shorter feedings are easier for baby to handle than long feedings. But a colicky baby may be soothed by lots of sucking, plus the extra cuddling that comes with nursing, so what do you do then? Try feeding him from one breast only during a two- to three-hour period. He may want to nurse a number of times during that time span; just keep to the "empty" breast. After two hours or so, switch to the other breast and again limit nursings to one side.

If your baby shows signs of colic, you'll want to be sure he gets nothing else but your milk. Avoid giving formula, juice, or water. Some babies also react to vitamins, especially those with added fluoride.

Occasionally, something the mother eats might be a possible cause of colicky symptoms in her baby. Some possibilities include certain vitamins, food supplements such as brewer's yeast, large amounts of caffeine or foods or drinks with artificial sweeteners. In some instances, a food such as milk (or foods containing milk) in the mother's diet can make her baby uncomfortable. (This is more likely to occur if there is a history of allergy in the family. It is explained later in Chapter 18.) Mothers who smoke cigarettes seem to have more instances of colicky babies.

Mothers of colicky babies have come up with a variety of ways to comfort and soothe them. Sue Nobriga Buckley of California talks about a "colic hold" that helped her daughter feel better:

Although Lara gained weight quickly and proved to be alert and healthy, every evening found us rocking or walking her back and forth for hours before her crying and wailing gave way to sleep. After five weeks of steady evening and occasional daytime crying sessions, we were hesitant to visit her grandparents. When we did visit, Lara typically acted pleasant during most of the day, only to start in loud and long in the early evening. As usual no one could comfort her until her grandfather picked her up, laid her astraddle his arm with her head slightly higher than her feet, and proceeded to immediately rock her to sleep. Amazed, we imitated his way of holding her whenever Lara began to act colicky, and almost every time the new way of holding her quieted and comforted her.

A soothing, pleasant bath proved to be a refuge for Judy Wesockes and her baby daughter, who live in Florida:

> When Amy has an attack of colic, usually between eight and
> ten in the evening, we go into a warm, deep tub and stay
> there for the duration of her attack. The moist heat, holding
> her, and relaxing all help. She gets almost immediate relief,
> but if we get out of the tub, the symptoms return. So we stay
> in, and I add more hot water as needed.

Knowing that your milk is the best possible food for your baby will help you to be relaxed and calm. It's one less thing to worry about, and baby will be spared the risks that come with changing formulas. The warm closeness of the nursing relationship and your gentle, loving care will help ease your baby through this trying time.

Some babies who are extremely fussy or seem to be colicky may actually be suffering from a birth injury or other physical discomfort. Be sure to have your doctor check your baby thoroughly to rule out a physical cause for baby's fussiness. Some fussy babies respond well to chiropractic adjustment, massage therapy, or other gentle, non-invasive treatments by practitioners who are accustomed to treating infants.

High need babies

As you read through this section you may be saying to yourself, "But I've tried all those things and my baby is still fussy." It may be that you have the kind of baby that Dr. William Sears talks about in his book, THE FUSSY BABY. He explains it this way:

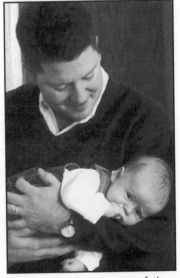

> In the first few days or weeks, parents begin to pick up on clues as to the temperament of their baby. Some parents are blessed with so-called easy babies. Others are blessed with babies who are not so easy....the term "fussy baby" is a bit unfair.... I prefer to call this special type of baby the high need baby. This is not only a kinder term, but it more accurately describes why these babies act the way they do and what level of parenting they need.

Dr. Sears assures parents that having a high need baby can be a blessing.

The colic hold is one way a father can help to comfort a colicky baby.

He points out that high need babies bring out the best in their parents. He says, "Those same qualities which at first seemed to be such an exhausting liability have a good chance of turning out to be an asset for the child and the family."

If you want to find out more, you can buy a copy of the revised edition of THE FUSSY BABY from LLLI's Catalogue, on our Web site at www.lalecheleague.org, at your local bookstore, or at your La Leche League Group. For details, see the Appendix.

Growth Spurts

Some time after the first week or two the baby who has been peacefully nursing every three hours may suddenly want to dramatically increase the number of times a day he is fed. No sooner does he drift off to sleep than he is up again, nuzzling the bedding or his fist, looking for something to eat. You may hear comments about your milk supply and some critics may suggest that breastfeeding doesn't seem to be working.

Tune out such remarks. This increase in the number of nursings is normal. More frequent nursing builds up the milk supply to meet the growing baby's increasing need. So settle in with baby for a few "frequency days."

Twenty minutes of fairly vigorous nursing every hour or so is more effective in building up your milk supply than less frequent, longer sessions at the breast. On the other hand, baby's nursing sessions should not be cut short. Most babies eventually settle into a fairly consistent pattern of nursing, one that is right for each particular child. These increases in frequency usually show up in relation to growth spurts. Like the rest of us, babies are hungrier at some times than others. Rather than check out the refrigerator, baby looks to mom. Baby's appetite temporarily gets ahead of his mother's milk supply.

Mothers commonly report such a fussy period coinciding with a growth spurt around two weeks and again around six weeks. If this happens, put baby to the breast as often as he wants to nurse. With extra nursings, it isn't long before your milk production steps up to meet his need. The interval between nursings will soon lengthen, and baby will be his old self again. The extra rest that comes to you with more frequent nursing may be exactly what the doctor would order. It may be that the tempo of all you are doing has picked up a little faster than is good for a new mother. Nature and your baby combine forces to help you get much needed rest.

When your baby is three months old, more or less, there is often another fussy period. It is probably due partly to a jump in appetite, and again, increased nursings will generally take care of this. If baby is healthy and gaining weight there is no reason to add any other food to his diet.

Another factor in the three-month fussy period, which you may or may not experience with your baby, is that he stays awake longer and is taking a greater interest in the world around him. Fussing at this age may indicate a need for company and activity. Keep him in the center of activity. Settle him near you in a safe spot on a blanket on the floor where he can really stretch out. He will enjoy music, movement, and people going by. As he gets older, he thrives on change and variety. As he becomes more aware of the world around him, the sights and sounds of the family group are wonderful stimulation for his senses. People often notice and comment on the early alertness and responsiveness of the baby who is part of the family group, who is talked to and sung to and smiled at often.

Nighttime Needs

During the early months, it is especially desirable for the baby to nurse during the night. Your young baby is growing at a phenomenal rate and has a physical need to be fed during the night. Also, your breasts can become engorged and uncomfortable if you go for six or more hours without a feeding, and in the morning your baby might have trouble getting started at the breast because of the fullness.

A study of nursing mothers in West Nigeria by Derrick and Patrice Jelliffe revealed that babies as old as ten months received at least twenty-five percent of their mother's milk at night. So it is not at all unusual for your baby to want to nurse at night.

In his book, NIGHTTIME PARENTING, Dr. William Sears points out that babies sleep differently than adults and he says that babies aren't designed to sleep through the night. Dr. Sears goes on to say, "Sleep problems occur when your child's night-waking exceeds your ability to cope."

One secret of coping with your baby's need for night feedings is to develop your skill at nursing the baby lying down. If you feel awkward when you first try to nurse in bed, continue to experiment with different positions and lots of pillows. Once you can feed the baby while comfortably stretched out, you've eliminated much of the work of mothering for about eight of the twenty-four hours in a day. In order to see what you are doing in the early weeks without turning on a bright light, consider keeping a small flashlight on the nightstand or under

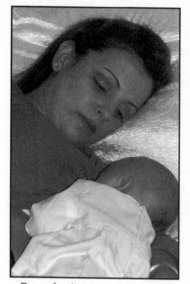

Breastfeeding is easier at night when baby sleeps close to mother.

your pillow. Or leave the light on in the closet with the door ajar. To change sides with a minimum of strain when nursing while lying down, simply hold baby close to you with both arms and roll over.

When your baby wakes at night, just tuck him into bed with you, start nursing him, and the two of you can drop off to sleep again together. It is quite safe—we have all done it, and so have mothers all over the world for centuries. The babies love the warm closeness and mothers say that they quickly develop a sixth sense about allowing room for the baby.

You may have heard stories of a parent rolling over on the baby in bed. Don't worry; your healthy, normal baby, even when very small, can move his head and in some way let you know if a blanket is over his face or if he is feeling closed in. Baby should sleep on his back or side to avoid getting his face buried in the bedding. If parents sleep on a water bed, keep it very full so it is firm and be sure there is no crevice between the mattress and frame. A free-floating water bed, without internal baffles, is not safe for baby.

Studies have shown that the risk of Sudden Infant Death Syndrome (SIDS) is reduced when babies sleep on their backs or sides. Of course, parents should not sleep with their baby if they are under the influence of drugs, alcohol, tranquilizers, or cold medications that may diminish their awareness of the baby's presence.

Recent research on SIDS shows that sleeping with your baby, along with breastfeeding, actually decreases the risk of SIDS.

In his book, *SIDS: A Parent's Guide to Understanding and Preventing Sudden Infant Death Syndrome,* Dr. William Sears summarizes his conclusions:

I believe that in most cases SIDS is a sleep disorder, primarily a disorder of arousal and breathing control during sleep. All the elements of natural mothering, especially breastfeeding and sharing sleep, benefit the infant's breathing control and increase the mutual awareness between mother and infant so that their arousability is increased and the risk of SIDS is decreased.

There are a number of ways to avoid the possibility that baby could fall off the bed. Pull his crib right next to your bed, leaving the side rail down and adjust the level of the mattress so it is the same height as yours. When close by, it's convenient to scoop him into your bed when he cries. You can also buy a special baby crib that attaches to the side of your bed or a guardrail that fits along the side of your bed to keep baby safe.

A resourceful mother in Pennsylvania, Pat Muschamp, uses a blanket to keep her baby from moving away from her after she has drifted back to sleep. Place baby's blanket diagonally on the bed, like a kite. You lie down with the inner corner under you and baby next to you on the blanket. Pull the outer corner of the blanket across baby's body and tuck it under your body. Your baby is wrapped snugly against you, and there is no worry about falling.

Some mothers wear a bra to bed at night. This is not necessary, but if you find you're more comfortable with some kind of support, choose a bra that is big enough or stretchy enough to allow for expansion if your breasts fill during the night hours.

When will he sleep through the night?

Probably the reason this question ever became so important is because of the inconvenience of nighttime bottle-feeding—getting up with the baby into what may be a chilly house, waiting while the bottle warms, fighting sleep, and being fearful that baby or bottle may be dropped. As a nursing mother, you are spared such inconvenience, so when you hear that a neighbor's baby sleeps through the night and yours doesn't, ask yourself, "Is it really that important?" Isn't the important thing that you can satisfy your baby's needs so easily at night as well as during the day? To a baby, it makes no difference whether the sun is up or the world is hushed in darkness. His need for mothering remains. It is no less important at night than during the day.

As to when he will sleep through the night, it's impossible to say. Babies are human beings, and each and every human being in the world is different from every other. Some babies will sleep through the night at an early age, and some will not. And not infrequently, the little one who sleeps through the night one week is waking the next.

Getting up in the night is never a favorite part of parenting. But there are ways to cope, to come to terms with the situation. How you react can make a considerable difference in how it affects you. We know the truth of this because many of us learned it the hard way. Pat Yearian of Washington says she gradually came to the realization that she stopped worrying about baby's sleep pattern by changing her atti-

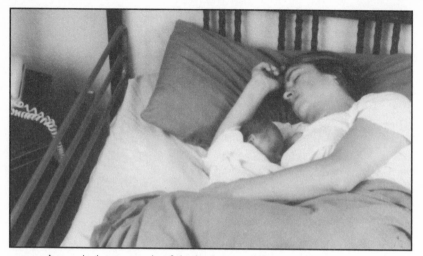

A guardrail on one side of the bed can protect baby from falling off.

tude. After all, a mother's reaction to interrupted sleep is up to her. Pat writes:

> If you resent the interruptions to your sleep, you will face each day more frustrated and trying harder and harder to fit the baby into your sleep pattern. On the other hand, if you can adjust your mental attitude to one of greater acceptance, you will find yourself able to enjoy those quite moments in the night with your infant who needs to be held and nursed, or with your toddler who just needs to be with someone. Acceptance of interrupted sleep doesn't come right away. In fact, for many of us it has taken a baby or two to fully appreciate their needs. When you begin to notice that your sleep can be interrupted many times a night, and yet you are able to face the next day with a smile, your attitudes are changing.

The late Dr. Gregory White, an experienced family practice physician, once commented on the subject of sleep in a talk he gave to parents:

> A lot of people think they are entitled to a night's sleep. Nobody's entitled to a full night's sleep and very few mothers get one. Many people do at one time or another during their lives, and I'm all for it. But no one's entitled to it, whether she's a new mother or not, if someone needs her. If a lazy, self-indulgent old man like me can get out of bed in the mid-

dle of the night to help people he hardly knows, certainly a
mother can do this for her own child.

Sharing Sleep

Rather than try to change their children's needs for parenting at night,
many families have decided to change sleeping arrangements. After all,
what babies and young children are seeking is not all that strange—
they just want to be closer to those who love them.

Dr. William Sears uses the term "sharing sleep" because he
emphasizes the fact that physical closeness causes mother and baby to
share sleep cycles. But he doesn't leave out fathers. He points out that
fathers report they feel closer to their babies when they sleep together.

The beauty of bedding down as a family is that it can be cus-
tomized to suit each individual family's needs. Some mothers choose
to return the baby to his own bed once he is fed and settled. In other
households, the crib and separate room for the baby are abandoned,
and an all-night family bed is adopted. Sleeping arrangements are as
varied as families.

Ann Parker's story is rather typical. This Indiana mother explains
that for the first six months after birth, baby Bryan slept in his parents'
room, but in his own bed. Ann writes:

> I kept going back and forth every few hours to nurse him, and
> one time I caught myself asleep, sitting on the side of the
> bed, with baby in arms. I could have dropped him, and that
> really scared me! From then on I nursed him in bed lying
> down, but as soon as he stopped nursing, I would take him
> back to his bed. That plan didn't work all the time, since I
> kept falling asleep while he was nursing. But in the morning, I
> felt better. I had slept longer and without as many interrup-
> tions. My husband's sleep wasn't disturbed that night either.
> So Bryan began sleeping with us every night.

By age two or so, many youngsters will proudly take to a conven-
tional bed of their own, although it will be easier for short legs to reach if
the spring and mattress are placed directly on the floor. With a full-size
mattress you can lie down next to your little one if he wakes up. It's less
disturbing for you to then move back to your own bed than it would be
to move him. For the child who is ready for his own bed, but still wants
to be near you once in a while, a sleeping bag or air mattress and blanket
can be stowed under your bed and pulled out to make a cozy spot.

Practical arrangements

When the big bed seems crowded (even though it may be almost the size of the room) because everyone is huddled over in one spot (yours), you may wonder if this time of intense togetherness will ever come to an end. It does, and your reaction at the time may not be what you thought it would be. Ann Backhurst of Michigan tells of her experience:

> Amy, age four, sleeps alone willingly all night. When Emily was about eighteen months old, she indicated an interest in sleeping in the crib. She now sleeps all night in it. Ken and I have our queen-size bed to ourselves again; to my surprise, I find that I really miss having the little girls sleep with us. While living through a difficult time with sleeping arrangements, I thought we would never see the end of this "family bed"—I couldn't wait. Now that it's over, we have cherished memories of a little person snuggling up on a cold winter night, or reaching out and putting an arm around one of us and knowing that all was secure.

Parents will find many practical suggestions on meeting their children's nighttime needs in the book we have referred to several times in this chapter—NIGHTTIME PARENTING by William Sears, MD. Copies are available from your local LLL Group, La Leche League International, or a bookstore. See the Appendix for details.

Babies, Beds, and Sex

You may be wondering—if baby's going to be sleeping in your bed, what happens to your marriage? Is there a survival plan for new parents?

We can offer some suggestions, but in the final analysis you and your husband are your own best authorities on what is the most loving, satisfying sexual relationship for you. Sex, like breastfeeding, is ninety percent mental attitude and ten percent technique. Both sex and breastfeeding flourish on the power of positive thinking. Needless worries can be counterproductive. The joy that you experience with the arrival of your baby will spill over into other areas of your life.

Common myths and questions

With the baby nursing so often and possibly sleeping in our bed, will there be any time for my husband and me to be alone together? Absolutely. We have all found opportunities. You will have to outwit the baby, but there are two of you. Consider a change of time and place. Where there is a will, there is a way.

Babies usually have one fairly long period of deep sleep. Take advantage of it. If your baby is easily disturbed, leave your bed (carefully) for the spare bedroom or the floor in the living room.

If baby is awake, you might try combining romance and distraction by lining up an array of lighted candles. Little babies are fascinated by the flickering lights. Some soft music is another possibility.

Few married couples can expect complete freedom all the time, without interruptions, to make love. There are the everyday outside demands from a job and from others who have needs. Restrictions do not go away as the children grow older and leave the parental bed. Ask any couple with teenagers. But you have a lifetime together to share your love. Tomorrow can be even better than today.

My breasts are tender, and it's uncomfortable when my husband touches them. Also, I'm concerned. Can sexual foreplay affect the milk? No. Your milk will be fine. Don't worry about passing germs from your husband to the baby on your nipples. Your baby is already exposed to family germs and there are special glands that keep your nipples free of germs when baby nurses. Nursing does not make your breasts off limits to your husband. The feeling of fullness and tenderness comes mostly in the early days of nursing and is temporary. You will notice it less if you nurse the baby just prior to making love. Your breasts will not be as full, and the baby will be more apt to sleep. But as one husband says, "Engorgement is gorgeous!"

At the time of a sexual climax, some women also have a milk letdown. The husband is often as surprised as his wife the first time it occurs, since the milk literally sprays out. The hormones that produce the let-down are also present at the time of an orgasm. Not all women experience this, and it lessens as the let-down reflex is better established. Keep a towel nearby for drying off in case it happens.

When breastfeeding, a woman has a greater interest in sex; OR: When breastfeeding, a woman feels less desire for sexual relations. The response to both of the above is "yes" some of the time and "no" at other times. There are no pat answers.

After childbirth one woman may enjoy a feeling of great responsiveness. Giving milk and making love are very natural and exciting parts of her life. Another woman may notice the opposite. Her desire for sexual relations could be better described as understated, although

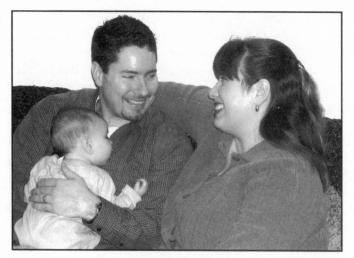

Loving husbands and wives want to please each other.

she loves her husband as much as ever and wants to be close to him; in fact, she needs the reassurance of his affection. Such different reactions are not unusual or abnormal. All men and women have highs and lows in sexual desire at different times in life.

As a breastfeeding mother, it can probably be said that you feel good about being a woman and are at ease with the way your body functions. Breastfeeding is the completion of a woman's sexual cycle. There are marked similarities in the way a woman's body responds during breastfeeding and intercourse. It is a fulfilling time in a woman's life.

Fatigue is probably the greatest deterrent to sex for any new mother. Fit in a nap after dinner, if you can. Sometimes, even when you're feeling more tired than sexy, an extra output of loving effort on your part at the right moment could produce results that are a delight to both you and your husband.

What about feeling "touched out"? A mother once wrote to us, "After having my baby or toddler in my arms most of the day, I feel as though I don't want one more person touching me. I'm annoyed when my husband approaches me. Is this unusual? Can you help me?" We replied to this mother by telling her she was not alone. Many a mother, after spending a good part of the day holding the baby and having little hands cling and pat, finds herself thinking that the last thing she needs is more body contact. She's "touched out."

Our cultural heritage probably shapes this response at least to some extent. The person who grows up in a society where people maintain a certain physical distance from each other, and even family members seldom hug, may find the almost constant contact with a baby a new experience, one that takes some getting used to. Add to this the fatigue that comes at the end of the day for most mothers of young children, and there may not be the energy or inclination to feel romantic.

The low estrogen level present during breastfeeding is often the cause of vaginal dryness. The solution to this is simple enough—a little more lovemaking ahead of time, supplemented, if need be, by a little lubrication such as KY jelly. An episiotomy can also cause painful intercourse, sometimes for many months.

You were a wife before you were a mother, so your husband should come before the children. This is very misleading. It isn't fair to put your husband and children in competition with each other for your time and affection. Whoever has the greatest need for love and attention at the time receives it. With maturity, gratification of want can be postponed for a time. Adults who are hungry can wait a while or find something to eat on their own. Babies cannot. With a little understanding, there needn't be a conflict. There is more than enough love to go around.

Dr. William Sears, pediatrician and author, reminds parents of the importance of their commitment to one another:

> **For mother-baby attachment to work in the way it was designed to work, it must be practiced within the structure of a stable and fulfilled marriage....the whole family works together—mother-baby, father-baby, and husband-wife....You should not make an either-or choice among these relationships. You need to work at all of them because they complement each other.**

This brings us back to the basic relationship. Loving husbands and wives want to please each other. They each try to respond to cues from the other. On one occasion, the wife puts forth an extra effort to respond to her husband's embrace, and on another, he puts her feelings and needs ahead of his own.

There's a time to give and a time to take. With mutual good will and good humor, it all works out. One word of caution: don't keep score. Once you do, you're sure to lose.

COMMON
concerns

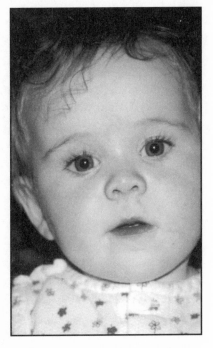

The early weeks of breastfeeding are a time of learning for both you and your baby. Most of the time the process goes smoothly, but once in awhile, problems develop that threaten to interfere with or interrupt breastfeeding. Some of those problems are covered here, along with information to help you overcome any difficulties and continue to enjoy breastfeeding.

Additional information on special circumstances will be found in later chapters. If you still have questions or concerns, we encourage you to contact your La Leche League Leader. More than likely she can offer suggestions and encouragement based on your specific situation that will help solve your problem and allow you and your baby to continue enjoying the benefits of breastfeeding. We can assure you that it is rarely necessary for a baby to be weaned because of a breastfeeding problem.

Avoiding and Treating Sore Nipples

Even though sore nipples can be very uncomfortable, they are certainly no reason for you or your baby to miss out on the advantages and pleasures of breastfeeding. It is normal to experience slight tenderness when baby latches on in the first three to five days after birth. After that, if proper positioning and latch-on techniques are used, you can expect little or no nipple soreness. If your nipples are sore or cracked, check the earlier sections of this book that explain the positioning and latch-on sequence.

Many mothers experience immediate relief from nipple discomfort when they begin latching the baby on correctly. It is worth taking the time to remove the baby from the breast and start again to latch him on correctly.

The way your baby grasps and releases the nipple is very important in avoiding sore nipples. The nipple should not be sucked in, but rather placed far back in baby's mouth when his mouth is open very wide. When removing him from the breast, always break the suction first using a finger to press down on your breast or pull back baby's cheek close to his mouth.

A mother who learned the importance of positioning her baby correctly to avoid sore nipples tells about her experience. Karen Price of British Columbia, Canada, writes:

> My daughter Katie nurses beautifully. We are truly a happy nursing couple now. But the first four months I suffered terribly from sore and cracked nipples. I hope I can offer some encouragement to other women who may be experiencing a similar situation.
>
> First of all, in my genetic makeup, no provision was made for protruding nipples. Before the baby came, I didn't even realize that this was unusual; I thought they would magically pop out when the baby was born. My next mistake was not attending La Leche League meetings ahead of time to see other mothers care for their babies.
>
> We had several problems following Katie's birth. She had a hard time grasping my nipple in her mouth; this combined with a weak sucking reflex caused much frustration for us both. A week later, extremely sore nipples became the main issue. I now know that I was not positioning her properly at the breast. Because of the way I was holding her, she was stretching the areola around the nipple causing me pain and

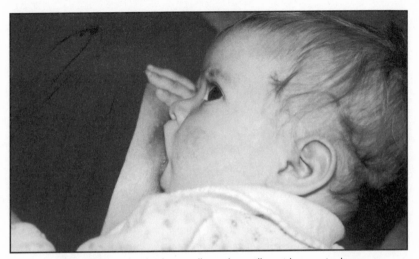

When baby is latched on well, mother will avoid sore nipples.

reducing the amount of milk she was getting. I dreaded each moment of nursing and cried through most of them because of the pain.

During that difficult time, I'd look down at the little being so helpless in my arms, whom I had wanted so badly, and somehow I was able to cope. This was one of the greatest sacrifices I have ever made, but the benefits are worth every moment of pain I experienced.

After learning to latch her on and position her correctly at an LLL meeting, the pain totally disappeared. Now I can't wait for each nursing moment. Love does conquer all, but sometimes the right information is needed, too.

Limiting feedings

If your baby is latched on correctly at the breast, there is no need to limit the length of his feedings. It can take several minutes before the "let-down" occurs and the milk begins to flow, so by taking him off after three or five minutes, as some recommend, the feeding could end even before it starts. If soreness persists throughout the feeding, your baby is not sucking correctly, and you need to get some help from someone who is knowledgeable about breastfeeding. Be sure that your baby is opening his mouth very wide and taking a large portion of breast tissue into his mouth, not holding the tip of your nipple between his gums. If baby is not latched on well, remove him from your breast by using your finger to break the suction and start over.

Allowing your baby to nurse frequently, as often as he seems to be hungry, will actually minimize soreness; he will tend to suck with more vigor if he is ravenously hungry. Babies should nurse at least every two to three hours during the day in the early months. Breastfeeding is a learned art and it is not supposed to hurt. Once you and your baby develop your own way to nurse effectively, the soreness will heal.

Flat nipples

Latching the baby on properly is very important if your nipples are flat and difficult for the baby to grasp. If the problem is caused by engorgement, the swelling that may occur when the milk comes in, it may help to hand-express a little milk ahead of time to bring the nipples out. (See other ways to treat engorgement in Chapter 4.) Be especially careful to wait for baby to open his mouth very wide before latching on.

Many experts believe that a baby who is latched on well can nurse effectively and draw out a flat or inverted nipple.

Ointments

Most ointments sold for the treatment of sore nipples are not useful and some may even be harmful. Avoid any product that needs to be wiped off before the baby nurses. Ointments containing steroids, astringents, or anesthetic agents are **NOT** recommended because they are potentially harmful to both mother and baby. In addition, numbing the nipples with ice may inhibit the let-down reflex. Antiseptic nipple sprays should also be avoided. Ointment can worsen soreness if it prevents the baby from grasping the nipple and areola properly.

Expressing a few drops of your milk after baby is finished nursing and rubbing it gently into your nipples will take advantage of the healing effects of human milk.

Moist Wound Healing

Drying sore nipples with a hair dryer and using a sun lamp are no longer recommended treatments. It has been shown that moist wound healing is more effective in treating nipple soreness as it allows healing to occur without the formation of a scab. Moist wound healing involves maintaining the internal moisture of the skin. It should not be confused with surface wetness which can cause chapping and further irritate the skin.

One way to retain this internal moisture and promote the healing of sore nipples is to apply a specially formulated type of lanolin, called modified lanolin.

Lansinoh Brand Lanolin for Breastfeeding Mothers® has been endorsed by La Leche League International for use in treating sore nipples. It is the purest and safest brand of modified lanolin. Other modified lanolin products may contain high levels of pesticides, along with free lanolin alcohols and detergent residues which have been identified as the cause of lanolin allergies.

Lansinoh Brand Lanolin for Breastfeeding Mothers® does not have to be removed before feeding the baby. You should be aware that similar products are available but they are not manufactured to the same levels of purity so they may not be as safe for your baby.

To treat sore or cracked nipples, gently pat nipples dry after feedings and take a pea-sized portion of Lansinoh, soften between clean fingers, and apply to each nipple. Use enough to maintain the moisture barrier and apply after every feeding. Gently pat it on; do not rub it in.

The use of Lansinoh may also relieve pain as it protects the nerve endings that signal pain. If the pressure of your clothing causes discomfort, apply Lansinoh and then use breast shells with large air holes, or tea strainers with the handles removed, to keep your clothing away from sore nipples.

Lansinoh Brand Lanolin for Breastfeeding Mothers® is available from many drug or discount stores in the USA and is also sold through LLLI's Catalogue, our Web site at www.lalecheleague.org, and many La Leche League Groups.

Nipple cleansing

Bathing with plain water is all that is necessary for your nipples. Avoid using soap on the nipples as it can remove the natural protective oils and predispose the nipples to cracking. (Use of soap on the nipples may be suggested if it seems that a bacterial infection is present.) Be careful, too, not to apply cologne, deodorant, hair spray, or powder near the nipples to avoid irritating the tender skin.

Avoid any kind of plastic lining in your bra or nursing pads. A plastic lining can cause trouble by keeping the nipples wet and causing chapping. Wearing a bra that is too tight can also put pressure on your nipples and cause soreness.

Sore nipples do heal

Frequent opportunities to nurse and cuddle your little one will help you cope until your nipples heal. Try napping during the day, eating nourishing foods, and drinking plenty of liquids. Limit visitors, especially those who may discourage or upset you, and accept offers of help with the household while you and the baby rest. Fortunately, sore nipples rarely last more than a few days, especially if you are following the suggestions given here.

If soreness persists, you'll want to check with someone who is knowledgeable about correct positioning and latch-on. A La Leche League Leader or a board certified lactation consultant may need to observe your baby as he is nursing. If your baby is not taking your nipple into his mouth correctly, there are techniques that can be used to help him learn to nurse more effectively.

In some cases, a mother's sore nipples are the result of baby's inability to suck correctly due to a short frenulum (tongue-tie) or a birth injury. Having the baby's frenulum clipped is a simple procedure that can be performed in a doctor or dentist's office without stitches or anesthesia. Babies who have suffered a birth injury, perhaps due to the use of forceps or vacuum extraction, may respond well to chiropractic adjustment, massage therapy, or other gentle, non-invasive treatment by a practitioner who is accustomed to treating infants.

There may be a relationship between apprehension on the part of the mother and sore nipples. Tender nipples may cause enough tension to hold back the let-down reflex. The delay in the milk may cause frustration for the baby and create greater concern on your part. What can you do about this? You can hand-express a little milk to start the flow, and you can make a deliberate effort to relax before nursing. You may want to ask your doctor to suggest an analgesic to relieve the pain while your nipples are very sore.

Some mothers have given up breastfeeding because of sore nipples. This is unfortunate because it isn't necessary. In a few very rare cases of extremely sore nipples, which might occur if baby has been sucking incorrectly for some time, it may be necessary to discontinue breastfeeding temporarily while the nipples are healing. During this time the mother may have to hand-express or pump her milk and give it to the baby from a cup or a spoon. As soon as the nipples respond to treatment, the baby can be put back on the breast, paying careful attention to positioning and latch-on.

Thrush

If you suddenly get sore nipples after several weeks or months of comfortable nursing, you and/or your baby may have contracted thrush. (Thrush can also occur in the newborn period.) If the nipple area gets itchy and feels very tender, or if the skin becomes pink and flaky, you may have thrush. Thrush is a fungus infection that thrives on milk. It may appear as white spots on the inside of your baby's cheeks, or on his gums. Your baby may also have a persistent diaper rash in connection with thrush, and you may have a vaginal yeast infection. Thrush can be related to taking oral contraceptive pills or an antibiotic. Mothers with diabetes may have a greater susceptibility to thrush. It is more common in warm, humid climates. You may have it on your nipples even when there is no sign of it in the baby's mouth.

Thrush may take several weeks to cure. Your doctor may prescribe medication or other forms of treatment. Be sure to treat both the baby's mouth and your nipples. Others in the family may also require treatment.

Wash your hands thoroughly after using the bathroom, as this will help keep thrush from spreading. You must be persistent about treating thrush but it is no reason to discontinue breastfeeding.

Sore nipples in later months

Another possible cause of sore nipples in later months is teething. Some babies' sucking pattern changes when their gums are sore, and this can temporarily cause nipple soreness. Try being more careful of baby's position at the breast and the way he is grasping your nipple. A change of nursing positions may help. Using Lansinoh Brand Lanolin for Breastfeeding Mothers® can also help.

Sometimes a mother will notice a small painful blister on the tip of her nipple. This is called a "milk blister" and could be caused by a plugged milk duct. Soak the nipple area in warm water several times a day and keep the area very clean. Try varying nursing positions so baby's mouth puts the least pressure on the blister. It may take a few days to heal completely, but resist the temptation to pop the blister yourself as this can lead to infection.

If you are nursing an older baby or toddler and suddenly notice that your nipples are sore, but none of the above reasons seem to be the cause, then there are some other questions that you can ask yourself. Has your little one been experimenting with unusual nursing positions which might cause nipple strain and abrasion? When he grasps or releases the breast, has he been sucking the nipple in or pulling off without first breaking the suction? Is it possible that you

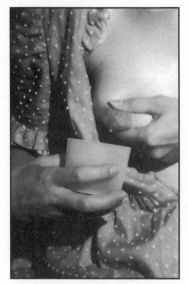

Learning to hand-express
your milk may be helpful in a
variety of situations.

might be pregnant? One or more of these situations might cause sore nipples in even a veteran nursing mother.

When you are experiencing sore nipples or any kind of problem it can be helpful to share your experience with another nursing mother, especially an LLL Leader. She may have additional insight into the situation. Sometimes, all you really need are support and encouragement to help you work through your problem or difficulty and see the brighter side of nursing your baby.

If your child tries to bite

When little ones start to get their first teeth, they sometimes try to experiment by nipping at mother's breast. This kind of behavior often indicates that baby is finished nursing and ready to play. Mothers sometimes react too strongly when this happens, and their startled response frightens a sensitive baby. Other times, baby doesn't get the message that mother's breast cannot be used for teething unless mother does take a stronger approach.

In the normal course of nursing, baby's teeth do not come in contact with mother's nipple at all. When a baby is sucking actively, the mother's nipple is positioned in the back of baby's mouth, not near his teeth. If a baby shows a tendency to bite down when he is finished nursing, a mother can be alert to signs that he is ready to end the feeding. She can keep a finger near his cheek, ready to insert it into baby's mouth at the first sign that he is ready to bite down. She should remove him from her breast immediately. This action, along with a firm, "No biting" is usually all that's needed to convince baby that this behavior is not acceptable. Having another more suitable teething object ready to offer him will reinforce the message.

If he is not convinced, and continues to try to bite, some mothers remove the baby from their lap, placing him on the floor, again giving the message, "No biting." Usually, baby gets very upset by this sudden interruption of his special time with mom and he needs to be picked up and comforted very quickly. You just want to let him know that it is unacceptable to bite at the breast.

Pumping and Storing Your Milk

When situations or circumstances occur that cause a mother to be separated from her breastfed baby, she'll need to know how to remove milk from her breasts by hand or by using a breast pump. She may also need information on how to safely store the milk she pumps so it can later be fed to her baby.

Some of the situations in which pumping will be needed include having a premature or sick baby who is unable to nurse, a mother planning to return to work or school, a need to relieve engorged or overfull breasts, or a situation where added stimulation is needed to increase a mother's milk supply.

Hand or manual expression

One of the best techniques to learn is hand or manual expression. This is the least expensive and most portable method you can use. It may require some practice in order to make it work for you. In some cases, watching another mother hand-express her milk is the best way to learn how to do it.

With practice, many mothers are able to express several ounces of milk very quickly. Wash your hands before you begin. The basic technique is to place your fingers on your breast with your thumb above and fingers below so they form a "C." Push back toward the chest wall while squeezing your thumb and fingers together rhythmically just behind the areola (dark area of skin that surrounds the nipple). In the case of a very large areola, fingers should be positioned about 1 to 1 1/2 inches (2 1/2 to 4 cm) behind the nipple.

Do not slide your fingers along the skin. Rotate your hand around the breast in order to reach all the milk ducts. Do this for three to five minutes on one breast; then switch to the other breast. Switching back and forth helps to increase the flow of milk. Use both hands on each breast in order to reach more of the milk ducts. Have a clean container ready to collect the milk.

The Marmet Technique of manual expression

Another hand-expression technique has been developed by Chele Marmet, a La Leche League Leader and lactation consultant who is the Director of the Lactation Institute in Encino, California. Many mothers who have been previously unsuccessful at hand-expression have found this method effective.

The key to the success of this technique is the combination of the method of manual expression and the use of massage to stimulate the milk ejection reflex. As with any manual skill, practice is important. This technique is explained in detail in the Appendix.

Breast pumps

Many breastfeeding mothers do just fine without ever owning or using a breast pump. When mother and baby are together most of the time, right from the beginning, and the baby is able to nurse often, a mother may have no reason to pump her breasts. If you learn hand expression, it can be used for the occasional times when you might need to save your milk or to empty your breasts. Before investing your money in a breast pump, you may want to consider whether it is something you will really need.

There are several types of circumstances in which a mother will want to use a pump. Mothers who plan to return to work when their babies are still very young can continue breastfeeding by pumping their breasts during their lunch hour and/or at midmorning and midafternoon breaks while at work. They can save their milk for feeding the baby later on.

A working mother will be looking for a breast pump that offers both ease and convenience. She may need to carry the pump back and forth to work with her and she needs to be able to use it quickly and efficiently. She also wants a pump that is easy to clean, perhaps even dishwasher-safe, to save time in her already busy day.

The mother who is pumping milk for a premature baby is in a situation where she needs to establish her milk supply for the future and to provide a specific number of ounces per day to meet her baby's present needs. However, she may not have the opportunity to actually nurse her baby for many weeks. She needs a pump that will closely simulate a baby's sucking action, in order to initiate a good let-down reflex and establish her milk production. A full size electric pump is best suited to this situation.

Some nursing mothers may decide they want to have a breast pump on hand just in case of a family emergency or other situation where they'll need to be temporarily separated from their baby. These mothers want to buy an inexpensive pump that just gives them the security of knowing it will be available even though it may never be needed. Breast pumps and other breastfeeding products are available from La Leche League International. See the Appendix for details.

Choosing a breast pump

"Bicycle Horn" Pumps. At one time years ago, this was the only type of breast pump available and it is still the least expensive. Suction is created by squeezing a rubber bulb, but sensitive breast tissue can be damaged as the suction cannot be regulated. In addition, these pumps cannot be adequately sterilized. They are not recommended.

Cylinder Pumps. Several different manufacturers offer piston-type cylinder pumps with a wide variety of adaptations. All consist of basically two glass or plastic cylinders. The

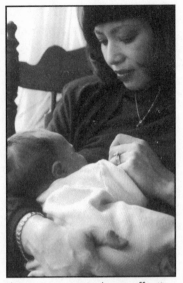

A pump can never be as effective as a baby who is nursing well.

outer cylinder usually doubles as a storage container and feeding bottle. Suction in these pumps is created by pulling the outer cylinder away from the breast. Many women report that this pump is comfortable to use and works effectively. Most of these pumps are small and lightweight, making them easy to carry with you, so they are convenient. Most are also dishwasher-safe.

Handle Squeeze Pump. A squeeze pump designed to be operated with one hand can be convenient to use when a mother wants to pump her milk from one breast while baby nurses on the other side. These pumps are lightweight, very portable, and relatively inexpensive. Most women report they are comfortable and effective.

Small Motorized Pumps. Small motorized pumps provide a combination of convenience and portability. They are small, lightweight, and relatively inexpensive. Suction is provided by a small motor that operates on electricity or batteries, saving mother the effort involved in using a hand pump. When a battery-operated pump is used regularly, the batteries need to be replaced often. A small motorized pump can be operated with one hand which is important in some situations.

Semi-Automatic Electric Pumps. These small electric pumps require the mother to regulate the suction and release but offer the advantage of an electric motor to provide the power. Some models are small enough to be very portable and moderately priced. A mother who plans to work part time and will need to pump her milk several times a week would probably find this type of pump effective.

Personal Use Automatic Pumps. These pumps are designed to be convenient and effective when a mother is separated regularly from her baby and needs to pump her milk several times a day. They operate automatically and closely simulate a baby's sucking pattern. Most allow the mother to pump both breasts at the same time. These pumps generally cost between $100 and $300, but a working mother who wants to provide her own milk for her baby would probably find this to be a worthwhile investment.

Fully Portable Pumping. A new type of breast pump is now available that offers a mother "hands-free" pumping. This pump is fully automatic and battery operated so the user can move around and perform other tasks while she is pumping her milk. Each pump unit is small enough to fit into your bra and the collection bags fit discreetly under your clothing.

Full-Size Automatic Electric Pumps. An automatic electric piston pump provides the most effective pumping action, automatically simulating the sucking action of a nursing baby. Most can be used for double-pumping (pumping both breasts at the same time). These are the pumps of choice for the mother who is pumping her milk for a premature or sick baby who is unable to nurse at the breast. Because these pumps are the fastest and easiest way to pump your milk, they provide the best stimulation for building and maintaining a good milk supply. This can be particularly important in a stressful situation.

Full-size automatic electric pumps are expensive, but they are widely available on a rental basis. In the case of a sick or hospitalized baby (or mother), health insurance will often cover the rental fees when the use of the pump is prescribed by a doctor. A working mother will find the cost of renting a pump less per month than the cost of buying formula for her baby.

Baby is best

No breast pump can match the effectiveness of a baby in stimulating a mother's milk supply and extracting milk. This is partly because mechanical suction cannot duplicate the synchronized action of the baby's tongue, jaw, and palate, but it is mainly because the mother's emotional response to her baby is an important factor.

Techniques for pumping

Learning the techniques of effective pumping requires patience and practice. But the rewards can be well worth your while if you are in a situation where you must be separated from your baby. Here are some tips that will help in any situation that requires you to pump your milk.

1. Follow the manufacturer's directions for any pump you use.

2. When using any kind of pump it's a good idea to moisten your breast before applying the breast flange. This improves suction.

3. Be sure to go easy at first and use the lowest setting or the least amount of suction to get started. It is possible to damage sensitive breast tissue, so heed the first signs of discomfort. Pumping should not be uncomfortable and never painful. Reduce the strength of the suction or the amount of time spent pumping. If discomfort occurs, check to be sure you are using the pump correctly. If necessary, switch to a different brand or type of pump.

4. Pumping in a quiet, relaxed setting will usually help the milk to flow more easily. Although this is not always possible in an office setting or a hospital nursery, it is worth the effort to try to find a secluded spot where you can pump undisturbed. Thinking about the baby, looking at a picture of him, or smelling an article of clothing he has worn can do wonders to encourage the milk to flow.

5. Be sure that your hands and the container you use to collect the milk are clean. Follow the pump manufacturer's directions for cleaning the pump. Bacteria can accumulate if dried particles of milk are left in the breast flange, tubing, or collection bottle. If you are pumping your milk for a hospitalized baby, there may be more specific precautions you need to take. Check with the nurses who are caring for the baby.

6. Research has shown that human milk can safely be kept for up to 24 hours if it is stored at 60 degrees F (15 degrees C), just below room temperature. An insulated cooler with ice packs will keep milk at this temperature. At 66 to 72 degrees F (19 to 22 degrees C), human milk can be stored for 10 hours. At 79 degrees F (25 degrees C), milk is safe from harmful bacteria for four to six hours. Human milk has a remarkable ability to retard bacterial

growth. You may need to be more cautious if you are expressing milk for a hospitalized baby.

7. Milk can be refrigerated for up to eight days (at 32 to 39 degrees F (zero to four degrees C) with no increase in harmful bacteria.

8. For longer storage, milk can be frozen and kept in a refrigerator-freezer for up to two weeks. In a separate door freezer it can be kept for three to four months. In a separate deep freeze that stays at a constant 0 degrees F (-19 degrees C) it can be kept six months or longer. Be sure to label and date frozen milk and use the oldest milk first.

9. It's a good idea to freeze your milk in small amounts varying from two to four ounces (60 to 120 ml). You can always thaw more milk if your baby needs it. Once thawed, human milk can be refrigerated for up to twenty-four hours but should never be refrozen. Do not let milk stand at room temperature to thaw. Instead, thaw it quickly by putting the container under running water, first cold, then gradually getting warmer until the milk is warm. Do not heat the milk on the stove or in a microwave oven. More information on storing your milk and feeding it to your baby can be found in Chapter 8.

To express milk for a milk bank

Because human milk has been found to be so important for sick or premature babies, nursing mothers are sometimes asked to donate their extra milk for these babies. In many hospitals, special milk banks have been established for this purpose. If you are asked to donate your milk, you will naturally consider your own baby's needs first, and you will probably pump or hand-express milk to donate only after feedings. If your baby is a little older, you might be able to express milk from one breast while the baby nurses at the other. This is less time-consuming, and can usually be done if you are using a pump that can be operated with one hand.

The milk bank will probably have its own set of instructions and may even provide you with a breast pump to use. If you are donating your milk for a sick or premature baby, you must be scrupulously clean in your techniques for expressing and storing your milk. If you, your baby, or any other member of your household has been ill, you should not donate milk until everyone has been well for twenty-four hours.

When the time comes that you are no longer donating milk, cut

down gradually on the pumping. If
you have built up a milk supply much
greater than your own baby's needs,
the sudden drop in demand might
cause engorgement, just as sudden
weaning would. Taper off gradually by
pumping out some of the milk whenever your breasts feel overly full and
uncomfortable. Or, see if your baby
will help out with an extra nursing
when you are feeling full. He'll probably be happy to oblige.

Breast Problems: Sore Breasts, Plugged Ducts, and Mastitis

A mother who is experiencing a
plugged duct or mastitis needs a
lot of rest.

It sometimes happens that a nursing mother notices a very tender spot
or sore lump in her breast. This can be a sign of a plugged duct or a
breast infection (mastitis). Knowing what to do about it can clear
things up quickly and avoid further difficulty.

Whatever the cause of a sore breast, there are three basic steps
involved in treatment:

Apply Heat; Get Plenty of Rest; and keep the breast comfortably empty by **Frequent Nursing.** These procedures may sound
deceptively simple, but immediate action can mean the difference
between a few hours of discomfort and several days in bed.

Plugged ducts

If a breastfeeding mother notices a very tender spot, redness, or a sore
lump in her breast, this may very likely be caused by a plugged milk
duct. What this means is that a milk duct has become inflamed
because the milk is unable to flow through it freely.

Plugged ducts may be caused by any of the following—improper
positioning of the baby at the breast, prolonged periods of time
between nursings, giving supplementary bottles or overusing a pacifier,
wearing a too-tight nursing bra or other clothing that constricts the
breasts. If an older baby suddenly starts sleeping through the night, or
nurses often one day and cuts way back the next day, a plugged milk
duct may occur. Occasionally a plugged duct is caused by dried milk
secretions covering one of the nipple openings.

Rest is essential at the first sign of a problem. If at all possible, you should climb into bed with the baby tucked in beside you for the remainder of the day. At the very least you should eliminate all extra activities and spend an hour or two relaxing with your baby at your breast and feet off the floor. A plugged duct or a sore spot on your breast may be the first sign that you are trying to do too much. You would be well-advised to heed this warning and get lots of extra rest for a few days after you've experienced a plugged duct.

In addition to rest, there are some other things you can do to treat a plugged duct:

- Apply wet or dry heat to the affected area, and remove any dried milk secretions on the nipple by soaking with plain warm water. Lean over a basin of warm water and soak your breasts for ten minutes or so three times a day, take warm showers, use hot wet packs, a heating pad, or a hot water bottle. Massage the affected area gently while it is warm, and nurse the baby or hand-express some milk immediately after treating the area with warmth. Getting the milk to flow while the breast is warm will help unplug the affected duct.

- Nurse the baby on the affected side frequently. Nurse at least every two hours including during the night, as long as the breast is tender or warm to the touch. Nurse first on the affected side at each feeding. Frequent nursings will keep the breast fairly empty so the milk flows more freely. Try positioning the baby so his chin is pointed toward the plugged duct.

- Loosen constrictive clothing, especially your bra. If possible, you may even want to discontinue wearing a bra for a few days. If you are more comfortable with a bra, try wearing one that is a size larger or a least change to one that has a different cut or style. This should relieve any pressure that the bra you usually wear may have been putting on the milk ducts. Some mothers try to get by without a regular nursing bra by wearing a stretchy type of bra and pulling the cup up or down for feedings. This could be causing pressure on the milk ducts with the result that they are not emptied properly. Some nursing bras with stretchy cups that pull down or to the side for nursing can have the same effect, putting too much pressure on some milk ducts.

- Check for other clothing or accessories that could be putting pressure on your breasts such as a heavy shoulder bag or baby carrier. The location of the plugged duct may give you a clue as to its cause.

- Check the baby's position at the breast. He should be on his side with his whole body facing you, and he should be able to grasp your nipple without having to turn his head. A large portion of the areola should be in his mouth. It is important for the baby to be positioned properly so that all the milk ducts are emptied at every feeding.

- Try changing nursing positions from time to time. Lie down, sit up, switch from the rocking chair to the sofa to a lounge chair. Try nursing with baby in the football hold. A variety of nursing positions will give the baby a better chance to reach all of the milk ducts and keep them emptied. (See Chapter 4 for details on various nursing positions.) One position that may be particularly helpful in clearing up a plugged duct is to place the baby in the middle of a bed or a quilt on the floor while you sit with legs crossed, yoga style, (or get up on your hands and knees) and lean over him to nurse, with the breast hanging freely from the rib cage. This position may not be the most comfortable for you, but it can allow a plugged milk duct to be opened more easily.

Breast infections (Mastitis)

Prompt and proper treatment of a plugged duct will usually keep a breast infection (mastitis) from developing. However, if you notice the type of soreness or lump that is usually associated with a plugged duct, and it is accompanied by a fever or flu-like symptoms (feeling tired, achy, or run-down), you probably have a breast infection. A breastfeeding mother will sometimes find herself developing a breast infection when other family members suffer from colds or other types of flu.

It is important that you begin treating a breast infection immediately. The treatment for a breast infection is the same as for a plugged duct: **Apply Heat, Get Plenty of Rest, and Nurse Often.** If this course of action is begun quickly, you may not need further treatment for a breast infection. However, if you still have a fever after 24 hours, and other symptoms persist, or if your fever is more than 101.5 degrees, you'll want to get in touch with your doctor. In this case, your doctor may prescribe medication. You'll want to continue getting lots of rest and nursing often while you take the medication.

It will not harm your baby to continue nursing when you have a breast infection. At one time it was standard procedure to recommend weaning if the mother had a breast infection. However, studies have shown that the infection clears up more quickly when the breast is kept empty. Also, the mother is much more comfortable than she would be after a sudden weaning. Antibodies in mother's milk protect the baby from the bacteria that may be causing the infection. Even temporary weaning is an unnecessary hardship at a time when you aren't feeling well in the first place.

If your doctor prescribes an antibiotic, be sure to take all of the medication that is prescribed. People sometimes stop taking a medication as soon as they start to feel better, only to have the infection reoccur in a few days. In the case of a breast infection, this would be hard on both you and your baby, so it's important to take the medication that is prescribed for you until it is gone. Most types of antibiotics are safe for a mother to take while she is nursing. If a doctor is wary about a specific antibiotic, ask him to prescribe one that has been found to be safe to take while a mother is nursing. Let him know how important it is for your baby to continue breastfeeding.

If you find yourself with a second breast infection within a few days or weeks of the first one, chances are good that the original infection didn't clear up completely. Repeated breast infections do occasionally happen, but they are almost always a recurrence of the first infection rather than a brand new infection.

If you do find that plugged ducts or breast infections seem to occur frequently, you may want to look into your general health, being sure you are eating a balanced diet and limiting extra activities so you have enough time to relax and enjoy nursing your baby.

Donna Sutton, a mother from Iowa, found that the advice she received from her La Leche League Leader helped her recover when she had a breast infection:

> After being home from the hospital for one week, I found myself with a sore breast and other symptoms of a breast infection. A consultation with a local physician produced the advice to stop nursing on the infected breast for at least four to five days, and express the milk by hand or breast pump. I knew that this was the wrong course to take, so after much deliberation I continued to nurse on both sides. My infection did not abate, and I could still feel a lump in my breast.
>
> I finally called my local La Leche League Leader. Her advice soon made all the difference in the world. After apply-

ing warm packs, nursing often (especially on the affected side), and resting, the lump in my breast began to disappear. I still remember my Leader telling me that nothing should be more important at this time than nursing my baby. I realize now that if I had consulted her initially, the infection would have cleared up more quickly and been less frustrating for Sarah and me. How many mothers have received the wrong advice and been forced to quit nursing?

I am grateful to my LLL Leader for her advice, and I'm a firm believer that breast is best!

Breast abscess

In very rare cases, a breast infection may develop into an abscess. This usually does not occur if prompt treatment is initiated at the first sign of a problem. An abscess is a localized infection that may need to be surgically opened and drained. Usually your doctor can do this in his office or perhaps he'll want to do it at the hospital on an outpatient basis. If this procedure should be necessary, you can continue to nurse on the unaffected breast with no problem, but you may need to pump or hand-express your milk from the abscessed breast for a day or so. Keeping that breast empty will promote healing, but the incision may be too close to the areola for the baby to nurse without causing discomfort.

Remember that any of these breast problems can be an indication that you should carefully evaluate other things that are going on in your life. These symptoms are often a nursing mother's first clue that she should be taking better care of herself. Conserve your energy by keeping extra activities to a minimum and spend as much time as possible just relaxing and enjoying your baby without regard to schedules and deadlines.

Breast Lumps and Breast Surgery

Most lumps in a nursing mother's breast are inflammatory, due to plugged ducts or a breast infection. Some are due to benign tumors (fibromas), a milk retention cyst (galactocele), and only in the very rarest of cases are they due to cancer.

If you have a lump that does not go away in a week with careful treatment for a plugged duct, we suggest that you consult a physician. Weaning is not necessary either for diagnosis or treatment of breast lumps. Mammograms, x-rays, and ultrasound tests will not interfere with breastfeeding. Mothers have had cysts removed, biopsied, and aspirated, without finding it necessary to wean. If your doctor is not familiar with the lactating breast, you may need to call his attention to this fact. It may be advisable to empty the breast by nursing the baby immediately prior to examination and/or whatever procedure the doctor may want to undertake. Nursing may be resumed again right after most diagnostic procedures, except after a radioactive breast scan.

If surgery is needed, care must be taken so that the fewest milk ducts and major nerves are damaged. Barbara Ann Paster of New Hampshire worked closely with her surgeon to be sure she would be able to continue breastfeeding after surgery:

Shortly after our second child, Sara, was born I noticed a lump in my breast just to the left of my nipple. I arranged to go in for the removal of the breast lump soon thereafter. Before the scheduled date of surgery, I sat down with my surgeon to discuss the nursing breast and how he could help me make my return to nursing go smoothly as soon as possible after the operation. While the surgeon had known I was nursing, he had never considered the problem of operating on a nursing breast. He agreed to be especially careful during the surgery to cut as few milk ducts as possible.

Because my lump was deep within the breast, my surgeon ruled out anything less than general anesthesia, claiming that it was too tender an area to manage otherwise. To minimize engorgement, we worked out a plan for me to nurse Sara immediately prior to surgery. We also decided on dissolvable stitches, which would absorb after healing.

Sara was put to breast on my unaffected side as soon as I regained consciousness. The incisional area was dressed with as small a dressing as possible so as not to alarm her. Within twelve hours of the surgery I was able to nurse on the affected side.

I won't say it was comfortable. I found that putting some pressure on the dressing helped allay the feeling that she would pull the incision or my breast apart. By the second or third day it was quite tolerable. Putting my baby to the breast was more comfortable than trying to hand-express or use a pump. My surgeon was amazed at how well the breast healed.

My incision line follows the curve of the outer edge of the areola. The surgeon went in from there and excised the lump from almost directly under the nipple. Luckily it was fibrocystic in nature which meant it was not life-threatening.

Another mother, Beverly Scott from Washington, found that surgery was not needed for her breast lump. She learned that the lump that formed in her breast when her son was ten days old was a galactocele, a milk-retention cyst. Fortunately, her doctor was familiar with this uncommon phenomenon and advised her to continue nursing and ignore the lump. However, by the time her son was twenty-one months old, the lump had enlarged to twice its original size and the doctor became concerned and suggested weaning. Beverly goes on to explain what happened:

> I was determined to continue with baby-led weaning. I decided to learn all I could about available options and then ask my doctor to proceed with treatment without waiting for Jesse to wean.
>
> I talked to my LLL Leader and received helpful information regarding surgery during lactation. I contacted my obstetrician, summarizing my conclusions in a letter and then calling him. We agreed that he would go ahead and remove the fluid from the cyst immediately for diagnostic purposes. If surgical removal of the cyst was indicated, I would arrange with a general surgeon to have the procedure done on an outpatient basis under local anesthetic with minimal interruption of breastfeeding. However, that did not become necessary, as a laboratory analysis of the fluid confirmed the original diagnosis: The cyst contained only milk.

A woman who suddenly finds a large breast lump soon after giving birth should ask her doctor about the possibility of a galactocele before submitting to invasive treatment such as surgery. Ultrasound and/or aspiration could confirm the diagnosis if there was any uncertainty.

Breastfeeding has been shown to reduce the incidence of breast cancer, nevertheless, there have been rare instances of a mother developing breast cancer while she is still nursing a baby. It is a good idea to learn how to do a monthly breast self-exam, and do it regularly. Any mother who discovers a lump in her breast that does not change or go away should have it checked by her doctor.

Previous breast surgery

Previous breast surgery usually need not stop a mother from nursing her baby even if she has had a breast removed because of cancer. Breastfeeding will not expose the mother to any greater risk of malignancy, nor will it harm the baby. And since milk production works on

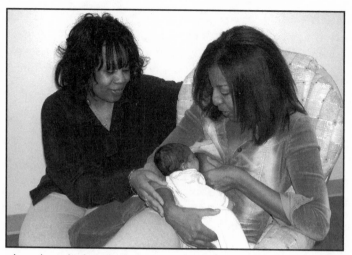

A mother who has doubts about her milk supply can get help from
a La Leche League Leader.

the basis of supply and demand, one breast can supply plenty of milk
for the baby.

If a biopsy was done or a lump or cyst removed from the breast a
mother may be uncertain whether or not milk ducts or major nerves
have been damaged. She will need to monitor her baby's wet and
soiled diapers as well as his weight gain to be sure he is getting enough
milk.

Breast implants

If a mother has previously had breast implants, there is sometimes
concern about how the surgery will affect her plans to breastfeed. If
the majority of milk ducts and major nerves have not been cut, breastfeeding should proceed smoothly. In some cases, even milk ducts that
were cut have been found to "recanalize" or grow back.

It is not always possible to know ahead of time whether or not a
mother who has had breast augmentation surgery can fully breastfeed
her baby. The best recommendation is to try breastfeeding and watch
carefully for signs of baby getting enough milk. If there is a problem,
and baby is not gaining well, a mother can continue to breastfeed along
with offering supplements with a cup, spoon, bottle, or nursing supplementer.

Some concerns have been raised about silicone leakage when a
mother breastfeeds with silicone breast implants. There is no evidence
that silicone used in breast implants can leak into a mother's milk or
harm the baby.

Breast reduction surgery

It was once thought that mothers who had previously had breast reduction surgery would be unable to breastfeed because major nerves and milk ducts had probably been damaged when large amounts of breast tissue were removed. Recently, La Leche League International published a book called DEFINING YOUR OWN SUCCESS: BREASTFEEDING AFTER BREAST REDUCTION SURGERY that tells a different story. Author Diana West has combined research and personal experiences of hundreds of mothers to show that breastfeeding after breast reduction surgery (BFAR) is something that is not only possible, but is becoming much more common.

One mother, named Jennifer, who is quoted in DEFINING YOUR OWN SUCCESS writes:

> I can't begin to describe how I feel about nursing. It is part of how I mother that I wouldn't trade for anything. Because the odds I got for breastfeeding when I first became pregnant were far less than 50 percent that I would be able to do this, I also feel as though my children and I are incredibly fortunate. I see breastfeeding as a gift that I have received, as well as one I can give to my children. I think the key to my success was a commitment to make it work, not giving up, and trying to fix any problems that came our way rather than seeing them as obstacles.

In some cases, a mother who has had breast reduction surgery will not be able to produce a full milk supply for her baby. But the benefits of human milk are worth the effort even if only small amounts of milk are available. And the benefits of feeding your baby at your breast go far beyond the actual milk. Another mother, Carol, who is quoted in Diana West's book, says:

> Through the use of galactogogues [herbal or prescription medications used to increase milk production], and by offering to breastfeed as often as every hour, I was able to increase my supply, so that by three to four months old, Kira was getting over 60 percent of her nutritional needs from me. The best part was that she was getting 100 percent of non-nutritional needs from our breastfeeding relationship. We had a closeness that is hard to explain.
>
> I may not have exclusively breastfed my babies, but by redefining my ideas of what breastfeeding means, from exclu-

sive feeding of my milk alone to a relationship that benefited us all, I realize I was having successful breastfeeding relationships. Breastfeeding is so much more than nutrition.

For more information, order a copy of DEFINING YOUR OWN SUCCESS from LLLI's catalogue. Or check out the BFAR Web site at www.bfar.org.

Is Your Baby Getting Enough Milk?

There is nothing quite like the delight that comes from seeing your baby thrive and grow on your milk. As his arms and legs fill out and his cheeks turn plump and rosy, you can't help but glow with pride...and marvel at how perfectly your body is continuing to provide for all of his nutritional needs.

A baby's need for milk and his mother's ability to produce it in just the right quantity have been said to be one of nature's most perfect examples of the law of supply and demand. Until the advent of mass produced artificial formula, the very survival of the human race depended largely on a mother's ability to produce a sufficient quantity of milk to adequately nourish her baby.

There is nothing mystical or magical about producing enough milk to satisfy your baby's needs. Establishing and maintaining an ample milk supply is easy when you understand how the milk supply is regulated and what kinds of things are likely to upset the balance between the amount of milk the baby needs and the amount of milk that is produced.

The more the baby nurses effectively, the more milk there will be. Understanding this "golden rule" of breastfeeding is the key to an abundant milk supply and a contented baby. Years ago, mothers were often told to wait four hours between feedings so that their breasts would "fill up." Many a mother and baby had a short-lived breastfeeding experience due to this well-intentioned but erroneous advice.

It is now well understood that milk is produced almost continuously, and that the more often and effectively the baby nurses, the more milk there will be. Thus, the mother of a baby who is nursing every two hours will usually have a bountiful milk supply, while the mother who is trying to "hold off" the baby and nurse only every four hours may have considerably less milk. Frequent and effective sucking at the breast signals the mother's body to produce a correspondingly increased amount of milk. Allowing the breasts to accumulate milk for a long period of time is interpreted as a signal to produce less milk.

In the first two days after birth, your baby will have only one or two wet diapers per day. After that, you can be confident that your baby is getting enough milk if:

- He has more than five or six really wet diapers and more than three bowel movements per day and is receiving nothing but your milk—no supplemental water or formula. (A baby older than six weeks or so may have fewer bowel movements and still be getting enough to eat.)

- He is gaining weight at an average of six ounces (170 grams) a week or about one and one-half to two pounds (680 to 906 grams) per month in the first three months. From four to six months, average weight gain for the breastfed baby is four to five ounces (113 to 142 grams) per week; from six to twelve months, average gain is two to four ounces (57 to 113 grams) per week.

  At your baby's first checkup, weight gain should be determined from the lowest weight the baby reached rather than his birth weight. Most babies lose five to seven percent of their birth weight and may take up to two weeks to regain their birth weight.

- In the first six months, growth in length of approximately one inch (2.5 centimeters) per month and growth in head circumference of one-half inch (1.25 centimeters) per month also show that baby is getting enough to eat.

- He is nursing frequently and is satisfied after each feeding. Most newborns nurse every two to three hours or eight to twelve times in a twenty-four hour period. This is an average, and some babies may nurse less frequently and still gain weight while others may nurse more often.

- He appears healthy—has good color and resilient skin, is "filling out" and growing in length, and is alert and active with good muscle tone.

"False alarms"

Some mothers think they do not have enough milk when actually there is no problem with their milk supply. They worry about symptoms which have other causes or they're unfamiliar with the variety of patterns that are normal in breastfed babies. If your baby is gaining well and has plenty of wet and soiled diapers, there is no need to worry if:

- Your baby nurses very often. Wanting to nurse frequently does not necessarily mean baby is hungry. Many babies have a strong need to suck and a need for a continuous contact with their mothers. Frequent nursing assures that your baby is getting enough milk. Human milk digests more quickly than formula and places less strain on a baby's immature digestive system, so that the breastfed baby needs to be fed more frequently.

- Your baby's nursing habits, weight gain, or sleep patterns don't compare with other babies you know. Each baby is an individual, and there are wide variations within the normal range.

- Your baby suddenly increases the frequency and/or length of his nursings. Babies who are very sleepy as newborns often suddenly "wake up" and begin nursing more frequently. Babies also go through occasional growth spurts (frequently around two weeks, six weeks, and three months). During these times they nurse more often than usual to bring in more milk for their expanding needs.

- Your baby suddenly decreases his time at the breast, perhaps down to five to ten minutes per breast. He may simply be able to extract the milk more quickly now that he is more experienced at nursing.

- Your baby is fussy. Many babies have a fussy period each day, often at about the same time of the day. Some babies are fussy much of the time. Fussiness can be caused by many things other than hunger, but often there is no discernible reason.

- Your breasts leak only a little or not at all. Leaking has no relationship to the amount of milk you produce and often stops after your supply becomes established and regulated to your baby's needs.

- Your breasts suddenly seem softer or smaller. This happens as your milk production adjusts to your baby's demand and the initial fullness or engorgement subsides.

- You never feel the let-down sensation or it does not seem as strong as it did before. This may occur as time goes on. (Some mothers do not feel it at all; it does not mean that they do not have a let-down.)

If your milk supply is low

If it seems that your supply is not meeting your baby's needs, then it is important to determine what is interfering with your production of milk. The following factors can cause or contribute to a lessened milk supply:

Supplementing. Supplementing with even an occasional bottle of formula, juice, or water can interfere with a mother's milk supply. Supplements fill up the baby and cause him to wait longer for the next feeding, thereby decreasing his sucking at the breast. The more formula he gets one day, the less milk the mother's body will make the following day. Supplementing causes a mother's breasts to produce less, not more.

Improper Latch-On. A baby can become confused by the use of any artificial nipple, as it requires a different type of sucking. If your baby is not sucking properly at the breast, he will not be able to stimulate your breasts to produce enough milk.

Pacifiers. Some babies are willing to meet their sucking needs with a pacifier, which may significantly reduce their sucking time at the breast.

Scheduled Feedings. Delaying the baby's feedings until the clock dictates a certain amount of time has passed can interfere with the supply and demand system of milk production. Following baby's cues and offering the breast when baby shows signs of being hungry is usually the best way to ensure an adequate milk supply.

Placid, Sleepy Baby. Some babies sleep most of the time and nurse only infrequently and for short periods. If this describes your baby, and if he is having few wet or soiled diapers and not gaining weight, it is important for you to awaken him regularly, stimulate him with gentle handling, and encourage him to nurse at least every two hours. You'll need to decide how often he should nurse until he learns for himself how to get enough to eat.

Cutting Back on the Length of Feedings. Allowing the baby to come off the breast on his own when he feels satisfied can help assure an adequate milk supply. Cutting feedings short can prevent your supply from increasing as your baby's needs increase. Also, the fat content of the milk increases later in a feeding. On the other hand, a baby who nurses almost continually and never seems satisfied may not be sucking correctly. A baby who is satisfied will end the feeding when he is full.

Offering Only One Breast per Feeding. After the milk is established, some mothers prefer to nurse at only one breast per feeding if baby is gaining well. If you are working to increase your supply, use both breasts but don't limit baby's sucking time at the first breast.

Mother care

A breastfeeding mother needs to take good care of herself in order to provide a good milk supply for her baby. Fatigue and tension can interfere with your let-down and contribute to an inadequate milk supply. Take the time to really relax every so often during the course of the day.

A poor diet can contribute to tension and fatigue and detract from your general well-being. Many mothers feel better when they eat five or six small meals every day rather than three big ones. Good nutritional intake, and eating more often, may be the answer for you. Eat fresh fruits and salads, whole grain bread, rolls, and crackers, meats, cheese, nuts, and fish. Avoid poor quality foods such as cookies, pastries, candy, fried snack foods, and the like.

Breastfeeding increases your need for fluids, as your body needs more fluids to make milk. Take a glass of water or juice with you each time you sit down to nurse the baby. If your urine is dark yellow in color and small in amount, you are not drinking enough liquids. What you drink is equally important. Water and unsweetened fruit juice are your best choices. Avoid excessive amounts of caffeine in coffee, tea, and colas.

Sometimes problems with a mother's health can affect her milk supply and her baby's weight gain. If you are having any health problems, check with your doctor about them. Most medications are safe for nursing mothers, but some can adversely affect your milk production. If a doctor prescribes any medication for you, be sure to mention that you're breastfeeding.

The use of hormonal contraceptives too early in the course of lactation can reduce milk production and affect baby's weight gain. There are no conclusive studies on potential long-term effects of hor-

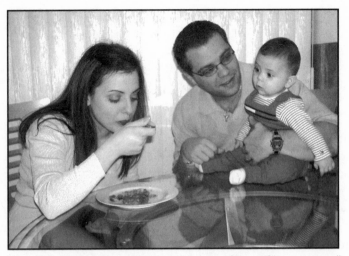

A breastfeeding mother needs to take care of herself by eating well.

mones that are passed on to the baby through the mother's milk. Non-hormonal methods of contraception do not have any potential effects on the baby or your milk supply. Breastfeeding delays the return of fertility for many months for most mothers. (See Chapter 19.)

Smoking may have a detrimental effect on your milk supply and your baby's health. Mothers who smoke may find that their babies gain weight better, are healthier, and seem less fussy when they cut down or stop smoking.

Increasing your milk supply

If you do find that some or all of the above factors have caused your milk supply to decrease, there are some positive steps you can follow to increase your supply of milk. If you are in a situation where you are concerned about your milk supply, it will be very helpful to get in touch with an LLL Leader or board certified lactation consultant. While we can offer you basic information here, she can supply additional insight based on your specific situation.

A slow gaining baby may be having difficulty sucking well because of a birth injury or other physical discomfort. This is something your doctor needs to check. Some babies who are not sucking effectively respond well to chiropractic adjustment, massage therapy, or other gentle, non-invasive treatments by practitioners who are accustomed to treating infants.

If your baby is not gaining weight at the normal rate, or if he is losing weight, you'll want to be sure to keep in close touch with your doctor. There is always a possibility that a health problem is causing baby's slow weight gain. A baby who is actually losing weight will need medical attention. You will probably need to supplement baby's feedings until your milk supply increases. In addition to going over the points listed here to improve your milk supply, be sure to read the section in Chapter 17 on "Slow Weight Gain."

Nurse Frequently for as long as your baby will nurse. Plan to spend twenty-four to forty-eight hours (or longer if your supply is quite low) doing little else but nursing and resting. A sleepy baby may need to be awakened and encouraged to nurse more frequently.

Offer Both Breasts at Each Feeding. This will ensure that your baby gets all the milk available and that both breasts are stimulated frequently.

Try Breast Compression. Once your baby is latched on well, breast compression can help keep him actively sucking for a longer time. To do this, hold your breast with one hand—thumb on one side, four fingers on the other—and watch the baby. Don't do anything if the baby is breastfeeding actively (the baby's jaw is moving all the way to the ear). When the baby is no longer actively sucking, squeeze the breast firmly and stay squeezed. The faster milk flow should cause the baby to start nursing actively again. Don't release the pressure. Keep squeezing until baby stops nursing actively and then release. Your baby may start breastfeeding actively again when you release. If so, wait until he stops to compress again. If not, rotate your fingers slightly around the breast and squeeze again. Repeat as needed on different areas of the breast until this technique no longer keeps baby active, then switch your baby to the other breast.

All Your Baby's Sucking Should Be at the Breast. Avoid bottles and pacifiers. Drinking from an artificial nipple requires a different type of sucking than nursing at mother's breast. Even though a supplement may be necessary temporarily, it can be given with a nursing supplementer while baby nurses or by spoon, cup, or dropper. (See the Appendix for information about the nursing supplementer.) Pacifiers can interfere with the extra nursing that is needed when you are trying to build up your milk.

Give Your Baby Only Human Milk, If Possible. Avoid all solids, water, and juice. If your baby has been receiving formula supplements you will not want to cut these out abruptly. You can gradually cut back on the amount of supplement as your milk supply increases, but you need to watch baby's wet and soiled diapers to be sure he is getting enough to eat. You need to be in touch with your doctor to monitor your baby's weight gain as you are cutting back on formula supplements.

Drink Plenty of Liquids and **Eat a Well Balanced Diet.** Eat a wide variety of foods in as close to their natural state as possible. Try to have a glass of water or juice with you each time you nurse. Most breast-feeding mothers keep a bottle of water with them at all times.

Get Plenty of Rest and Relaxation. Your milk supply will increase faster if you are relaxed and rested. Plan to do as little as possible for a while. Cut out all non-essential tasks, and get help with the essential ones. Take naps with your baby as often as possible. For relaxation, try a warm bath, soft music, exercise, a walk outdoors, or whatever works best for you. Try to spend at least a few minutes each day doing something special to pamper yourself.

After reading through this section, if you have any further questions or concerns be sure to get in touch with your La Leche League Leader. Being in touch with other breastfeeding mothers through your La Leche League Group will offer you the support and encouragement you need. Your happy, healthy breastfed baby will soon provide the reward for your efforts.

The Baby Who Is Pleasingly Plump

If your breastfed baby is a round little fatty, some may say he's gaining too much. While he may weigh more than the average shown on the doctor's charts, the baby on human milk alone will not be overweight. A totally breastfed baby who is "overweight" is not necessarily overfat or obese. Still, in a weight-conscious world, even baby fat is suspect, and the mother of a plump, fully breastfed baby may be told that her child should be put on a diet.

Heredity plays a definite role in determining a child's growth pattern, as became obvious in the Nixon family in Florida. Baby Alena weighed almost eighteen pounds at three-and-a-half months, and her mother, Janice, was told that the development of a large number of fat cells in infancy would cause Alena problems later in life. This was Janice's first child and she was understandably upset. "But I thought back over all I had read or heard at the LLL meetings I had been going to since my eighth month of pregnancy," Janice recounted. "Was Alena

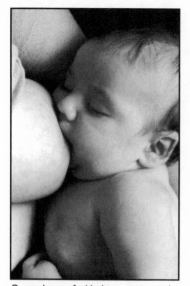

Some breastfed babies gain weight quickly but this does not lead to weight problems later in life.

happy and alert most of the time? Yes. Was she developing well in all other aspects? Yes."

Janice also remembered her mother telling her that she herself had been a very large baby, and she and her mother searched the family album for baby pictures. "A picture of my mother when she was a baby also showed her to be extremely chubby, and she was completely breastfed." Their findings were meaningful because neither has had a weight problem as an adult.

At the four-month checkup, Alena weighed in at almost nineteen pounds and was twenty-five inches long—way above the norms. Janice showed the doctor the family pictures:

When the doctor saw the pictures, he was so impressed that he called in another doctor to look at them. They talked about the loopholes in the "fat cell" theory, and the obvious fact that fat babies do not always become fat adults. They both agreed that there was no reason for me to alter Alena's present care in any way. Absolutely no diet!

There are hazards in limiting growth by putting a baby on a diet. The young child is a dynamic body builder, producing cells of all kinds, brain and nerve cells as well as fat cells. Researchers have observed that the flesh of the breastfed baby is firmer than that of a baby who is not breastfed. There are no "empty" calories in human milk, as there are in highly processed foods.

It must be remembered here that fat accumulated in the relatively inactive pre-toddler state is preparatory for the highly active time when the busy toddler hardly has time to eat. It is not unlike the extra weight that a woman puts on during pregnancy in preparation for the extra demands of motherhood. We have found that by age two or three, the heavyweights among the tiny tots usually slim down beautifully.

Some babies who start out tiny and petite at birth surprise everyone with their rapid gain. Ann Tutor from Japan tells how she handled critics with the comment, "We grow them big at our house!" She writes:

Although Melanie weighed in at six pounds ten ounces at birth, by the time we left the hospital she was six pounds even and seemed to me the tiniest, prettiest little baby girl I had ever seen.

We attended our first La Leche League meeting when Melanie was one month old. She weighed nine pounds at her two-month checkup, and by the second LLL meeting we attended I began to notice that while Melanie had started out smaller than some of the other babies, she had caught up and even passed a few of her little friends. When she was about three months old, people began to casually mention how big my "dainty little girl" was getting, and at her four-month checkup I was surprised to find out that she weighed eighteen pounds.

When at six months Melanie weighed twenty-four pounds, she became a real conversation piece. While I was proud to have a healthy, happy baby, I began to worry about and even resent some of the comments about my baby's weight. Thank goodness my La Leche League friends and my wonderful doctor kept assuring me that as long as Melanie was totally breastfed we were doing great! My doctor even paraded Melanie around to his colleagues at one visit to show them this lovably round, totally breastfed baby.

Melanie is seventeen months old now and weighs thirty-one pounds, and while she doesn't yet have to worry about being called skinny, she has slimmed down considerably. We still get comments about her weight once in a while, some of which still aggravate me, but I don't worry about it anymore. We're in no hurry to end our nursing days. While I hope that Melanie doesn't keep that cute round tummy and those dimpled thighs forever, I know she has had a wonderful start in being breastfed.

Weight problems in later years

While some people may be concerned that too much weight gained in infancy will lead to obesity later on, the truth is that many factors contribute to weight problems in adults. Some aspects that are related to eating habits in childhood are automatically avoided when you breastfeed your baby and follow the guidelines included in this book.

As a breastfeeding mother, you are not going to fall into the anxiety trap of monitoring how many ounces of milk your baby takes. You will not get into the habit of coaxing him to finish the last few ounces in a bottle. When you start solids, your child will probably be at least six months old. You will have bypassed the unnatural situation that comes when solids are given to the younger child, who automatically pushes out whatever is spooned into his mouth, making it difficult for a mother to know if her baby is hungry or not.

Breastfeeding is the first preventive measure against obesity in adult life. In fact, research has shown that breastfeeding protects against later obesity. Children who were breastfed have been found to be less likely to be overweight in adolescence.

Good eating habits do start early, and you can be assured that your baby is receiving the very best nutrition available if he is breastfed.

Did You Ever Hear of a Nursing Strike?

Occasionally a young baby will suddenly refuse to breastfeed for no apparent reason. This can be a real puzzle, especially if the baby is under a year old and probably not at all ready to be weaned.

A situation like this is called a nursing strike. It's a baby's way of communicating the fact that something's wrong. It usually lasts from two to four days and requires some motherly ingenuity to figure out exactly what the problem is.

How can you tell whether your baby has gone on a nursing strike or has just decided to wean himself? A baby who is really ready to wean will usually be well over a year old, will be eating lots of solid food and drinking liquids from a cup, and will gradually lose interest in one nursing at a time. A baby who is on a nursing strike may not be eating much or drinking from a cup at all. He nurses fine one day and abruptly refuses to nurse at all the next day. He also shows signs of being obviously unhappy about the whole situation. He wants you to figure out what's wrong and solve the problem for him.

Consider the following possibilities: Is your baby teething? Does he have a cold, sore throat, or stuffy nose that prevents him from nursing easily? Does he have an earache that makes it painful to nurse? Are you anxious or upset about something? Babies respond to their mothers' feelings.

Has nursing become a stressful time, with too many outside interruptions or distractions? Have you been deciding when the baby should nurse and when he should stop, instead of letting him lead the way? Has the baby become dependent on a pacifier or his thumb, so that he routinely sucks quite a bit on either?

Has some recent change in your nursing pattern confused the baby? Has he had too many bottles? Been left with a sitter? Been repeatedly put off when he cries to nurse? Have you gone back to work, or are you worrying about what will happen when and if you do have to leave the baby?

Sometimes a nursing strike occurs after baby bites mother a time or two, and your understandable reaction has upset him. He bites, you jump or let out a startled cry. Baby is frightened, cries, and won't resume nursing for fear of another jolt or yell.

Sometimes the unexpected can cause a baby to refuse to nurse. Mary Shumeyko of New Jersey writes:

> The other day our twenty-month-old, Jonathan, bumped his chin. His mouth seemed to be bleeding a bit, so we wiped it off, I nursed him, and he continued playing. I went back to what I was doing. Several hours later, after happily nursing to sleep, Jonathan awoke crying in obvious pain. I offered him my breast. He tried to nurse, then drew away, crying harder. This continued all night, with Jonathan waking every half hour or so, and my husband or I walking the floor with him since he wouldn't nurse.
>
> The next morning he seemed to feel better and tentatively asked to nurse. When he opened his mouth I discovered the problem: he had cut his tongue when he bumped his chin, and (after the initial numbness wore off) nursing obviously had been quite painful. My heart went out to him. Not only had he injured himself, but his standard "cure-all" hurt even more. Fortunately the mouth heals quickly, and he's once again nursing regularly. The episode was a good reinforcement for me, though. After one night of not nursing, I'm more aware than ever of how precious this beautiful relationship is.

Even if you are not sure why the baby has gone on a nursing strike, you will want to help him get back to regular nursing as soon and easily as possible. Try nursing him when he is very sleepy, or already asleep. Many babies who refuse to nurse while awake will nurse when they are drowsy or asleep. Some babies are more likely to nurse if mother is walking about rather than sitting still. In any case, plan to devote yourself almost entirely to the baby for a few days. Lots of cuddling, stroking, and skin-to-skin contact may help. Relaxing together in a warm bath may help. Maybe some time spent just with you away from the hubbub of the rest of the family will calm the baby and encourage him to start nursing again. Rethink your priorities. You will both be better off and happier when things get back to normal again.

A mother from Guam, Becky Hallowell, found that calling her La Leche League Leader helped get to the bottom of her problem:

> We were on our third day of six-month-old Todd's refusing to nurse when I decided that something had to change. We were at our wits' end, and I was in pain from engorgement. My husband had been very supportive but was finding the situation increasingly difficult as I became more and more upset. He begged me to call Linda, our La Leche League Leader. "She'll be able to help you," he said.
>
> Linda and I talked it over, and she suggested the possibility of a nursing strike. I had been too close to the situation to recognize the problem, but soon realized we had all the usual causes and then some.
>
> 1. We all had bad colds.
>
> 2. Solids had been introduced on a trial basis and seemed to upset him.
>
> 3. We were all very tired and in a new situation with extra stress. Todd's grandparents, whom we hadn't seen in a year, were visiting us for a month. During their visit, Grandpa ended up in the hospital. There had also been two recent deaths in our family.
>
> 4. Todd had been biting me due to teething, and I had reacted strongly.
>
> Our solutions were to relax and try to nurse him as often as possible, especially when he was sleeping. We also kept in close physical touch by my carrying him around the house in his usual nursing position.
>
> After we began to try these solutions, the strike continued one more day (a total of four) and then nursing became easier. But it did take time to get back to normal. We found during this transition time that the swimming pool was perfect for relaxed nursing. Todd is a swimmer and loves the water. It took another week, but thanks to La Leche League and Linda, we're a happy nursing family once again.

Carol Strait, an Iowa mother, sheds some light on another reason why some babies may refuse to nurse:

When my two-and-a-half-month-old baby girl began refusing the breast, a thousand thoughts ran through my mind—I must be eating the wrong foods, maybe she was teething, I was probably too nervous (what nursing mother wouldn't be nervous when her new baby suddenly refused to nurse?), perhaps she was weaning herself—and even the fearful thought that she didn't like me! Quite by accident I discovered the answer to our problem. My first clue was that Christie always seemed fussier and wouldn't nurse just after I had showered and applied spray deodorant. I'm not sure what ingredients in the spray were responsible, but my problem was easily solved by simply switching from a spray to a solid stick deodorant. Now my little girl and I are a happy nursing couple again.

Holiday weaning

Another disruption in the normal course of breastfeeding that sometimes catches mothers by surprise is the "holiday weaning syndrome." It occurs when holidays or other especially hectic times, such as moving, result in our getting so busy that we overlook our baby's needs. It's easy to put off that nice quiet moment of nursing when there are so many other demands on our time. In the midst of cooking, entertaining, shopping, and such, the leisurely closeness of the nursing relationship is temporarily or even permanently lost. Solids or bottles may be tried to tide baby over, or perhaps he's "good" and consents to wait—and wait—for nursing time to come around. And then suddenly, no one knows quite how, baby is weaned. Toni Pepe from Connecticut describes holiday weaning:

A unique season in the private life of the baby has been cut short, and later, in the long days at home, come the regrets. Guard against holiday weaning. In the seasons of the world, these days of celebration return again and again—but the special season of nursing comes only once in the life of a child.

PART THREE

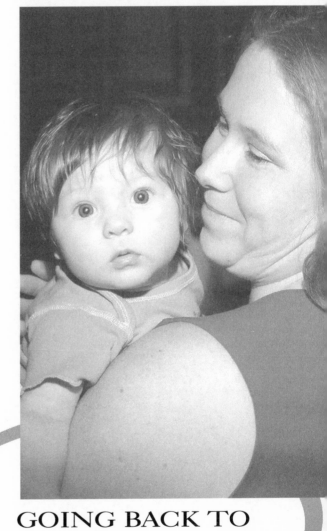

GOING BACK TO
work

CHAPTER EIGHT

BREASTFEEDING AND
working

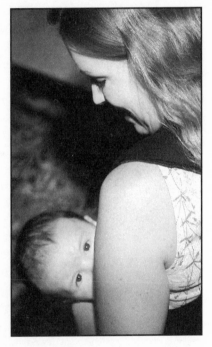

If you plan to return to your job soon after your baby is born, you may be wondering if you should even consider breastfeeding your baby. By all means, you can look forward to being a nursing mother. Breastfeeding is the best choice for you and your baby. Usually, a quiet time with baby at the breast is the last thing on the agenda before mother goes off to work and the first thing she does when she returns home.

Once you are aware of the benefits of human milk, you will probably want to furnish your baby with all the milk he needs while you are gone. You may be thinking, "All right, but isn't breastfeeding difficult when a mother has to miss feedings?" It does take some extra effort, and it requires that you plan ahead, but isn't that true of most worthwhile things in life?

Benefits of Breastfeeding

In many ways breastfeeding simplifies life with a baby. When at home there are no bottles to prepare, disruption of sleep can be minimized, and the one-on-one attention every baby needs is practically guaranteed despite the other demands of the household. The protection from illness that human milk provides is an advantage that is especially important to a working mother.

149

The breastfeeding relationship may be particularly precious to the mother who is regularly separated from her baby. The emotional closeness can contribute to the special bond between mother and baby, helping to compensate for their time apart. As one working mother said, "I love being able to make the shift from the workaday world to the world of family with the closeness of breastfeeding." Another mother added, "I wish I could tell all working mothers how much easier, special, and joyful it is to breastfeed. I am surprised to find that some people feel sorry for me and others think it is so courageous to do the perfectly natural thing."

Charlotte Lee Carrihill from New York works full-time as a stock broker but she was able to breastfeed her son Colin and is now nursing her daughter Laura. She writes: "The bond that we have built through these nursing experiences will be with us always. Through breastfeeding, I have learned more about mothering. I have learned to put 'people before things.' Nursing isn't only a way to feed your baby, it's a way to comfort and love your baby, too."

Gale Pryor, co-author of the popular *Nursing Your Baby* and author of *Nursing Mother, Working Mother*, writes:

Looking back, I realize that continuing to breastfeed while working tied the two halves of my life together and helped me make sense of myself as a mother.

Survey findings

To find out more specific information about how employment affects breastfeeding, Kathleen Auerbach, PhD, a lactation consultant, La Leche League Leader, and former editor of the *Journal of Human Lactation,* surveyed 567 married and single employed nursing mothers.

When these women's responses were tabulated, certain patterns emerged. Of the factors Dr. Auerbach analyzed, how soon after the baby's birth a mother returned to work seemed to have the most influence on the course of breastfeeding. This affected breastfeeding even more than the number of hours a week the mother worked. Mothers who rejoined the workforce when their babies were at least sixteen weeks old typically nursed longer than those who returned to work sooner. This may be because their milk supplies were solidly established and they had had more experience breastfeeding.

Whether the mothers worked full-time or part-time also affected how long breastfeeding continued. A greater percentage of the mothers working part-time nursed their babies for at least a year. The longer a mother waited to return to work and the fewer hours per day she worked, the longer she was likely to nurse.

Another variable that influenced the course of breastfeeding was whether or not the mothers expressed their milk when they missed a feeding. Eighty-six percent of the mothers surveyed expressed milk by hand or pump while they were away from their babies and forty-nine percent fed their babies only human milk until they were ready for solids at about six months. Mothers who chose to express their milk were more likely to nurse longer than those who did not.

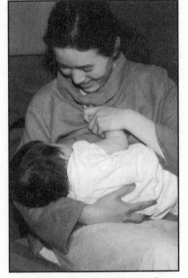

Expressing milk offered five main advantages:

The breastfeeding relationship may be especially important to a working mother.

It helped maintain the mothers' milk supplies;

It provided human milk for their babies, avoiding the risk of sensitizing them to allergies through formula;

It prevented or relieved uncomfortable fullness;

It minimized leaking; and

It helped prevent plugged ducts or breast infections, which may develop if the breasts remain overly full.

Pumping or expressing seemed to accomplish its purpose best when it was done every three hours or so. For the mother who was away from her baby for six hours, two pumping sessions were usually sufficient. If mother and baby were apart for eight to ten hours, three pumping sessions seemed to be needed.

When mothers experienced breastfeeding problems such as leaking, engorgement, and breast infections they were often able to solve them by expressing milk at work if they were not already doing so, or expressing their milk more often. Some mothers solved their problems by revising their priorities—making more time to be with their families and learning to leave work at the workplace.

When asked if they would combine breastfeeding and working with future babies, the responses were overwhelmingly in favor of breastfeeding. Eighty-two percent of the mothers said they would again choose to combine breastfeeding and working; eighteen percent said that with future children there was no doubt they would breast-feed, but they would make other choices regarding work, such as giving it up entirely, delaying their return until their children were older, or reducing their work hours.

Proceed Slowly

The length of time a mother is able to spend at home with her baby before returning to work is an important factor in assuring success at breastfeeding. Also, a mother and baby have a great need to be together in the early months. Once you hold your baby in your arms you'll probably decide you want to delay returning to your job for as long as you can so you and your baby can enjoy this precious time together.

Bargain for as long a maternity leave as you can possibly manage. If at all possible, arrange to be home at least six to eight weeks after your baby is born. One study found that women who returned to work before their babies were two months old had more breastfeeding prob-lems and weaned earlier than women who returned to work later. Three months at home with your baby is better yet. If you can stretch the time to six months, you will probably have seen him to the time when he begins to take other foods. The longer you can stay home with your baby, the longer both of you will enjoy the benefits of being together.

Stretching your maternity leave may mean using vacation time or accumulated sick or personal leave. Sometimes this leave will be paid, other times it will be an unpaid leave with an understanding that your job will only be held for a certain number of weeks or months. Some companies are willing to add an unpaid leave of six months or so onto a standard maternity leave. Policies are changing as more and more peo-ple, both men and women, request provisions for extended leaves for a variety of reasons. It is worth your while to look into the company's past treatment of employees who have received personal time off for whatever reasons.

Mothers and babies need time to be together in the early days and weeks. This is a special season in the life of a child, a time when mother and baby establish a relationship meant to last a lifetime. Whatever your plans for the future months, take time now to nurture this new being.

In *The Baby Book*, Dr. William Sears discusses the importance of making the most of your maternity leave:

Don't dwell upon the day you will return to work, lest the preoccupation rob you of those precious weeks of connecting with your baby. During the weeks or months at home with baby, let your baby develop your nurturing skills. Enjoy the time spent with your baby as you let mutual giving bring out the best in both of you.

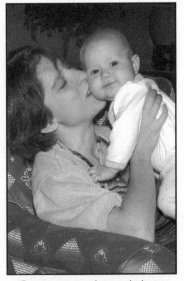

Connecting with your baby is important in the early weeks.

Delay introducing the bottle

Many mothers who are planning to return to work may be tempted to begin using bottles early "to get the baby used to them." But there are several reasons why this can bring a quick end to breastfeeding. If the bottles contain formula, this can interfere with a new mother's milk supply. The amount of milk a mother produces is determined by how often her baby nurses and how much her baby takes from the breast. Giving formula during the adjustment period sometimes short-circuits this "demand-and-supply" process, reducing the amount of milk produced.

Even if the mother pumps her own milk, giving bottles too soon can cause nipple confusion. Nursing at the breast requires more active participation from a baby than taking liquid from a bottle. If both breast and bottle are given during the impressionable early weeks, a baby may try to suck the breast as he sucks the artificial nipple. Babies may learn to suck less efficiently at the breast and may not gain well or may refuse to nurse altogether. A pacifier sometimes produces this same effect. Once a baby is three to four weeks old and has had lots of practice nursing, he is more likely to be able to switch back and forth between the different feeding methods.

Remember, too, that if baby does refuse to take a bottle when you are separated, feedings can be given by cup or spoon until baby gets used to the change.

Try working "mother hours"

When the time comes that you can no longer postpone making a decision about returning to work, try to begin with a part-time schedule. Returning to work for three days a week will be easier on you and your baby than five days a week. Being separated for just six hours a day can make it easier to continue breastfeeding than being gone for eight or nine hours a day. Keep an open mind about such options. If you have specialized skills or years of training, your employer may be willing to make adjustments rather than losing you entirely.

Some Practical Hints

If you plan to combine breastfeeding and working, you'll want to learn how to pump or express your milk. The milk you collect while separated from your baby can be given to him the next day. Expressing your milk will continue to stimulate your milk supply and avoid overly full breasts. Some women are reluctant to ask their employers for time to pump during their work hours. Studies have shown that breastfeeding provides benefits to employers because working mothers who breastfeed have healthier babies and take less time off. Because of this, it is becoming more common for large US corporations to offer corporate lactation programs. In Minnesota, legislation was passed in 1998 protecting a mother's right to pump her milk during her workday.

Saving your milk for your baby

No other milk or formula is as good for your baby as your own milk. Many mothers are able to provide enough milk to satisfy all their baby's needs while they are away. This involves knowing how to pump your milk as well as how to store it. You'll want to be sure your sitter is aware of how to handle the milk you leave for your baby.

New research has shown that human milk can safely be kept at room temperature (66 to 72 degrees F [19 to 22 degrees C]) for up to ten hours because of its remarkable ability to retard the growth of bacteria. Milk can be kept refrigerated for eight days. For longer storage, it can be frozen. Frozen milk can be kept up to two weeks in the freezer compartment of your refrigerator, three to four months in a separate door freezer that is opened frequently. It can be kept six months or longer in a separate freezer that stays at a constant 0 degrees F (-19 degrees C). Once the milk is thawed, it cannot be refrozen; if the freezer defrosts for any reason, the milk must be used or discarded.

After pumping or expressing your milk into a clean container, transfer it into a glass or plastic storage container, baby bottle, or plastic milk storage bag. Use a separate container to refrigerate the milk each time you pump or express. These cooled batches can later be combined for a feeding or for freezing. You can add refrigerated milk to milk that is already frozen, just be sure the amount you are adding is smaller than the amount already frozen so it does not thaw the frozen milk. Allow room for expansion when filling containers for freezing. Do not tighten caps until milk is completely frozen.

Freeze the milk in small amounts varying from two to four ounces (60 to 120 ml). There will be less waste this way as the sitter can choose the amount according to a baby's hunger or usual feeding pattern. Always label each container with the month, date, and year. If your milk will be used in a situation where more than one baby is being fed, you'll want to add baby's name on each container.

You can freeze your milk in either glass or plastic storage containers. Some mothers store their milk in plastic nurser bags designed for feeding babies. Freezing milk in these less-durable bags can be risky because the seams can split as the milk freezes. If you do use these, it is a good idea to use them doubled. Squeeze out the air at the top, roll down to one inch above the milk, fasten, and place the bag into a container which will hold it upright until it is frozen solid. These bottle liners are not recommended for long-term storage.

Collecting your milk

There are a number of inexpensive manual breast pumps available today, but many mothers find that hand-expressing their milk is easy and convenient. (See Chapter 7 for more information on pumping or hand-expressing your milk.)

Don't be discouraged if the amount of milk obtained is small at first. With practice many mothers are able to pump three or four ounces (90 to 120 ml) in fifteen or twenty minutes. Most pumps allow you to pump both breasts at once which saves pumping time. It is normal for the amount to vary from one pumping session to the next.

Follow the manufacturer's directions in caring for any type of pump. Usually it is necessary to clean the parts carefully after each use and sterilize the pump occasionally. Talk to other mothers about the types of pump they find effective. The type of pump that requires squeezing a rubber bulb to draw out the milk is not recommended because the mother has little control over the amount of suction and these are usually not very effective.

When and where to pump

Some mothers start pumping and storing their milk ahead of the time they will be returning to work in order to have a reserve supply available. Others pump only while they are away and have enough for the baby's feedings on the following day. Some mothers pump extra milk in the morning or evening to be sure baby has enough to eat when they

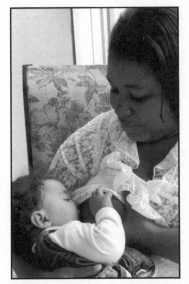
Baby will be eager to nurse as soon as mother arrives home from work.

are gone. Some mothers find it easy to pump an ounce or two (30 to 60 ml) after baby has nursed in the evening or early morning.

The number of times you'll need to pump or express your milk while you are away from home will depend on the total length of time you are away from the baby as well as baby's age. It's usually best not to go more than three or four hours without removing milk from your breasts. If you are leaving a very young baby who has been nursing more often, you may need to pump or express your milk more frequently at first so your breasts do not get uncomfortably full or start to leak.

If your breasts start to leak at an inopportune time, apply firm pressure directly on the nipple for a minute or two. This can be done discreetly by folding your arms across your breasts. You don't want to do this too often, though, as it is better to relieve the fullness by removing some milk. You can purchase nursing pads to wear inside your bra to absorb this leakage. Some working mothers keep an extra blouse, sweater, or jacket at work in case their milk leaks. After a while, your breasts will adjust to your new schedule and you will have fewer problems with leaking.

Finding a suitable location for pumping or expressing your milk will depend on each individual situation. If your company doesn't have a pumping room for mothers to use, you may be able to use a private office, an isolated storeroom, or the women's lounge. If you'll be using an electric pump you'll need access to an electrical outlet. You'll want someplace where you can relax and have some privacy. Some mothers find leaning over a sink helps avoid milk dripping on their clothes and makes use of gravity in removing the milk. Wearing two-piece outfits will make your pumping sessions easier.

As you prepare to pump or express your milk, think about your baby and visualize an outpouring of milk. It's a special gift only you can give your baby.

If you prefer to keep your milk cool and no refrigerator is available where you work, you can use an insulated thermos or small cooler. Put ice into the thermos in the morning to get it cold, then pour out the ice and add your milk. You can keep ice packs in the cooler and add the containers of your milk throughout the day. You can also use one of these methods to keep your milk cool on your way home.

Giving your milk to the baby

Your milk can be given to the baby by spoon, cup, eyedropper, or bottle. You don't need to introduce the bottle in baby's first few weeks just because you'll be returning to work later on. Some babies refuse to take a bottle from mother when they know the breast is right nearby, but they soon become accustomed to taking a bottle from the sitter. Explain to the sitter that your baby may need some persuasion in learning to accept a bottle. Since you'll want the baby and the sitter to get to know each other before you actually return to work, these get-acquainted visits can be a good time for the sitter to get the baby used to taking a bottle.

The sitter needs to know that you plan to leave your own milk for the baby and how to handle it. Also be sure to emphasize that you do not want the baby given formula or other foods without your permission and that your baby should be held while he is being fed. Stress that you don't want your baby left to cry.

Mothers sometimes wonder how much milk they need to pump for each feeding they will miss. Breastfed babies normally take between two and four ounces (60 to 120 ml) of milk eight to twelve times a day. No one can predict ahead of time how much milk an individual baby will take, but it is unlikely that a breastfed baby would consume an eight-ounce (240 ml) bottle of human milk at one feeding. Storing your milk in two to four ounce (60 to 120 ml) quantities allows the sitter to prepare just enough to satisfy your baby without wasting any milk.

Other supplements

Mothers usually instruct the sitter to give only human milk if it is available. Any other supplement, if needed, should be prescribed by the baby's doctor. If your baby is older than three or four months, and seems to need more milk than you can pump, consider asking your doctor if you could start some mashed banana as a supplement instead of introducing formula.

Feeding Tips for the Sitter

You'll want to share the following tips with the person who will be caring for your baby:

- Refrigerated human milk will separate as it is not homogenized. It may look spoiled or sour to someone who is not familiar with it. Shake gently to mix the fat particles into the watery portion. If milk has been refrigerated in small batches, you can mix these together for a feeding. To warm the cold milk, hold it under warm running water for several minutes until it reaches room temperature or immerse the container of milk into a pan of water that has been heated on the stove. Do not heat the milk itself directly on the stove or in a microwave oven as valuable components of the milk can be destroyed if it gets too hot.

- To thaw frozen milk, hold the container under cool running water and gradually add warmer water until milk is thawed and warmed to room temperature. If hot running water is not available, heat a pan of water on the stove and immerse the container of frozen milk into the warm water. If necessary, remove the container of milk and reheat the water. If more than one container is being thawed, you can combine the milk for a feeding.

- You can also thaw frozen milk in the refrigerator overnight. An unopened container of human milk that has been frozen and thawed can safely be kept refrigerated for up to twenty-four hours.

- It is not known whether or not leftover milk should be discarded after baby has taken some of it from the bottle. Recent studies have shown that human milk actually retards the growth of bacteria so it may be safe to refrigerate unused milk for later use. Thawed milk should not be refrozen.

- If baby seems hungry just before mother is due home, try to keep him satisfied with just a small amount of milk because mother will want to nurse the baby as soon as she arrives.

- Be sure all bottles, nipples, cups, or spoons used to feed the baby are kept clean. Washing your hands is important before feeding the baby and after changing his diaper.

Encouraging baby to take a bottle

Most babies take a bottle easily no matter when it is first introduced; others take a while to get used to a new way of feeding. Some ways that have worked to encourage a baby to take a bottle include:

- Try running warm water over the bottle nipple to bring it up to room temperature.

- Instead of pushing the bottle nipple into the baby's mouth, try tickling baby's lips with it and allow him to draw the nipple into his mouth.

- Try different types of nipples and different sizes of holes.

- Try feeding the bottle in different positions, such as: with baby sitting on the caregiver's lap, facing outward, or try feeding the baby while walking or swaying from side to side.

- Remember that baby can be fed in other ways. Try using a cup, spoon, or eyedropper if baby is reluctant to take a bottle.

Establish a Routine

Time will be a most precious commodity in your life. When a woman combines mothering and working, she must be a miser with her time. Don't overlook the trusty baby carrier or sling to help you catch up with household work and keep the baby close to you. It has proved a blessing to all of us at times. And don't be surprised if your baby becomes something of a "night owl," wide awake, bright-eyed, and busy in the center of family activities during the evening hours. Some working mothers tell us that they deliberately encourage an up-at-night, down-during-the-day sleeping pattern for the baby. If the baby sleeps for longer periods while mother is away, he will need fewer feedings during the day and be more eager to nurse in the evenings.

Try setting your alarm for at least twenty minutes before you have to get up. Nurse the baby during this time (even if he's still half asleep) so that he's more likely to be contented while you dress and prepare for the day. Then nurse again just before you leave. It'll calm you both and make separation a bit smoother.

If you and your baby are separated for a considerable length of time, give special attention to your homecoming. Plan on sitting (or lying) down and nursing or playing with the baby for the first thirty minutes after you arrive home. Everyone will be more relaxed and dinner preparation won't be so chaotic. Plan ahead and keep nutritious snacks on hand for both you and the family.

Drink plenty of fluids and eat a nutritious diet of simple wholesome foods. Get most of your daily liquid in water or juice. The biggest problem mothers face is fatigue. This is especially true for employed breastfeeding mothers. Adequate rest will make life smoother and alleviate many problems.

Starting a new job, or even taking up where you left off in the old one, is very tiring for a new mother. One suggestion is to start back to work on a Thursday instead of a Monday so you'll have the weekend to recuperate before facing a full workweek.

Many working nursing mothers are able to nurse their babies full time on their days off or on weekends with no problem making the adjustment. If you have been pumping regularly while at work, your milk production will be about the same. (You can refrigerate or freeze the milk you pump on Friday for the sitter to give the baby on Monday.) Even if baby needs a supplement during your absence, frequent nursing on the weekend will supply him with plenty of milk, probably much more than you can remove by pumping. In this case, you may experience some fullness on Monday because of the increased stimulation over the weekend. It will make your pumping efforts easier.

A mother from Indiana, Leslie Koczan, tells this story of her experience as a working breastfeeding mother:

I knew that I had no choice but to return to work shortly after Laura's birth, although I would have dearly loved to stay home with her. I returned to work when Laura was only seven weeks old. She was so tiny and precious, and it was so very difficult to leave.

Our nursing relationship sustained us and strengthened our bond, despite the daily separation. For mothers who must work, I would strongly encourage breastfeeding. For me the major advantage was this: It was the one thing that I could do for my baby that the sitter could not do. It was a special bond between my baby and myself.

By seven weeks of age, Laura's need to nurse followed a fairly regular three-hour pattern. So, depending upon when she had last nursed in the morning, the sitter gave Laura a bottle of my milk about three hours later. I took my lunch hour to coincide with her next feeding and nursed her while eating my sack lunch. The sitter gave her another bottle three hours later, and I nursed her immediately after work. For each missed feeding, I pumped my breasts, collected the milk in disposable bags, marked them with the amount and date, and stored them in a refrigerator at work. Each evening, I took the day's milk to the sitter's to be stored in her refrigerator or deep freeze until needed.

There were several important factors contributing to our success.

- I found a sitter close to my workplace, so I could be with Laura each noon. This also gave us an extra hour together driving to and from work. My sitter, coincidentally, had been very active in LLL and therefore was very supportive of my nursing.

- Laura was given a bottle only by the sitter. No bottles were ever given at home.

- My job was sufficiently flexible to allow me time to pump twice a day and to take my lunch hour beginning anywhere from 11:00 AM to 2:00 PM. Knowing that the need to pump would end as Laura got older made it more acceptable to my supervisor. It also helped keep up my morale when I became tired of pumping. After about three months, I was pumping only once a day and in another month, not at all.

- I became active in my local LLL Group and its members were very supportive and encouraging.

Last, but definitely not least, I had lots of help from my older daughter and husband, who fixed sack lunches every morning, started dinner in the evening, changed diapers, and entertained the baby.

Nighttime nursing

Be prepared for more evening, nighttime, and early morning nursings. Bringing the baby to bed with you is a definite plus.

Lori Brewster, a mother of two from Michigan, found nighttime nursings very special. She and her husband worked opposite shifts in the automotive industry so one of them was home while the other was at work:

The first time I was pregnant, I was sure that I wanted to nurse. I breastfed Matthew for eight weeks but weaned him when I had to return to work. I found out later that weaning was not necessary.

When I was pregnant for the second time, I knew that I wanted to breastfeed once again. This time instead of just turning to books, I contacted my local La Leche League Leader. That turned out to be the best phone call of my family's life.

Since the birth of Amy Rose five months ago, she and I have nursed happily. I returned to work after eight short weeks of leave, but brought my breast pump and cooler with me. While I am at work, I pump my breasts three times a day. On Friday I freeze bottles for Monday. While at home, I nurse on demand and love it.

The nights are very special for Amy and me. People think I am crazy when I tell them she nurses four or five times during the night. They wonder how in the world I can survive. They do not understand that she sleeps right next to me. Nighttime is my favorite time of the day.

After breastfeeding Matt and then going to bottles, I knew that I did not want to do that again. Bottles are such a hassle. Now when I get home, I just have to clean my pump and wash a few bottles and I have the rest of the evening for my family. If you have never breastfed, you can't appreciate the convenience. Take it from one who has done both, "Breast is best."

I would encourage any mother to read all she can but also contact La Leche League for the support needed. If you are working full-time, don't let that stop you from nursing your baby.

Who Will Take Care of the Baby?

The most important task you will face before you go back to work is finding the best person possible to care for your baby while you are gone. Can you arrange for a family member to take over this responsibility? The baby's father is an obvious first choice, if he is available. The element of change for the baby will be minimized. A loving grandmother or an aunt who is already familiar to the baby are also high on the list of choices. A motherly neighbor may be interested in caring for your little one during the day.

Most people, though, are not fortunate enough to have a family member or friendly neighbor available as a caregiver and must look fur-

ther. They must then concern themselves with references and inter-
views. If the caregiver is new to the baby, by all means have her come
to your home or visit hers a few times with the baby so the two of
them can get acquainted before you begin working. Be sure to tell her
that you are breastfeeding and explain in detail how you want the baby
fed, what his likes and dislikes are, what his sleeping pattern is, and,
most important, the fact that you do not want your baby to be left to
cry. Let her observe your interaction with the baby so she can see how
he is accustomed to being handled. And you can watch how the caregiver and the baby relate to one another to be sure she is the right person to care for your baby.

Think about finding a caregiver who lives close to your place of
work rather than close to where you live. This would make it possible
for you to visit the baby at lunch time or perhaps have the caregiver
bring the baby to you.

When choosing a caregiver, look for someone who will give your
baby as nearly as possible the same single-minded devotion and care
that you give him yourself—someone who knows babies—who understands their needs. Will she sing to him? Talk to him? Rock him gently
to sleep? Keep him dry and comfortable and always close by?

Constancy in nurturing is the means by which a child learns to
trust others. A baby needs a loving, nurturing person, and this person
should be the same someone, not an often changing parade of new
faces and personalities. While a working mother naturally hopes to find
such a reliable, loving substitute, she should also be aware that over a
period of time, her baby will inevitably grow to love this "other
mother."

You must also face the possibility that the patient, kind caregiver
you have this morning may announce at nightfall that she is moving
away or taking another job. Such a disruption can be a serious loss for a
young child.

Because of the unpredictability of finding and keeping a private
caregiver, working mothers may consider a day-care center as a solution. While there is a degree of permanence in using a day-care center,
day-care workers may come and go. And while the decorations may be
charming, children under the age of three may not adjust well to a
group situation. A young child was not meant to compete for attention
with a large number of children of similar ages. Often a child will enjoy
short play sessions in a preschool setting, but all-day care may become
a threatening situation. Group care in a day-care center falls far short
of meeting a baby's or toddler's needs to relate to one person, to count
on one person for loving attention at any time. The chances of illness

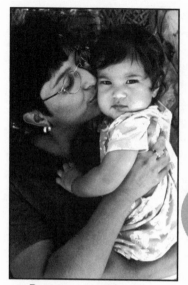

Being separated from her baby is often difficult for a working mother.

and infection are also considerably greater when children are in a group setting. If your child is in a day-care setting, providing your milk will help to protect him from such illnesses.

In the *New York Times Magazine*, Sally E. Shaywitz, MD, had this to say about mother substitutes:

We do not know enough about nurturing to be able to tell mothers that if they find a person or an institution that meets such-and-such standards that this will be an adequate mother substitute. We can list people's credentials, pinpoint the standards for a day care center, but just as human milk cannot be duplicated, neither can a mother. We cannot put mothering into a formula and come up with a person who has the special feeling for your child that you do.... Just as everyone but a mother is excluded from nursing a baby, so they are also excluded from those immense feelings of satisfaction and inner unity with the child.

Coping with the separation

For many mothers, separation from the baby turns out to be the hardest part of returning to work. Lisa Bicknell Casey of Oklahoma tells what happened to her:

I was allowed only two short months off after Jason was born. I spent most of those two months recovering from his cesarean birth. It seemed I was no sooner on my feet being the kind of mother I wanted to be, when it came time to return to work.

After contacting my LLL Leader, I purchased a breast pump, and the week before I went back to work, I dutifully pumped my breasts. It seemed so slow and awkward. I doubted I could ever pump enough to feed my beautiful boy. Thank goodness it got easier.

That first week of work I cried every day after leaving Jason at the sitter's, but I was blessed with an excellent sitter whom Jason took to immediately. This only upset me more. After all, every day I was replaced by a bottle and a sitter. Would my baby need me?

Things proceeded well in spite of my fears. Then one day the sitter had to give Jason almost eighteen ounces of my milk. I was ready to give up. How could I possibly keep up with his demand? Fortunately, this only happened once. Before long Jason had adjusted his nursing so he was taking only eight to ten ounces during the day and nursing frequently at night. I did not hesitate to take Jason in bed with us from the start, so I slept through many feedings and was never really sure just how frequently he nursed at night.

Jason refuses his bottle if he knows I am around, which reinforces my confidence as a mother. I know now that my baby does need me. Jason and I are able to share this kind of physical closeness that working might have denied us. For a mother who reluctantly returned to work, breastfeeding has been a godsend.

A mother who plans to combine breastfeeding and working would do well to find the time to attend La Leche League meetings. Breastfeeding mothers who are separated from their babies regularly need the important support that comes from being with other nursing mothers. Your baby is welcome at LLL meetings.

Is it all worth it? Would it be easier to give up breastfeeding if you plan to return to your job? One working mother who had bottle-fed a previous baby and is now breastfeeding puts it this way. "Breastfeeding simplifies many things for me, plus it helps to ensure that when I am home, I am spending time with my children." Another mother says: "My child benefited both physically and emotionally from the time we spent as a nursing couple!" And many others add: "I didn't want my baby to miss out on the benefits of breastfeeding just because I had to return to work."

CHAPTER NINE

MAKING A
choice

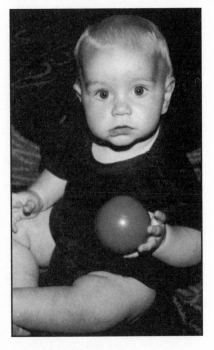

C hoosing whether or not to work outside your home after your baby is born is a complex decision. You'll want to take your time and evaluate your options before you reach a conclusion. Author Kaye Lowman talks about making this choice in her popular book, OF CRADLES AND CAREERS:

A woman today is able to choose to be single or married, to pursue a career or to stay at home, to raise a family or to remain childless, to combine motherhood with a career or to make raising her children a full-time commitment. But make no mistake: the availability of so many options is a mixed blessing.... Implicit in the freedom to choose is the obligation to choose wisely.

The Mother-Child Relationship

There are many important factors to be considered when you make the decision about returning to work after your baby is born. Let's take a look first at the mother-child relationship. This subject has fascinated the scientific community for a long time. A child's early years

167

hold the clues to his future behavior as an adult. Society stands to gain or lose, depending on the soundness of mother-baby attachment.

La Leche League is strongly committed to the belief that babies and mothers need to be together in the early years. We are convinced that a baby's need for his mother's loving presence is as basic as his need for food. Mary Ann Cahill, one of La Leche League's co-Founders, writes:

> No one can replace you as mother. From all evidence, from all that is known about how babies grow and learn to live and to be competent adults, it can be said that a mother is the one most perfectly suited to be nurturer in the early years.

Scientists hold that a child's initial one-to-one relationship with his mother is the foundation for emotional growth. From the security of the baby's ties to his mother he learns to relate to others. "The only true basis for the relationship of a child to mother and father, to other children, and eventually to society," Dr. W. Winnicott, a pediatrician from Great Britain, says, "is the first successful relationship between mother and baby."

Separation brings anxiety

In her book *Oneness and Separateness*, Dr. Louise Kaplan, psychologist and Director of the Mother-Infant Research Nursery of New York University, explains that an infant does not have an identity of his own at birth. Based on her work in mother-infant research, Dr. Kaplan states, "From the infant's point of view, there are no boundaries between himself and mother. They are one. The child must negotiate the move from oneness with his mother into separateness and a sense of individuality. It is a second birth that unfolds gradually in the first three years of life. Maintaining the early mother-baby relationship is extremely important to the successful completion of this journey."

And Selma Fraiberg, a professor of child psychoanalysis who wrote *Every Child's Birthright: In Defense of Mothering*, states her views very emphatically:

> It has been determined that children who do not have the benefit of a single, sustained contact with a loving mother or mother-figure for at least the first three years of their lives, will—depending upon the degree of deprivation—manifest a diminished capacity to love others, impaired intellectual powers, and an inability to control their impulses, particularly in the area of aggression.

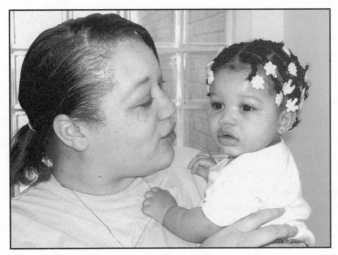

Motherhood is a special season in a woman's life.

A Canadian, Donna K. Kontos, PhD, consultant psychologist, comments, "There is at present no known substitute for a family environment for childrearing.... Prolonged maternal separations cause distress to the child. All the research and all of the literature tell us that the best thing for an infant is to have a consistent good mother around most of the time."

Another psychologist, Dr. Joyce Brothers, recognizes the pressures on mothers to work, yet notes, "I realize that the economic necessities of life often force us to do things differently than we would like. But when it comes to child raising, I am convinced that a woman should make every possible effort to spend the first three years with her child. It does make a tremendous difference."

In their book, *The Irreducible Needs of Children: What Every Child Must Have to Grow, Learn, and Flourish,* T. Berry Brazelton, MD, and Stanley I. Greenspan, MD, state this emphatically:

In the first three years, every child needs one or two primary caregivers who remain in a steady, intimate relationship with that child.... The lion's share of a baby's time needs to be with caregivers who are going to be an ongoing part of the child's life and have the child's trust. The depth of one's intimacy and feelings for others depends in part on the depth of feeling one experiences in ongoing relationships.... Becoming dependent on primary caregivers who disappear does not breed in a baby an inner sense of security and consistency.

The young child who is separated from his mother exhibits all of the classic symptoms of grief. He may cry unconsolably or withdraw into unnatural quietness. Regarding this separation anxiety, Humberto Nagera, Professor of Psychiatry at the University of Montana, points out:

> When the child is confronted with the mother's absence his automatic response is an anxiety state that on many occasions reaches overwhelming proportions. Repeated traumas of this type in especially susceptible children will not fail to have serious consequences for their later development.... No other animal species will subject their infants to experiences that they are not endowed to cope with, except the human animal.

Staying at home—for now

How does a mother reconcile her own need for a healthy sense of self-esteem, achievement, and self-confidence with the needs of her baby? Many young women today are opting to put their careers "on hold" when the baby arrives. They see motherhood as a special season in their lives, one that they do not want to miss. The working world will still be there two or three, five or ten years from now. Stay-at-home mothers of young children often see themselves resuming their working careers once their children are older. They view the time at home as a short-period, "a sliver of time" when gauged against the many years that they can, and probably will, work outside the home.

Mary Ann Kerwin, one of LLL's co-Founders, is a good example of this. After spending more than twenty years as a mother at home, deeply involved in caring for her large family, she found there was still "plenty of time for another career." Mary Ann began attending law school when her youngest child started high school. She adds:

> Our children teach us much more than we realize. Being a mother taught me patience, perseverance, self-discipline, and hard work. After coping for twenty-four hours a day with children, no task seemed too hard.

Judy Kahrl of Ohio appreciates the fact that it takes courage for a woman to stand in the face of society's pressure and say, "At this time in my life, and with this new person as my responsibility, I am going to use my resources of time and physical and emotional energy in the most effective way possible for the nurturing of that new life."

Does it pay to work?

Perhaps you would like to stay home with your baby, but you can't see how your family can manage without your paycheck. Home is where your heart is, but a job is where the money is—or is it?

Many women discover that it is not realistic to think of one's take-home pay as "pure profit." Often the costs involved in working are overlooked. Some quick calculations of expenses versus income yield surprising results. There is the cost of a working wardrobe and transportation expenses getting to and from work each day. When you spend the day on the job, you probably prepare more convenience foods or eat out more often. And then there's the cost of child care. Sit down and estimate how much money these things add up to and subtract this amount from your income. You may very well find that there will be little net gain if you continue to work after the baby arrives.

When tallying up the funds that will be available to you if you stay home, consider the likelihood that you may drop into a lower tax bracket (in the United States) after you stop working. The tax savings alone may be substantial. Many mothers find that it doesn't "pay" for them to work outside the home.

Jonathan Pound of Financial Planning Information, Inc., from Boston, writes:

It may not pay for both parents to work.... First of all, in the USA the government takes about 40% of the second income right off the top. For example, if you are earning $25,000, $10,000 is eaten up in taxes. Child care, at $150 a week (and that's a low estimate) costs $7500; commuting, clothes, meals, and so on, cost another $2500. Therefore, $20,000 of your gross pay of $25,000 is gone before any of that second income reaches home. Only $5000 (20% of the gross) is left to spend. If more women knew that, I'll bet they'd think twice before going off to that job.

Earning extra money

What if your family's financial situation is such that you feel you absolutely have to bring in some extra income? Happily more and more mothers have been able to combine working and keeping their babies with them.

Many kinds of work can be done just as well at home, so you might be able to interest your employer in having you do part-time work at home, coming into the office just for planning or meetings. With computers, modems, faxes, and email, this kind of flexibility in the working world is becoming more available to families.

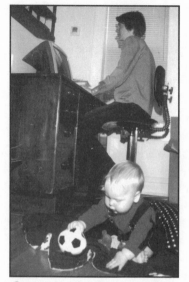

Some job skills allow a mother to work from home keeping her baby nearby.

If you have a computer, get in touch with several different companies or placement services about freelance computer work from home, or run an ad in the newspaper. If you have a specialty like art, writing, photography, or public relations, you can develop a freelance clientele and work out of your home. Giving music lessons is another good option. Or, if you are a teacher, contact local schools about tutoring in your home. Taking care of other mothers' children is another way to bring in extra income.

Another possibility is to take baby along with you to your job. Given the right circumstances, an increasing number of women find that mothering the baby is compatible with their jobs. They may not spend as much time in the office as they would if they left the baby behind, and their paycheck may be adjusted accordingly, but the bottom line compares favorably to full-time work and paying for child care.

Kymberlie Stefanski, from Illinois, tells how she has been able to work flexible hours and meet her daughters' needs:

I do computer programming and when my daughter, Moriah, was seven months old I started working two days a week and she came with me to the office. I had a private office and I brought toys and books for Moriah to play with while I worked at the computer. When she needed a break from being in one room, we took the opportunity to walk around the building and connect with others I needed to be in touch with. She usually nursed herself to sleep and took a long afternoon nap, which helped me get my work done.

When I was pregnant with my second baby, I proposed working from home after my maternity leave. Because I had already proven my abilities and productivity, this was considered an option. With a toddler and a baby to care for, I wasn't sure that I could dedicate two full days a week, so I suggested working for three hours every afternoon from home. This way Moriah can take her nap and I can focus on my work and the baby.

So far, this arrangement works well for us. Moriah doesn't always nap the whole time, but with a videotape of a children's show or some of her toys, she usually does okay with minimal supervision while I work. She stays in the same room as me so I can keep an eye on her. I am trying to adjust the baby's sleeping times to encourage her to also nap while I work.

I have to go into the office sometimes for meetings and I take both children with me. I reserve some toys for the office so Moriah doesn't get tired of them as quickly. I also take snacks for her that she may not normally get at home (to make it a treat). Explaining ahead of time what we are going to do helps her know that I expect her to play quietly and stay near me.

And Debi Drecksler from Florida adds, "I've been able to take my children along with me whenever I needed to work outside the home. My most recent job was a Youth Director. I ran a day camp, and, during the school year, an after-school enrichment program."

Jo Montgomery, from Washington, tells how she found a way to stay at home after her baby was born:

Elizabeth was born on leap year day. I had planned on returning to work full time when she was three months old. By the time she was six weeks old, we had developed a solid nursing relationship. When I investigated day-care options, I became depressed. I felt cheated at the thought of leaving my precious baby.

I talked to my husband about my feelings. He was very supportive, and we both decided that I wouldn't return to work in June. I told my employer that I thought I might possibly return in September, but I couldn't make any promises.

I had been working in the graphics field for six years, so I entertained the idea of putting my skills to work for myself at home. On July 1st I started my own business retailing wedding and baby announcements. Through referrals, my business has blossomed to include some commercial accounts, too.

Taking your business home won't work for everyone, but it's worth thinking about. I am so glad I have gotten to know my daughter, Elizabeth, "full time."

In the practical context of mothering a young child day after day, of changing and feeding him, returning his smiles, applauding his efforts to reach a toy, distracting him at times, or consoling him when tears appear, the mothers we have talked to make no distinction between the quantity and quality of time they spend with their babies. Mary Ann Kerwin, a co-Founder of La Leche League, has observed, "Babies need quantities of quality time."

Take One Step at a Time

If you are awaiting the arrival of your baby, you are probably thinking about what you should tell your employer regarding your future plans. From experience, many mothers insist: "Do not make any commitments before your baby is born." If at all possible, keep your options open.

You do not want the specter hanging over your head of having to return to a job by a certain date because of an agreement you made while still pregnant. Most businesses offer a maternity leave, and will hold your job for you for a specified period of time after the baby is born. By all means take advantage of whatever leave is available to you, and give yourself that time to assess how you will feel about leaving your baby. For someone to expect you to promise away your future and that of your baby before you even have a chance to meet is tantamount to signing a blank check—no, it is worse.

Shirley Callanan, a mother from Utah, planned to work on a part-time basis. But after her baby was born, she wrote, "I really didn't know what to expect of motherhood or how I would feel, and it's hard to describe the feelings that flowed through me those first few days, weeks, and months of my daughter's life. I was needed by this tiny person; I knew I could not leave her with someone else, no matter how loving."

Exploring options

In OF CRADLES AND CAREERS, Kaye Lowman explores many aspects that are available to women who refuse to make an "all-or-nothing choice" between their careers and their families. Her book includes stories of women who have "reshaped the workplace in order to make it more responsive to their need to work and their desire to have a family." She goes on to explain:

> Whether a woman's need to work is financial, social, or emotional, the desire to be a parent may be equally strong.... The career woman today understands her baby's need for her and

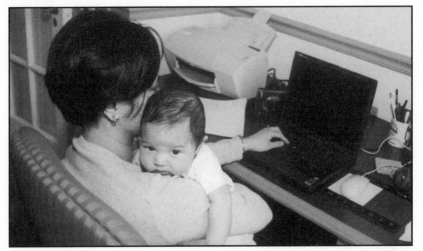

Some mothers are able to adjust their work hours so they can be home more.

the importance of being a meaningful part of her baby's life. And she realizes how much she herself will lose if she misses out on the opportunity to mother her own children.... Careers can be put on hold; babies grow up and are gone. It was a wise and thoughtful Mother Nature who brought babies into the world needing to be breastfed and cared for, reminding us that mother and baby are very much a unit for many months after birth and that they need to be together. To try to ignore or circumvent this physical and psychological need is to tamper with one of the most fundamental and basic elements of human nature.

Some women make one decision before their babies are born and find their attitudes change once they become mothers. Such was the case with Joy Cohen of New York:

I have worked with children for eleven years: as an early childhood teacher, as a teacher and therapist in a therapeutic nursery, and as a psychotherapist caring for seriously disturbed children and their families.

When I was pregnant, I believed that I would be ready to resume my part-time psychotherapy practice after three or four months. I couldn't have known then the power and intensity of my baby's and my need for each other. I wanted to give myself totally to this new and wonderful adventure called mothering. Slowly but surely I did just that.

Those first few months passed quickly, and I began to feel pressure to resume my practice. The children and families with whom I had been working were anxious to continue. My friends and family encouraged me not to give up my career.

My own cultural stereotype of the woman who can easily manage family and career during her children's early years was being challenged. The only stimulation I felt I needed was the stimulation of my baby nursing at my breast. I wanted to savor every minute of my new life and this delicately unfolding new relationship. I felt a crisis of the heart upon me.

Fortunately, I did not have to work for economic reasons, and my husband said that he had confidence in me and that he would be supportive of any decision that I made.

I had previously arranged to have my mother care for Michael during my sessions. When I told her that I didn't want to go back to work and felt the baby strongly needed me, she told me that I was making a big mistake. I was pained that my mother couldn't be as supportive as I would have liked, but if I have learned anything from helping people know their feelings, it was to acknowledge and trust my own.

After much soul-searching, I decided to stop working with my clients. The separations were difficult and sad for everyone. I tried hard to stay connected to my own heart and knew that what was best for me would ultimately be best for all concerned. When I knew I would no longer have to be away from Michael, I breathed a long, deep sigh of relief. The internal and external work had been difficult, but as I nestled in to nurse my baby with the knowledge that I would not have to be away from him until we were both ready, I knew that it had been necessary work from which I had grown deeply as a mother and as a person. I knew that I had made absolutely the right decision.

For some mothers, even working part-time interferes with their ability to mother their child. Elizabeth Golestaani, from Iran, is one such mother:

Until recently, I had always thought part-time work—say two hours three times a week—was the ideal for the mother of a small child. Add to this the great demand for my English-teaching skills here in Iran, and I was under a lot of pressure to return to work. So I did—and what a mistake. It took me a long time to accept the fact that I'm not Superwoman and that in my case working even part-time is too much. I kept thinking that soon I would get more organized or my toddler, Sa'id, would need me less, and then all would be well.

The idea of "giving up my career" was so scary! I kept wrestling with my thoughts and emotions. Then I received the January-February issue of NEW BEGINNINGS. In it, I read an article by a mother who had been in exactly the same situation. She wrote about how important it is for one to acknowledge and trust one's feelings, and that helped me enormously.

I was finally able to decide to do what I believed was right for me, which was to stop accepting teaching commitments while I have a small child. I still had to finish out the university semester, but just having made the decision changed my attitude so much.

After just two days, I realized my feelings and behavior toward Sa'id had changed. I was less irritable, more loving, and the angry scoldings were replaced by hugs and listening and eye contact. Life seemed so good again.

I hadn't realized my teaching had such a bad effect on my mothering until my decision to stop. It was hard telling everybody "no more," but I kept reminding myself "Sa'id first." For me, staying home allows me to be the kind of mother I want to be.

Choosing to Stay Home

"Becoming a mother is unlike almost any other experience, and it is impossible for a woman to know beforehand how deeply the experience will affect her. Until your baby is born and in your arms, nursing at your breast, you cannot know what it means to have a child, and then to leave a child." These words reflect the thoughts and emotions of mothers who have decided to stay at home full-time while their children are small.

One mother, Pat Smith from Pennsylvania, was faced with a difficult choice during pregnancy:

Of course I would return to work after having our baby! This was a foregone conclusion during the several years my husband, Skip, and I tried to conceive a child. We had rarely, if ever, considered otherwise, because the reasons for my continuing to work were so compelling: finances, lifestyles, careers.

In many ways we followed the young suburban working couple lifestyle. As happy consumers, we weren't quite ready to relinquish some of our material well-being. Among our peers, a mother's right to work after childbirth wasn't questioned.

Then there was the matter of careers. I had a promising future with a fine corporation owned by the major stock exchanges. In fact, I was due for a promotion into middle management that would mean relocation to New York at the company's expense.

Five months into my pregnancy, the New York promotion offer came, and it proved to be the undoing of my finances, career, and lifestyle. The offer was a fork in the road, because it brought into focus the commitment the new job demanded. Although the rewards were positively tantalizing, it didn't take me long to realize that I'd have little time or energy left for anything but part-time mothering if I were to pursue this career path.

Did I want to be a future vice-president of this corporation, or did I want to be a full-time mother? This was the question I had to answer once I accepted the premise that I couldn't be both. As I considered the question, images of the baby started invading my thoughts. They were fleeting, fragmented images at first, but when the images formed this scenario, I stopped cold: I saw myself wrapping the baby in blankets, taking him to the babysitter's house, holding him in my arms, then handing him over to someone else for the day. I knew right then and there that I would not go back to work after he was born.

For me, this was an irrational way to make a decision. I had a list of every rational reason to work, and at one single thought—separation from my little one—I tossed the list right out the window. I resolved that I would do whatever was necessary to stay home with the baby.

Colin was born three years ago, and we have been almost inseparable ever since. In retrospect, my worries at the time seem trivial now. After all, we now own a home in a friendly, family-oriented town, a car, and all the comforts we really need. A real worry, as I see it now, is how I would ever had made it through a working day without my baby.

My ex-boss called me about a year ago and offered me my old job. I was delighted to decline. I told him I wouldn't even consider it.

A sense of worth

The value of good parenting is never denied, but all too often it is unsung. Jobs in the marketplace have a highly visible rating system, usually, the higher the pay, the greater the prestige. The at-home mother has only one title, and there are no periodic raises telling her that she is doing a good job. The rewards are there, right in the family, though they are much more subtle.

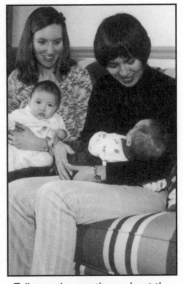

Talk to other mothers about the choices they have made.

A California mother, Emily Holt, discovered unexpected enjoyment in mothering. She reflects on the changes in her life that came with the birth of her baby. "I sit holding our five-month-old daughter, who is nursing so sweetly at my breast. I watch my husband's face light up with joy as she grabs his beard, laughing aloud. Oh yes, my job was wonderful as jobs go, but in these five short months, I have seen myself grow in a hundred ways, reaching for what is best in me to greet this beautiful new life. Sharing every delightful moment of Sarah's discovery of our world, I realize how blessed I am to be a mother."

Carolyn Keiler Paul of New York doesn't think she's wasting her time by staying home with her children. She says, "I think it's time we stop apologizing for being 'just a mother.' Childrearing is not a menial job. It calls for all our talents and resources. My college education isn't going to waste, because it has enriched me so that I may in turn enrich the lives of my children."

A major investment

Other mothers' stories can be inspiring and informative, but no one else can tell you what is the best course of action for you and your family. We can tell you about a baby's needs, we can tell you what works best to ensure successful breastfeeding, we can tell you how mothers have combined breastfeeding and working. And we can tell you about mothers who have discovered unexpected personal growth and fulfillment in staying home. But only you can make the decision that best reflects your own family's needs.

We encourage you to learn as much as you can, explore all the options that are available to you, and discuss these questions with others who have been faced with similar decisions and choices.

Attending La Leche League meetings can be a helpful source of information and encouragement. Talking with other mothers who are in situations similar to your own can reinforce the choices you make. Whether you are an employed or at-home mother, you can look to La Leche League for support in breastfeeding your baby. We will not hesitate to answer your questions, delight in your progress, and stand by you in your decision to breastfeed whether or not you return to work.

Be as cautious in your decision-making about returning to work as you would be with a major investment—the investment here is a critical period in your life and that of your baby. The early months and years set the course for the rest of your child's life, and they can never be recaptured. And as Dr. Marilyn Bonham, a psychiatrist who wrote *Laughter and Tears of Children*, reminds us, "The outflow of (a mother's) love and affection for the very young child is pure gold in the bank."

PART FOUR

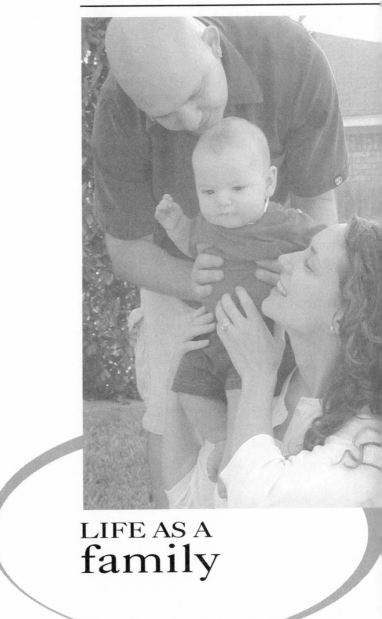

LIFE AS A
family

CHAPTER TEN

THE MANLY ART OF
fathering

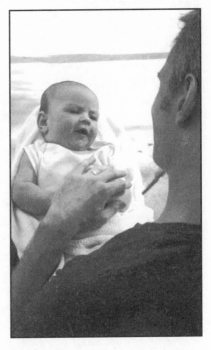

A father's unique relationship with his baby is an important element in the child's development from early infancy. From our experience, we know without a doubt that breastfeeding is enhanced and the nursing couple sustained by the loving support, help, and companionship of the baby's father.

Nowadays, men no longer fit the stereotyped image of the father in the waiting room of the hospital, pacing the floor, while his wife delivers their baby surrounded by strangers. A father today is more often next to his wife during childbirth, supporting her and sharing the unforgettable emotions of this event. From the moment of birth, father and baby begin to get acquainted. The more a man can participate in the birth of his son or daughter, the more powerful and meaningful it will be. Just ask a new father who was at the birth of his child and be prepared to listen!

The metamorphosis that makes a man a father does not happen overnight. He usually acquires the title "father" much more quickly than he captures the spirit of fathering. In fact, men can't even count on the natural assistance of hormones that aid the mother. It has been said that when a baby is born, so is a mother. Fathers emerge more

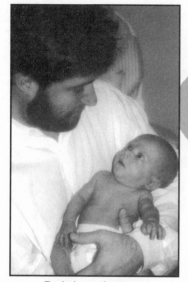

Dads have their own special ways of interacting with their babies.

gradually, as Dr. William Sears, pediatrician and author points out:

Although mothers do indeed have a hormonal head start on developing their intuition, I believe that fathers also have natural nurturing abilities, and, if given the opportunity to develop these abilities, fathers can indeed participate in the care and comforting of their babies.

Sue LaLeike, from Florida, tells how father and daughter developed a special relationship:

There is no way a father can take over a mother's role or vice versa—breastfeeding sees to that. But a nursing mother needs the baby's father to do his part by giving love to them both. The baby may not experience the closeness of nursing with Dad, but going for walks in the front carrier, laughter and nuzzlings, the family bed, and even burping and diapering can all contribute to very intimate relationships at a very early age. Charlie's role has been important since our baby's conception. He has helped all along—he didn't wait. He caught and prepared fresh Rocky Mountain trout for me in the first weeks of pregnancy. He supported my views on birthing and nursing. He read and discussed and went with me to doctor's appointments and birthing classes. And then he held and cradled our beautiful daughter moments after her birth in a way that made me know that he was the only person in the world I trusted her with.

He made all the first moves, and it sure does show in the way our daughter cries, "Daddy—home—happy!" when she hears him opening the gate at the end of our driveway.

Fathers Get Involved

While more and more men are recognizing that breastfeeding is the natural and ideal way to feed the baby, some first-time fathers don't realize how much they can be involved during the breastfeeding period.

After birth, the intimate relationship between mother and baby continues. They are still a unit, and for some time mother will be the baby's sole source of nourishment. In language that is irrefutable, biology makes it clear that the mother-baby relationship is primary and should not be set aside. This relationship is unique and the prototype of all other relationships throughout life. A father's contribution is equally important, but it is different. Babies thrive on both.

Chris Phillips, from New Jersey, describes one way a father can spend time with his child:

> A lot of new nursing mothers seem to worry that Daddy will feel left out if he can't help feed the new baby. Not so! Actually, I think just the opposite is true. The lack of bottles seems to encourage a father to become more active in other areas of an infant's care and upbringing. My husband, Ronny, took on the job (or should I say joy?) of bathing our firstborn son, Nicholas, starting with his very first bath.
>
> Everything went smoothly until Nicholas was about five months old and began to outgrow the kitchen sink. We discovered that bending over the tub was too much of a back strain for Ronny. He missed his special time with Nicholas. Thankfully, we came across a solution when someone told me about her husband taking their kids in the shower with him. What a terrific idea! It had never occurred to me that a baby would enjoy a shower, but why not? Nicholas had always loved the water; we would give it a try.
>
> That was over a year ago and Nicholas still loves the shower. Of course, there are a few adjustments to make when showering with a baby, but all in all, bathtime became a joy again and Ronny enjoys being an important part of his baby's life.

In BECOMING A FATHER, a book written especially for dads, Dr. Sears encourages them to get involved with their children:

> Speaking as one father to another, let me share a secret with you: Babies are fun, kids are a joy, and fatherhood is the only profession where you're guaranteed that the more effort you put into it the more enjoyment you will get out of it.

Some fathers take a while to grow into a nurturing relationship with their baby. Sally Thomas from Wisconsin writes about the changes as her husband developed more interest in their son:

> During my pregnancy, Eric, my husband, had surprised me with his interest and delight in my diet, exercise, and our growing baby. He was so supportive and interested in making our birth the kind of experience we wanted.
>
> However, after we got home with our son, Eric didn't seem as involved. He'd hold Joseph only with my prompting and only for a very short time. He kept saying "He doesn't do anything."
>
> When Joseph was a couple of weeks old I was talking to a friend about my concerns, and she told me that her husband had had a hard time relating to a tiny baby, too. She suggested I let Eric blossom as a father in whatever way that he felt comfortable.
>
> As the months went by and Joseph became more alert, Eric began to take more and more of an interest in his son. When Joseph became mobile and learned to like roughhousing, there was no holding Eric back. Soon Joseph seemed to prefer his daddy, and his face would light up at Eric's appearance.
>
> I am thankful every day for our now fourteen-month-old toddler and his wonderful and supportive father. And I love to watch my two favorite fellows playing as Eric—the tough-guy father—leans over and whispers in Joseph's ears, "I love you so much. What would we ever do without you?"

Fathers and Breastfeeding

Of all the sources of encouragement a woman may receive in breast-feeding, the support of her baby's father is the most meaningful to her. But for some women, support from the baby's father is not easy to come by. Perhaps a mother is a single parent and she is alone with her baby. She may need to look for support from friends or relatives. Or it may be that a married woman has a husband who is uncomfortable with the idea of his wife breastfeeding. A mother who faces these situations can still have a satisfying breastfeeding experience. A mother who feels all alone can especially benefit from regular contact with women in a support group, such as La Leche League.

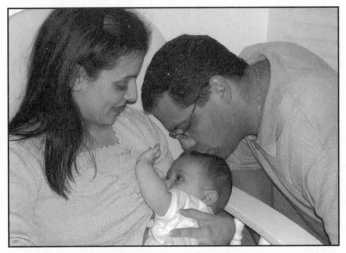

Breastfeeding mothers appreciate the support and encouragement of their husbands.

Sometimes a father who has misgivings before the baby was born learns to accept breastfeeding as he sees his baby thrive on mother's milk. A mother's enthusiasm for breastfeeding often sparks a father's interest. A father who is hesitant can only begin to support your decision to nurse the baby if he understands what it means to you.

Dr. Sears encourages fathers to support their wife's decision to breastfeed. He writes:

> I am absolutely convinced of the superiority of human milk for human babies. I want to convey to new fathers a feeling from the bottom of my heart: Do everything within your power to encourage and support the healthy breastfeeding relationship between your wife and your baby. Breastfeeding is more than just a method of feeding. It is a lifestyle choice. Providing understanding and support for the breastfeeding pair is one of the most valuable investments you can make in the future health and well-being of your family.

Men are sometimes surprised at the intensity of their reaction to seeing their wives breastfeed their babies. Archie Smith, a father from Texas, recalls his first impression:

> Before becoming an expectant father, I had never given much thought to breastfeeding. When my wife, Sheri, asked me what I thought about it, without hesitation I said I thought it was a good idea. It seemed to be the natural way. We talked more about it, and Sheri was eager to try breastfeeding.

> After Angie was born the nurse handed her to Sheri and
> she began to nurse. Standing a few feet away I could feel the
> emotions flowing from one to another. Then seeing the smile
> of satisfaction on my wife's face, I knew we were a family. It
> was an experience I will long remember.

And another father, Dean Cook, also from Texas, adds his
thoughts:

> Before our baby was born, my wife, Kathy, and I discussed
> breastfeeding, and we agreed our baby would be breastfed for
> at least six months, preferably as long as he needed it. I have
> long felt that there is no better way to nurture a child.
> However, I soon discovered after reading the materials that
> Kathy brought home from her LLL meetings that I knew only a
> few of the benefits of breastfeeding. And after gaining some
> experience as an active father of a nursing baby, I was amazed
> at my own intense emotional involvement with nursing.

What Can Fathers Do?

Though mother is the only one who can nurse the baby, there are a
number of things that no one else can do quite as well as a loving
father. Have you ever watched a mother try to soothe a fussy baby by
nursing and rocking and patting, and just about everything else she can
think of, and then watched in amazement as the baby's father lifts the
little one out of her arms, hoists him onto his shoulder, and promptly
puts the baby to sleep! It is a trade secret known only to fathers; we
don't know if it's the broad shoulders, the large, strong hands, or the
deep baritone voice that does the trick. But no matter—we know that
it works, and clever nursing mothers are the first to take advantage of
this ability.

Babies are often their fussiest late in the day, mother is tired after
a full day of baby care, and perhaps there is the added pressure of hungry children awaiting dinner. When dad arrives home, whatever difficulties he may have experienced at work are now behind him and he
can welcome walking into an entirely different environment. So he is
able to approach the baby in a more relaxed way at the moment than
the mother can. Many fathers take advantage of this to establish their
own special relationship with their babies.

In BECOMING A FATHER, Dr. Sears describes a special form of baby-
soothing that only works for dads—he calls it "the Neck Nestle." Dad

puts baby in a sling or baby carrier on his chest and lifts him up a bit so baby's head nestles under dad's chin. Dr. Sears explains:

> In the neck nestle, father has a slight edge over mother. Babies hear not only through their ears, but also through the vibration of their skull bones. By placing baby's skull against your voice box in the front of your neck and humming or singing to your baby, the slower, more easily felt vibrations of the lower-pitched male voice will often lull baby right to sleep. An added attraction of the neck nestle is that baby feels the warm air from your nose on his scalp. Experienced mothers have long known that sometimes just breathing onto their babies' faces or heads will calm them. They call this "magic breath." My children have enjoyed the neck nestle more than any of the other holding positions.

What do fathers most enjoy doing with their babies? There are probably almost as many answers as there are fathers, but over the years we have observed that fathers seem to have a special gift for playing with even very young babies. While mother is often preoccupied with cuddling and feeding, father is likely to tickle baby under his chin, hoist him into the air, or bounce him on his knee. A caution may be needed about shaking a baby as this can be harmful, but movement and exercise are important to the baby's overall development. Babies thrive when provided with both gentle nurturing and lively activity. As Louise Kaplan, PhD, explains in her book *Oneness and Separateness*, "Fathers have a special excitement about them that babies find intriguing.... Fathers embody a delicious mixture of familiarity and novelty."

Fathers need to spend time with their babies in order to get to know them better and get "tuned in" to their needs. Watch for cues that baby is ready for some fathering interaction. A hungry baby won't be at all interested in playing. But once baby has nursed his fill, dad can take over the burping, diaper-changing, singing, rocking, and cuddling. Some fathers

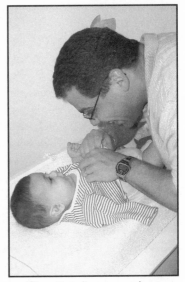

Changing diapers can be a time to have fun.

enjoy bathing the baby—or bathing with the baby, soaking together in a warm tub. A gentle massage can be another form of interaction between father and infant and don't overlook the sling or baby carrier. It's not just for mothers.

Learning about the usual stages of a baby's development in the first year can help a father enjoy his baby more. It's important for him to know when his son or daughter is ready to play peek-a-boo, when to expect reaching and grasping, and when to encourage crawling and climbing. A father can play an important role in these stages of development and proudly watch his child's growth and advancement. Another book by Dr. William Sears, GROWING TOGETHER: A PARENT'S GUIDE TO BABY'S FIRST YEAR, explains baby's stages of growth and development. See the Appendix for details.

Husband and Wife—
A Parenting Team

A husband and wife are a parenting team—each has an important and unique contribution to make to their child's development. They need to trust each other, respect each other's unique role, and help each other in times of stress. The most important thing you and your husband can do for your baby is to love one another.

The fact is that babies both expand horizons and rock boats. Your marriage will never again be the same. But it can be even more loving and it need never be dull. The silver and gold of future anniversaries are waiting. A prerequisite to attaining that treasure is putting your heads together now to chart your course.

There's a need to talk through the feelings that come with any important junction in life. We have referred to the emotions that a new mother often experiences, and it is just as reasonable to expect the father to react emotionally to his new responsibilities. A father and pediatrician, Jerald Davitz of California, tells fathers: "A very difficult feeling that most fathers have shortly after the new baby arrives home from the hospital is the unsettling sensation, 'Am I sure this is really what I want?' or 'Things were better before.' You need to understand you've got some reason to feel jealous and threatened at first, but these feelings will soon go away."

Communicate your feelings

While talking with other young mothers, Martha Hartzell of Georgia found that communication between husband and wife about what is important to each can go a long way toward improving their relationship.

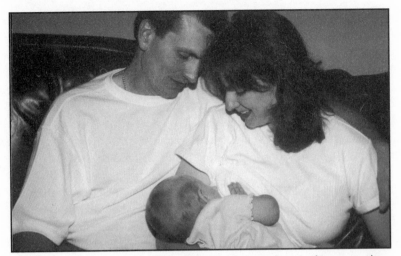

Communication is important as mother and father adjust to their new roles.

Mothers often find themselves totally immersed in nurturing and caring for their tiny baby. Some women have described their feelings about having a newborn as "like falling in love all over again." As one mother recalled, "I found everything about her endlessly exciting and fascinating. I could hardly think about anything else. My feelings were so intense for several weeks that there seemed to be little room in my life for anything else."

Such a new and powerful emotion could well upset the equilibrium in a marriage. A husband may find himself feeling like a jilted lover and, to make matters worse, his wife is too preoccupied with the baby to even notice!

It helps to remember that today's intense involvement will become tomorrow's comfortable, easygoing relationship. A baby must be loved and cared for in order to survive, and this initial intensity between mother and baby is designed to assure that the baby's needs will be met. With plenty of time, and ongoing communication about their needs and feelings, mother, father, and baby will eventually settle into a new relationship that is comfortable and satisfying for all three of them.

First-time parents are often intensely involved with their new responsibilities. Both husband and wife are putting out a tremendous effort. They must be careful not to let their concentration on these new responsibilities isolate them from each other.

Psychiatrist Lucy Waletzky of Georgetown University, Washington, DC, found that husbands often experience some jealousy because of the closeness of the nursing mother and baby. She advises: "Effective communication between husband and wife should be encouraged before, during, and after birth." Motherhood and fatherhood are new roles that need to be talked over and learned together. Time spent together during the first few weeks after the baby's birth can add a new dimension to a husband and wife's love for each other.

The rewards are great

Being a parent is not easy, but it can be extremely rewarding. Dr. David Stewart, father of five from Missouri, has this to say:

> Parenting is not easy. It can try us to the point of frustration. But this frustration can be productive because it is the symptom of growth and expansion. I sometimes think that nature gives us children to force us to grow up ourselves....
>
> Parenting is the greatest opportunity we normally receive to make good in this world. Your job may be important. Your volunteer activities may be important. But few of us do anything so important as to make much difference in society a hundred years from now. But the way you treat your children will matter a hundred years from now. The attitudes you pass on to them will be passed on to their children, who will pass them on to theirs....
>
> Parenthood works in two directions: good parenting makes for happy children; but it also makes for happy, fulfilled parents. It is not possible to give happiness without receiving it.

Men seldom have the opportunity to get together and share their ideas about being fathers. This can be just as important for them as it is for mothers. La Leche League Groups are not just for mothers—activities are often scheduled when fathers can get together and compare notes about their role. Couples' Meetings and Area Conferences provide these opportunities. In some local areas, fathers are invited to attend regular LLL Group Meetings. Check with your La Leche League Leader for details.

The book we've quoted throughout this chapter, BECOMING A FATHER: HOW TO NURTURE AND ENJOY YOUR FAMILY, by William Sears, is also a wonderful source of encouragement for fathers. Revised in 2003, copies are available from La Leche League Groups and La Leche League International. See the Appendix.

To quote David Stewart, "Ever uncertain, ever unreliable, ever unpredictable—most of life's offerings are fickle. Fatherhood is forever."

CHAPTER ELEVEN

MEETING FAMILY
needs

Throughout this book we talk about a mother meeting her baby's needs as though she and her baby were alone on a desert island. In reality, there are probably other family members whose needs must be met as well as household tasks that somehow must be accomplished. Faced with these responsibilities, you may be wondering just how you can keep things running smoothly while spending so much time breast-feeding and caring for a newborn.

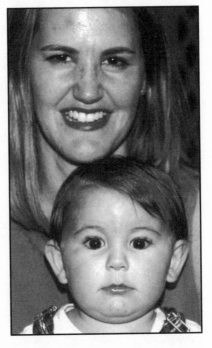

Over the years, La Leche League mothers have developed some techniques and tips that may help you. A basic recommendation is to always put people before things. Meeting the needs of family members should always come before immaculate housekeeping or caring for material possessions. Along with this, you'll want to remember that your family's priorities may not be the same as those of your next door neighbor or your favorite cousin (who doesn't have any children). Other people's standards or values may not be the ones that work out best for you and your family. Babies are small for such a short time. It would be a shame to waste those precious months trying to please others instead of enjoying your baby and meeting his needs.

Housework and a New Baby

Top household efficiency and a new baby mix about as well as oil and water. Meeting baby's unscheduled needs makes a strict household schedule pretty much a thing of the past. This is not to say that a well-ordered life automatically becomes chaos at the moment of birth, but it is fair warning that you may want to reorganize your approach to household chores.

The key to survival is to simplify. Pick an afternoon to take a walking tour of your home, critically examining each room for items that should be removed, rearranged, or discarded. Do you hate to see the knickknacks on the bookshelf covered with dust? Then put them away and replace them with a fresh new plant that will brighten both the room and your spirits. How about that overstuffed closet where everything from ski gear to broken lampshades seems to end up? If you take the time to clean it out while you are pregnant, it won't get on your nerves later. Discard the things that are beyond repair or that you no longer need—don't just move them somewhere else or they will soon be in your way again. Box up the things you want to keep and store in the attic or basement.

Whatever the season, do as much "spring cleaning" as you can before the baby is born. Light household chores are good exercise, and having them done will be a godsend later when you'll want to devote your time and energy to the baby. This sudden zeal for cleaning and readying the house so often felt by mothers during the last months of pregnancy is referred to as the "nesting instinct."

Give some thought to rearranging your cleaning supplies so that they are readily accessible (but stored in a childproof area). You'll want your supplies to be handy so you can quickly clean a bathroom mirror or scour a sink if you have a moment before stepping into your shower or while keeping an eye on a three-year-old in the tub. Your bathroom will be clean in minutes following bath time if you quickly wipe a mirror (already fogged), take a swipe over the sink and counter, and wipe up the water on the floor with a large towel, one that was already consigned to the laundry hamper.

In households where there is a baby, housework is nearly always done in quick snatches—a series of mini-cleaning spurts. Five to ten minutes at full speed in the kitchen, devoted to whatever is most bothersome to you—perhaps the breakfast dishes on the table or the grubby floor in front of the sink or refrigerator—will improve the looks of the house and give you a sense of accomplishment. Picking up the clutter near the door or around your husband's favorite chair may be a worthwhile priority. Throughout the day, center your attention on

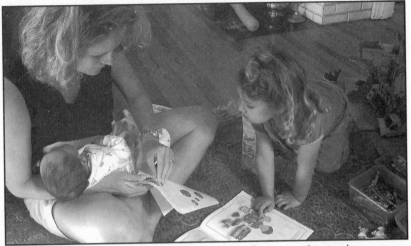

Sitting on the floor to nurse the baby allows a mother to also
pay attention to her toddler.

what you have accomplished, beginning with the all-important work of
nurturing your baby, rather than dwelling on the tasks that still need
doing.

Make your bed or not, as it pleases you. Plumping up the pillows
and tossing the covers back to air is a time-honored custom. Without a
spread in place, you'll probably lie down to nurse the baby more often
during the day. Keeping up with the dishes is about as easy as keeping
up with the Joneses. If baby is not agreeable to having you do the
whole job when the meal is over, fill the sink with hot soapy water and
let everything soak until you can get back to it later on or the next
morning. If you have a dishwasher, reload it during those times when
baby is wakeful and wants to be held in your arms or snuggled in his
baby carrier. Babies usually love the constant up-and-down and back-
and-forth motions that accompany the loading and unloading process.
Don't rush it. Some babies are soothed by the sound of running water.
And many a fussy baby has fallen asleep in a baby carrier while his
mother vacuums.

Little people and clutter seem to be inseparable. But clutter can
be picked up and put out of sight quickly if you are equipped with a
clutter-catcher—a cardboard box or other suitable container to carry
with you as you whiz through each room depositing all the odds and
ends that have been scattered about. This system enables you to de-
clutter an entire house in fifteen minutes or so. The contents of the
box can be sorted later when you have more time, but for now the
house looks fairly straightened, and a visitor will be able to walk in the
door without fear of skidding on a stray truck. Concentrate on immedi-

ately putting away the especially important items such as car keys, which will drive you frantic when misplaced. Always putting your keys on a handy hook just inside the door could be one of the best habits you could develop. For safeguarding other small, valuable items picked up around the house during the day, the pockets in your jeans or an apron are indispensable.

Early in the morning, perhaps while you're relaxing with your baby for an after-breakfast nursing, make a list of the "must do" tasks for that day. Further refine your choices by selecting one, or possibly two, of the most important. Box off these top-priority items and plan on getting to them at the first opportunity, before you get caught up in another project or just the everyday chores. If it's something you can't do until later in the day, set your alarm clock or oven timer to ring at the appropriate time. Getting just one "top-priority" item crossed off your list every day will give you a feeling of accomplishment no matter how many things are left undone. Beware of going all out for cleaning, cooking, and scrubbing whenever the baby is taking a nap. Give some of that time to the other children, take a nap yourself, or relax with a project you enjoy.

Meal planning

When there is a new baby in your life, mastering the art of advance meal preparation is as vital as knowing how to relax in a rocking chair. Many women prepare double recipes of stews, casseroles, spaghetti sauce, chili, and the like during the last weeks of pregnancy and put the extra portions in the freezer. We've heard of thoughtful friends giving the mother-to-be a "casserole shower," presenting her with meals which they have prepared and frozen in disposable pans, complete with instructions for cooking or reheating. And the lovely practice of bringing a meal to the new baby's family has certainly not lost its appeal.

After the baby arrives, let simplicity in menu planning be your watchword. Make a list of your favorite one-step, no-fuss meals and be sure to keep the necessary ingredients on hand. A dessert or snack of fresh fruit is always quick and nutritious. Hard-boil several eggs in the morning so they are available for lunch or a quick snack.

If you don't already have a slow cooker or crock-pot, put it at the top of your list for the next gift-giving occasion. These marvelous cookers allow you to prepare your meat, potatoes, and vegetables at any convenient time during the day, and it's all ready to eat at supper-time with no fuss or bother when you're tired and the baby is most likely to need your undivided attention. If you have a microwave oven, foods can be prepared quickly or cooked ahead of time and reheated when everyone is ready to eat. An inexpensive item that is helpful for a mother whose attention is often distracted from cooking is a metal plate that fits between a cooking pot and the stove burner and keeps the food from burning.

For help in meal planning, you will find many ideas in La Leche League's cookbooks, WHOLE FOODS FOR THE WHOLE FAMILY and WHOLE FOODS FROM THE WHOLE WORLD. Both are collections of mother-tested recipes with an emphasis on good nutrition and easy preparation. For details, see the Appendix.

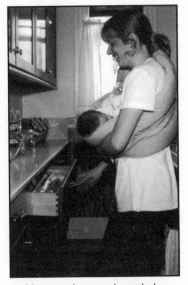

Using a sling can keep baby happy while you handle some household tasks.

Power snacks

Nursing mothers should eat at regular intervals, and active children also need to eat often. To keep young temperaments soothed and tummies satisfied until mealtime, consider introducing salad snacks. Simply assemble an assortment of fresh, raw vegetables and fruits. (Note that raw carrots and nuts should not be given to toddlers because small chunks can be aspirated instead of swallowed.) Preschoolers can be happily occupied in the preparations by washing and tearing greens, pulling the strings from celery stalks, breaking the cauliflower or broccoli florets, shining the apples, and arranging them all on a platter. Prepare these early in the day and keep in the refrigerator for quick munching later on. The addition of cheese, slices of hard-cooked eggs, or strips of cooked meat will add protein and staying power.

Sitting down for a few minutes for a snack is a positive measure to divert youngsters when they're tired and hungry and perhaps getting irritable. You can create a happy atmosphere with music—a favorite recording, or better yet, a sing-along with mom. The songs from your childhood are fresh and dear to your children and can become a part of their heritage. Children especially like to hear their names inserted into the songs you sing.

Laundry

We are all amazed at how much laundry a new baby can generate and how quickly laundry stacks up once a baby joins the family. Before the baby arrives, try to be sure that all of you have the most ample supply of clothing that your budget will permit, particularly underwear and socks, so that you won't have to do laundry every day or two. Another item mothers like to stock up on is a dozen or more lightweight, inexpensive washcloths ("seconds") that often come packaged in bundles. They're handy for all kinds of mop-ups and since they are thinner than regular washcloths, they are convenient to use when washing behind delicate, small ears and in the creases of chunky arms and legs.

Eventually the laundry has to be done, of course, and your own approach undoubtedly will depend on the kind of facilities available to you. Whether you depend on the neighborhood laundromat or have your own equipment, enlist your husband's help. If your husband isn't already familiar with the intricacies of a washer and dryer, the hour is at hand for him to learn! When you are doing the laundry, you can use a sling or baby carrier to good advantage. Whether it involves trips to the laundromat or doing the laundry right at home, baby will be held and comforted, and you'll get clean clothes!

Consider using two to three inexpensive plastic buckets to soak clothing that might stain. Then you can run it through the washer at a time that is convenient. Some system of pre-sorting laundry is a great help, too. As a container fills, you can quickly see when you have a load of white or colored items, and you can drop them into the washer as time permits.

Your toddler will love to be in on the action of transferring laundry from the dryer to the basket and then helping sort the clothes. Long ago, many of us decided that a considerable amount of laundry is just as serviceable when left unfolded. Undergarments, in particular, can be sorted—tops and bottoms—and put away in a drawer, in plastic bins, or on a shelf. Clean socks can be sorted into two baskets—one for white and the other for colors—and the older members of the family can each match their own pairs.

If you're in the habit of ironing some things, now would be the time to give it a second thought. Taking shirts and blouses out of the dryer immediately and putting them on hangers saves a lot of wrinkles. Try the ten-minute test. Wear an ironed piece of clothing for ten minutes and notice how it takes on a more lived-in, rumpled look before too long. The same item probably looks just the same after a ten-minute wearing even if it has not been ironed! You'll wonder if it's worth the time and energy to take out the ironing board.

As you make plans for keeping up with the laundry, concentrate on ways to lessen it. To start, you may find that the large bath towels that are used for drying when jumping out of the tub can be recycled if they're spread out and hung to dry instead of bunched on a small towel rack. A towel can be fastened around a towel bar with a large safety pin or gripper snaps, so children can use it to dry their hands without having it end up on the floor and then inevitably in the hamper.

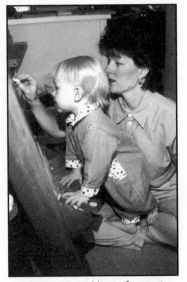

Little ones need lots of attention to keep them out of mischief.

Time for the Other Little Ones

You will find that generous portions of love and reassurance will go a long way toward helping your older child, the ex-baby, accept the demands that the new baby is making on your time. When the baby is fussy you can remind an older child, "Mary, when you were little and hungry, I always asked Elizabeth to be patient and wait because you needed to be fed (or rocked, or held, or whatever)." The child loves the idea of once having been the "star," and it's a happy thought that can be reinforced with a hug. When feeding the baby, a nursing mother usually has an arm free for quick hugs or other important tasks.

There's peace of mind in keeping your older child near you when you're nursing the baby, rather than having him off somewhere on his own. A popular suggestion is to arrange a nursing corner that accommodates at least three—mother, baby, and an older brother or sister. Have an extra chair or stool next to your rocker, with some interesting play items nearby. Change the assortment regularly; surprises are always fun. One creative mom, Marge Bazemore of Georgia, added a small table for a work surface, and she and son Russ enjoy a variety of activities while the baby nurses. Marge describes their favorite choices:

- A cassette tape recorder. It's easy to operate and Russ enjoys hearing his voice as well as Phil's cooing.
- Simple puzzles.

- Playdough. I also keep a cookie cutter handy.
- Finger puppets.
- Crayons, paper, pencil, and coloring book.
- Pegboard. I made one out of a piece of ceiling board and we use golf tees for the pegs.
- Viewmaster and slides.
- Books and family photo albums.
- Spools and a cord for stringing.

From time to time, sit on the floor while nursing. You'll be at eye level with your toddler, and the whole floor is the play area. It's great for building with blocks or rolling a soft ball. This is especially helpful when the ex-baby is looking for extra attention. Jealousy toward the new baby often shows up when the baby is three or six months old, if it hasn't happened sooner.

The mother who is expecting her second child sometimes finds it hard to imagine that she will feel as close to the new baby as she does to the little one who is already here. Can there be the same strong love the second time around? The miracle of mother love is that it increases with each new birth. It is not diminished, not limited. It is not a pie that must be sliced into smaller pieces to accommodate extra plates at the table. With the new baby comes a resurgence of love for all of the family.

Little helpers

Toddlers love to help, and clever mothers find lots of things for their little ones to help with. If you use nonbreakable dishes, your little one may enjoy setting the table, carrying one item at a time from the stack of dishes set out. Young ones never tire of the repetition of walking back and forth, especially when a smile and "thank you" accompany each dish that is delivered to the table. Shining the glass in a low window that has been sprayed with cleaner (or plain water) is another enjoyable pastime for little ones who want to help.

Many toddlers seem to be fascinated with a hand brush or whisk broom and dustpan, so put yours to work under the kitchen table or some other open area. Old mittens and socks make great dusting mitts for little hands. If mother helps, too, even children who are barely walking will learn to put toys back in the toy box when it's time to clean up.

Preschoolers need lots of stimulating learning activities to keep them happy and out of mischief. A wonderful resource book, published

by La Leche League International, is PLAYFUL LEARNING, by Anne
Engelhardt and Cheryl Sullivan. Written for parents who want to
organize an at-home preschool for their little ones, it can also be used
on an individual basis. Craft projects, simple recipes, music and number activities, story-telling, and reading readiness are all included. The
information about a preschooler's development can help you better
understand your child's needs. For details, see the Appendix.

Dads can help

An understanding husband is one of a nursing mother's most treasured
assets. He can step in to provide you with a welcome respite when he
is home, and your older children will thrive on the extra attention.

Dads are often masters at keeping toddler minds and hands busy
when mother needs some time alone with the baby, or when she
decides to take advantage of baby's naptime for a relaxing bath or
some much needed rest. Father and toddler will both enjoy a round of
toddler-size roughhousing, and who but daddy can add such excitement to stories by putting in all those low, rumbling noises?

Fathers and their little ones often develop a new and very special
relationship when a new baby joins the family. Let your husband know
how much he is needed and appreciated, encourage him to spend
some extra time with your toddler or preschooler, and be prepared to
watch the two of them become the best of friends.

Older children

If you have older children, you're also probably wondering, "How can I
possibly have enough time for them after the new baby arrives?" You
ask if there won't be times when an older child will want your attention, and the baby will also need you. More than likely there will be,
and this is when—and how—the mutual love and understanding that
cement good human relationships are fostered. Learning to consider
the needs of someone who is helpless before one's own needs is a valuable lesson for the older children. It is something that you will want to
help them understand as much as you can.

In discussions about the arrival of the new member of the family,
ask your older children to help you think of ways of managing and
helping each other. Encourage them to remember that the new baby
will be the only member of the family who is completely dependent on
you—just as they were at that age. When thought of in this way, it's
easier for a young person to recognize (if not always accept) that
baby's needs must certainly come first.

The period before your new baby arrives is an excellent time to teach the older ones some new household skills. Select chores that match each one's ability and continue to work along with your child whenever possible. The children will learn from you, and humdrum chores, such as doing the dishes, can be transformed into special moments for sharing youthful hopes and problems. Children do not make appointments with their parents to talk over their deeply felt concerns. Such sharing takes place in the context of normal activities, during times when parent's and child's hands are busy, but their minds and hearts are in touch with each other.

Don't be surprised if your young helpers are less than enthusiastic at times. That's normal. Pour on the praise and be patient with your apprentice. We all need to feel needed, and children benefit from knowing that the family is depending on them to carry out their assigned jobs. We parents overlook a golden opportunity if we don't help our children learn to accept responsibility and to enjoy the self-esteem that comes with being expected to do a job and doing it well.

School-age youngsters in the family are generally very accepting of a new baby. They enjoy babies, and vice versa. Potential problems usually come from a variety of outside activities in which this age group is often involved and which demand a parent's participation. These often include driving to and from games or lessons, attending programs, or working together on special projects. Such a pace can be hectic for a mother who also has a new baby.

You will have to be realistic and firm in setting limits for the time being. Do only those extras that you and the baby can honestly manage. Your husband can be a big help here, spending extra time with the older children's activities whenever possible. If a particular activity is very special to an older child, and neither you nor your husband can participate, be assertive in asking another parent to help you. For instance, a friend or neighbor could drive to and from functions for a few weeks; you can reciprocate later.

If you will be driving with the baby along, an infant auto safety seat is a must. If you use it faithfully, beginning with baby's first ride (usually the trip home from the hospital), you and your baby will soon accept the procedure as a matter of course. The safest place in the car for baby or toddler is the back seat. Plan to nurse the baby before starting out in the car, so you and baby will be more relaxed. If baby does need to nurse before you arrive at your destination, pull over in a safe location and tend to his needs. What better excuse could you have for being late?

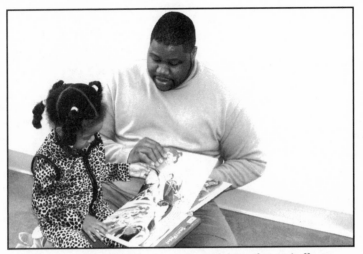

Dads can add excitement to stories with lots of sound effects.

When it comes to getting your husband and older children off to work or school on time, advance planning can save the day. Betty Wagner, one of the LLL co-Founders, managed by setting her alarm for about twenty minutes earlier than usual. Still resting in bed, she'd reset the clock for the regular time and nurse the baby. When she had to get breakfast and help the older children, she at least knew the baby would not be hungry in the midst of the morning rush.

You will be proud of your older children as they grow to understand the helplessness of the baby and accept the sacrifices they are asked to make. It has been gratifying to many of us to find that a crying baby is almost always disturbing to older children. They sense that something is not right, and they are happy again only when baby is happy. Looking ahead, you'll find that cheerfully putting the needs of the baby first, as a matter of course, is an example of caring for others that benefits everyone. It's a good way to educate your children for their future roles as loving parents.

Developing a Parenting Style

Parents find themselves making many decisions as their children grow and family needs change. We all grow up with some idea of what it means to be a parent and raise children. Perhaps we were brought up in a loving, caring family and we choose our own parents as role models when we have children. Or possibly, our childhood was not a happy one and we want to offer a more secure environment to our children.

Either way you'll want to make an effort to learn as much as you can about parenting, child care, meeting children's needs, and child development. You'll find books listed in the Appendix that offer practical information on these topics. Also, discussing these matters with other parents with values and concerns similar to your own can prove invaluable. La Leche League Groups offer this opportunity. Although the basic meeting topics are related to breastfeeding and young babies, additional topics are often discussed at Couples' Nights, Chapter Meetings, or informal get-togethers that are planned.

La Leche League Area and International Conferences offer further opportunities to expand your understanding of parenthood. Check with your local La Leche League Leader or the LLLI Web site for details of upcoming events you may be interested in attending.

NUTRITIONAL
know-how

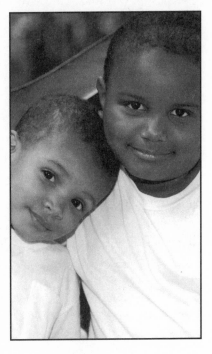

If you already have good eating habits, there is no reason for you to make any major changes while you are breastfeeding. On the other hand, if you know that your eating habits need improvement, pregnancy and breastfeeding are good incentives to do this. Your baby's development during pregnancy depends to a great extent on good nutrition; your own health and well-being are also at stake. Your investment in your baby's welfare should provide strong motivation that will make it easier for you to change your eating habits.

Your baby will get off to a fine start on your milk. You will want him to build on this good start by giving him healthful foods when he is ready for them and by teaching him nutritionally sound eating habits that will become lifelong practices. The best way to accomplish this is by being a family in which everyone has good eating habits.

In this chapter, we include some general principles of food selection to help you learn how to choose the foods you and your family need to maintain good health. We urge you to pursue this topic further, reading other books on good nutrition and keeping up-to-date on current dietary recommendations from knowledgeable sources.

La Leche League's basic approach to good nutrition is to recommend eating a well-balanced and varied diet of foods in as close to their natural state as possible. With few exceptions, the more a food is processed the more nutrients are lost. To help you prepare tasty and nutritious meals for your family, La Leche League publishes a series of cookbooks that include mother-tested recipes and tips on good nutrition. WHOLE FOODS FOR THE WHOLE FAMILY is a complete cookbook that can be used by beginning cooks as well as experienced family chefs. The recipes use only whole unprocessed foods with minimal amounts of salt and sweeteners. WHOLE FOODS FROM THE WHOLE WORLD is a collection of family-tested recipes from La Leche League families all over the world. WHOLE FOODS FOR BABIES AND TODDLERS by Margaret Kenda provides information about starting solids and includes basic recipes that can be used for family meals. WHOLE FOODS FOR KIDS TO COOK offers simple recipes for children that use natural and wholesome ingredients. These cookbooks are available from La Leche League Groups, the La Leche League International Catalogue, and on our Web site at www.lalecheleague.org. See the Appendix for details.

The Basic Approach

Some of the following suggestions originally came from the late Dr. Herbert Ratner whose sensible approach to good nutrition was based on selecting foods in proper balance in order to meet all of our nutritional needs. His basic approach to healthy eating was to:

- Eat a variety of foods
- Eat a variety of animals and plants
- Eat a variety of the parts of animals and plants

People instinctively seek a variety of styles and colors to decorate their homes and their bodies. The inner body also thrives on a diversity of foods with a wide range of flavors, colors, even textures—chewy, soft, firm, juicy, crisp. All the different textures, colors, and flavors of food reflect different food elements and values needed for the body.

In selecting foods, don't concentrate on four-legged animals, like the cow, to the exclusion of two-legged animals, like the chicken; or land animals to the exclusion of water animals.

In fact, don't limit yourself to animal sources of protein. When you think "main dish" consider recipes that include beans and other legumes (lentils, peanuts), nuts, seeds, and grains. Many wonderful

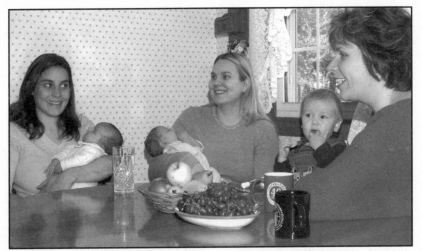

Getting together with other nursing mothers can be a
good opportunity to share tips on family nutrition.

traditional meals feature these healthful foods, sometimes combined with small amounts of meat or cheese. Your family—and your food budget—will benefit.

In the plant kingdom, don't restrict yourself to the tried-and-true vegetables and fruits. Besides green vegetables look for orange and yellow vegetables—squash, sweet potatoes or yams, varieties of peppers. There are different parts of plants, too, that are edible. The parts don't have to belong to the same plant. There are leaves, including greens that go into a salad, as well as Swiss chard, collards, beet greens, kale, and cabbage. There are roots, like carrots, beets, turnips, and onions. There are stems and tubers, including asparagus and potatoes, and the fruits of a plant, such as corn, beans, and tomatoes, as well as apples, oranges, grapes, bananas, and melons.

With such a variety to choose from there is no need to limit yourself to eating the same two or three vegetables for the rest of your life. This would deprive your body of healthful nutrients each has to offer.

Fats are needed in the cooking and preparation of some foods and they supply us with energy. There are animal fats and vegetable fats, solid fats and liquid fats, saturated fats and unsaturated fats. Animal fats include butter, cream, lard, and chicken fat. Vegetable fats include margarine and vegetable oils. Research has linked high-fat diets to heart disease and other ills, and nutritionists tell us that many people today consume too much fat in their daily diets. Some fats are better for health than others. Any fat that is solid at room temperature (butter, margarine, vegetable shortening) should be eaten in moderation. Olive oil and fish oils from certain fish (tuna, salmon, whitefish) are better for you and will add variety and flavor to your family's diet. Safflower oil, canola oil, and soybean oil also contain the kind of fats that are important for your health.

You can lower the fat content of your favorite ground beef recipes by substituting lean ground turkey for all or most of the ground beef. When seasonings and other ingredients are added, there is little difference in appearance or taste. Another way to cut back on animal fat is to decrease the amount of foods you eat that come from animals and to rely more on plant sources for protein.

Vary your meals

As you plan your family's meals, you'll want to provide a variety of foods. You can respect your own likes and dislikes as long as your dislikes aren't too numerous and as long as you do not impose your likes and dislikes on the rest of the family. After all, you don't want your children to grow up with restricted eating habits unless there is a reason for restrictions.

Margaret Kenda, nutritionist and author of WHOLE FOODS FOR BABIES AND TODDLERS, writes:

> Good nutrition is a matter of balance. You balance each meal with foods that interact to fulfill a wide range of physical needs. The greater the variety of good foods, the more you can be assured of complete nourishment.

If there is a particular food you or other members of your family dislike, there is always a substitute. Cheese and yogurt are good substitutes for milk. Eggs are a good alternative to meat and fish, as are combinations of whole grains, nuts, dried peas, beans, lentils, and brown rice. This demonstrates one rule of nature. There are so many different kinds of foods that every culture in every age on every continent has had a varied selection of foodstuffs available to eat. This has resulted in a wondrous variety of national cuisines. Modern transportation and mechanization make possible a varied selection of foods throughout the year by sharing the productive seasons and rich bounty of other parts of the world with all of us.

Eat natural foods

Generally speaking, the further one gets away from the natural state of food, the less nutritional value is left in the food. Fresh foods are usually better than frozen and frozen foods are preferable to canned. Since cooking is one step removed from the natural state, some foods are better raw than cooked. This is especially true of fruits and vegetables, with a few exceptions. For example, vitamin A is more available in cooked carrots. Most protein foods need to be cooked. Under-cooked foods, with due allowance for digestibility, are better than over-cooked foods. The stir-fry method permits food to be cooked quickly and to retain many of the nutrients and flavor found in uncooked foods.

By partaking of the many digestible parts of the living whole, and by concentrating on natural foods, you will get all of the known nutrients in proper and natural proportions. You will get all of the essential nutrients that have been discovered by science, and you should get those that have yet to be discovered; not only the vitamins and minerals of today, but the vitamins and minerals and other nutritional factors still undiscovered. If you eat a wide variety of foods daily, any need for vitamins and other supplements will be lessened. This approach to nutrition is more economical, and it doesn't require a science course. It will protect you against ill health and at the same time supply you with a variety of choices to please everyone in your family.

What to avoid

Chemical additives. The fewer the additives the better! A large number of chemicals are in common use today in the food industry. They are added to enhance color or prolong shelf life. Much more study needs to be done to determine just how safe these chemicals are. In the meantime, since some of the chemicals have not been properly tested and their safety is uncertain, it seems wisest to avoid them. Read the labels on bottles, cans, and packages and choose those items that have the fewest artificial flavors, colors, and preservatives. Better still, whenever possible, prepare your own food from the freshest products available.

Sugar. One of the chief offenders in confusing our appetites is sugar. Used excessively it can dull the palate for the delicate flavors of fresh, natural food. Sugar can be easily misused and is especially bad for infants and young children, primarily because it satisfies hunger and displaces healthful, natural food. Sugar is obvious in many desserts, candies, and soft drinks. But there is also an amazing amount of "hidden" sugar found in many other commonly used packaged and/or bottled foods. It is very important to your good health that you acquire the habit of reading the list of ingredients on every packaged or bottled food item you buy. Corn syrup, corn sweeteners, fructose, sucrose, and dextrose are other names for sugar.

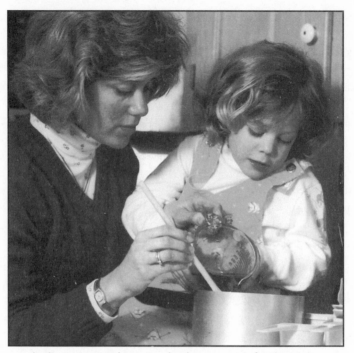

Little ones enjoy being involved in preparing family meals.

Many of the best cooks in La Leche League have learned to cut out sugar entirely or greatly reduce it in as many recipes as they can. They have found that even in dessert recipes a sharp reduction in the amount of sugar called for works equally as well, and does not detract from the flavor. If your little ones are served fresh fruit as dessert from the beginning, they'll love it. As you and your husband wean yourselves from too much sugar, your taste buds will begin to appreciate the flavor of natural sweetness.

Salt. Salt (sodium chloride) can be another offender in our diet. Like sugar, it is often overused in an attempt to enhance the flavor of our food. This may result in an excessive intake of salt, which can be harmful. Overuse of salt is linked to high blood pressure in some individuals. (Hypertension can lead to stroke—a leading cause of death in many parts of the world.)

Salt was originally added to foods as a preservative and to cover up the unpleasant taste of foods that were spoiling because of lack of refrigeration. We are better off if we reduce the amount of salt we use. Many excellent cooks have found other ways to enhance flavor; they use a variety of herbs, spices, and other seasonings.

Highly processed cereals and grains. These products provide another source of confusion to our appetites. Processing robs cereals and grains of important minerals and vitamins. To make up for the loss of natural nutrients they must be enriched. This prevents obvious nutritional deficiencies that can develop when people eat nothing but refined foods (white flour instead of whole-wheat, white rice instead of brown, etc.). But the enrichment is only an enrichment of an inferior product; many other valuable nutrients are lost, including fiber.

Whole grains and cereals are excellent sources of fiber, as are many fruits and vegetables. In the long term, a high-fiber diet may help prevent certain kinds of cancers. For the short term, fiber is important in preventing constipation, a problem for many women during pregnancy and postpartum. Processing removes fiber from foods, along with flavor and texture. Serving whole-grain breads, whole-grain cereals, both hot and cold, and other grains such as brown rice or barley will boost the fiber in your family's diet and add interest to your meals.

How to Eat Well

By following the basic approach we have outlined so far, and adding the art of making foods tasty and attractive, you'll bring the joy of eating to the family table and you and your family will benefit nutritionally. Here are some practical tips to help you and your family eat well.

Read the labels

Acquiring the habit of reading the list of ingredients on food packages, cans, and bottles is most important. This will help you select foods that provide the most wholesome ingredients and avoid those that contain too much sugar, salt, fat, chemical additives, artificial colors, or ingredients to which you or other family members may be allergic.

It is important to read the list of ingredients because other information on the label can often be misleading. A can labeled "fruit juice drink," for example, is actually just a fruit-flavored drink, with lots of sugar. It is not pure fruit juice. By calling it a "drink" the company has stayed within acceptable labeling standards and has probably led some people to believe the product is better for them than it really is. Another confusing term is "fortified." Sometimes the company lists the vitamins they've added, but these "fortified" foods usually offer less food value than the real thing—and at a greater cost.

Don't be deceived by the term "wheat flour" in a list of ingredients on a bread label. "Wheat flour" refers to white flour. It must say "whole wheat" or "whole grain" to indicate the grain has not been processed. You should also know that ingredients are listed in descending order of amounts found in the product. For example, if flour is the first ingredient listed, it means there's more flour in the product than anything else. If the second item is sugar, dextrose, or corn syrup, that means that next to flour there is more sweetener than anything else, and so on down the line. (Of course, when several types of sweetener are listed separately, it might be that sugar is really the main ingredient when you add them all up.) The chemicals are usually listed last, but some highly processed items may have more chemicals than food: for example, coffee-cream substitutes, some pudding desserts, and some ice creams contain more chemicals than any other ingredient.

Changing food habits

Food habits don't change overnight. Introducing new foods requires tact, patience, and imagination. In the beginning you'll want to choose alternatives that resemble familiar foods. When you are shopping and reading labels, don't even bring home the foods you don't want your family to eat. If the adults in the family continue to snack on cookies and chips, the children will want to follow their example.

Creative approaches can make new foods more appealing. Melted cheese on whole-grain bread may look better to a toddler if it is in the shape of a triangle or a butterfly. A melon slice on salad greens can be a sailboat salad. Tickle your toddler's imagination by calling a crunchy slice of apple an apple "cookie." Colorful sliced vegetables with dip have eye appeal. Even unusual containers can pique children's interest. Serve snacks on toy dishes, in special cups, or in a toddler's very own lunch box. Try a blender drink of bananas, milk, some ice, and a little vanilla. If it's served in a fancy glass with a straw, what child could resist?

Using whole grains

Introducing whole grains to your family can be an enjoyable change because there are hundreds of ways to use them. If your family doesn't like oatmeal for breakfast, try cornmeal, either as a cereal, good old-fashioned fried cornmeal mush, or nice hot corn bread. Some recipes use a combination of cornmeal and whole-wheat flour, others use cornmeal only. Kasha is an old standby from people whose origins are in the Middle East and Eastern Europe. It is both nutritious and easy to cook. It can be used hot or cold, much like rice. The smell of spicy raisin-bran muffins baking will draw people to the table. A hot muffin is hard to resist, and muffin recipes are easily changed to include whatever ingredients you have on hand—apples, nuts, blueberries, grated

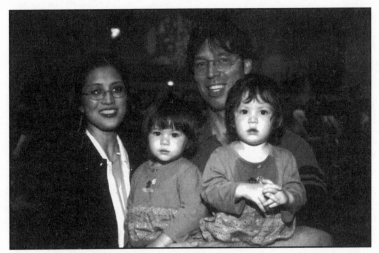

Providing a variety of healthful, nutritious foods for your
family is worth the extra effort.

carrots, etc. What a pleasant way to get your family off to a good, ener-
getic start for the day! Try using granola, too. Granola recipes abound
and it's fun to make your own, since the commercial varieties are often
heavy on sweeteners and fats.

Husbands and older children have been known to balk at the
introduction of whole-wheat bread. One suggestion is to offer them
"half and half" sandwiches for a while—using one slice of whole-wheat
bread and one slice of white. Very young children whose tastes have
not had time to become conditioned usually like the whole grain bread
right away.

If you enjoy baking, you can introduce whole-wheat flour gradually
into your baked goods. Just substitute whole-wheat flour for part of
the white flour you usually use in the recipe. This is especially easy to
do in homemade breads and muffins. Many mothers have found that
baking their own bread is great fun and a lot easier than they expected.
If you gradually increase the amount of whole-wheat flour to the white
flour over a period of months, eventually you'll be making a one hundred percent whole-wheat bread that no longer tastes "strange" to
your family. It may even become more desirable than the white bread
they used to like, especially when it's hot from the oven!

If you do use white flour in your recipes, be sure to use
unbleached flour, so as to avoid the extra chemicals used for bleaching.
For extra nutrition, place one tablespoon of soy flour in each cup of
white flour. Soy is high in protein, so it will add to the food value of
the baked goods and will not be noticed in the final product. Dried
skim-milk powder is also a nutritious supplement if milk allergy is not

a problem. A tablespoon or two can be added to various cake, bread, muffin, or pancake recipes without changing texture or flavor.

Use nuts and seeds in recipes

Plain raw nuts and seeds are too full of goodness to overlook. Even when roasted they are still nutritious, though less so than when raw. You can increase the food value in your potato salad, or chicken or tuna salad, by adding a tablespoon or two of sesame seeds. They are so tiny and bland in flavor that even the pickiest member of your family won't notice them. A sprinkle of hulled raw sunflower or sesame seeds over breakfast cereal or yogurt will increase food value and add both flavor and a bit of crunch. In just about any kind of batter you make, you can add sesame seeds or finely ground nuts, and no one will be the wiser. Nuts and seeds are delicious in waffles, pancakes, muffins, and breads.

Nuts and seeds packaged by the ounce and sold in the grocery store are relatively expensive, as well as often stale. Look for one of the new, "old-fashioned" stores where you can scoop nuts, seeds, and dried fruits from big bins and buy them by the pound. These usually offer considerable savings over the packaged variety, and they are likely to be fresher and better flavored. Store them in the freezer to keep them fresh longer.

A caution is needed about giving nuts to children under three or so. The young child may not chew them well and there is a danger of small chunks being inhaled into the lungs instead of going down the throat.

Eat less meat

If your family is accustomed to eating only beef and chicken, try this easy way to prepare fish. Start with fillets, about one-inch thick, completely boned, either fresh or frozen. Broiling is the easiest and quickest way to cook them, and the shorter the cooking time the more nutrition is retained. Spread a thin coating of melted butter or olive oil on the fillet and broil about five minutes on each side, longer if frozen or if fillet is more than an inch thick. Before serving, sprinkle with dill weed, paprika, curry power, or whatever spice you prefer, then squeeze on some fresh lemon juice or place lemon slices on the serving plate as a finishing touch.

Between-meal snacks

Make between-meal snacks nutritious and not just something to fill up on. If you or the children are ravenous and supper isn't ready, try raw vegetables or fresh fruit. If the apple or orange you offer a hungry little one is sliced, peeled, and cut into small portions, even the most finicky little eater is unlikely to refuse. Even if a light eater's appetite is somewhat lessened by the before-meal snack, it really doesn't matter as long as the snack is nutritious. Just consider it part of his meal. Many times a nutritious morsel is gobbled avidly when handed out beforehand when it might have been scorned had it appeared cooked on a dinner plate. This reminds us of a mother who routinely cooks only half of the vegetables for a meal, serving the remainder raw at the table so each child can take his choice. You'll have to be careful of raw carrots, though, for the child under three. They may not be chewed properly, and can be inhaled rather than swallowed. Young children can usually handle other raw vegetables and fruits quite well.

Frozen snacks have special appeal in hot weather. While toddlers are teething, frozen foods can also be soothing to sore gums. Some nutritious frozen snacks are: yogurt and fruit juice popsicles, frozen blueberries, strawberries, grapes, slices of peach or pear, and even frozen green peas. Frozen bananas on a stick are much better for your children than ice cream bars.

Dried fruits, including raisins, are nutritious, but should not be eaten as a daily snack. They are hard on the teeth because of the high natural sugar content. Because of their sticky texture they also tend to stick in the crevices of the teeth, evading the toothbrush and thereby contributing to tooth decay. In addition, many dried fruits have been dipped needlessly in honey or rolled in sugar. Sun-dried fruits with no sugar or honey added, make excellent sweeteners for cakes, cookies, or muffins made from whole-grain flour. Used in baking they are less harmful to the teeth.

Quenching your thirst

Unsweetened fruit and vegetable juices provide food value as well as quench your thirst. There are many varieties of canned or bottled apple, grape, tomato, grapefruit, and pineapple juices that are unsweetened, with no chemical additives. Mixed flavors of juices are popular now, too. Frozen orange, apple, grape, and mixed juice concentrates are also available in unsweetened brands. Freshly squeezed orange or grapefruit juice is delicious when available. Try adding carbonated mineral water to fruit juice for a bubbly treat.

If you begin having these juices on hand, chilled and ready, your family will learn to enjoy their natural sweetness. Of course, you'll want to completely avoid buying colas and other soft drinks or sodas. If they aren't even in the house, the natural drinks will be more appealing.

Don't forget water! To really quench one's thirst there is nothing like it! Sometimes when it comes from the refrigerator or from a brightly colored container, it may seem more appealing   than if it is just "plain old water from the faucet." A slice of fresh lime or lemon in a glass of ice water on a hot summer day both looks and tastes refreshing. Because of the pressure to serve soft drinks, parents have to be patient and persistent in resisting, and imaginative in providing substitutes. The currently popular practice of carrying a bottle of fresh water everywhere is one that should be encouraged.

Grow it yourself

One of the best suggestions we can offer is to plant your own vegetable garden. If you have space in your yard, so much the better. If not, see if your local park district offers small plots of land to would-be gardeners. Or see if a friend or neighbor would like to lend you space in return for a few fresh fruits and vegetables.

There is something very special about the smell of a garden growing—the pungent scent of tomatoes, the sweet-sharp smell of carrot tops. And most of all, you'll have a great feeling of pride and satisfaction when you discover that the seed you planted is now a full-grown vegetable or fruit waiting for you to eat. Children will often eagerly eat the food they've picked from the garden which they would otherwise refuse to try.

An advantage of growing your own vegetables is that they will be free of the chemicals commercial growers use in the soil, as well as free of the pesticides that are sprayed on the plants during various stages of growth. Unfortunately, some of these chemicals remain on the skin of the fruit or vegetables and cannot be washed off. When you peel them to get rid of the chemicals, you also lose some valuable nutrients. With homegrown produce, it's a choice you don't have to make.

Special Hints for Nursing Mothers

We stated earlier that if you have good eating habits, there is no reason for you to make any major changes when you are breastfeeding. You do have to remember to eat enough to keep yourself in good health. Eating well is part of being a good mother.

A few reminders

Nursing mothers just naturally feel the need for extra liquids and should drink enough to satisfy their thirst. You can drink water, fruit and vegetable juices, milk, soup, or other liquids. In the excitement and bustle of caring for a new baby, you may not always notice that you are dry and thirsty. Some mothers take a drink of water whenever they sit down to nurse the baby and carry bottled water with them when they go out. If you are eliminating large amounts of pale yellow urine, you are probably drinking all you need.

Constipation (hard, dry stools) may be a sign of inadequate fluid intake. If you get constipated, increase your liquid intake as well as your consumption of fresh fruits and raw vegetables. And be sure you're getting enough whole grains (breads and cereals). Avoid commercial remedies. In fact, it is better to try to prevent the problem by starting during pregnancy to see that your kitchen is well stocked with high-fiber foods and fruits and vegetables so that it is easy to eat the right foods. Many new mothers have

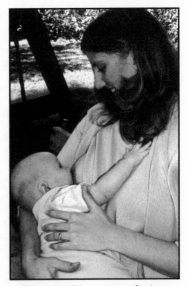

Eating well keeps you feeling good so you can enjoy nursing your baby.

found that raw pears are especially effective for keeping bowels loose. Prunes, raw or cooked, and prune juice are also helpful. Some find a good helping of cooked greens is all that is needed.

Milk products and other sources of calcium

You don't have to drink milk in order to make milk for your baby. If you are allergic to milk, you don't have to drink it at all. Cow's milk is a good source of calcium but it is also a very common allergen. If there is a history of allergy in your family you might want to cut down on or eliminate milk during your pregnancy as this is when some babies become sensitized to it. The reaction shows up after the baby is born.

Even if you are not sensitive to cow's milk, you may not care for it. It is good to realize there are other products that will provide the calcium you and your baby need. Yogurt, hard cheeses (such as cheddar, Swiss, and Parmesan), and cottage cheese are good sources of calcium. Many people with milk allergies can tolerate at least small amounts of these. Blackstrap molasses and calcium-enriched tofu, a soybean product that is becoming more widely available, are also good sources of calcium, as are bok choy, broccoli, collards, and kale. Sesame seeds are especially rich in calcium. They can be added to baked goods, muffin or pancake batter, or sprinkled on salads or cereal.

Generally, meat and nuts are not good calcium sources, but three exceptions worth noting are liver, almonds, and Brazil nuts. In the fish family, very high calcium is found in canned sardines and canned sockeye red salmon, both of which are normally eaten with bones. These bones, unlike the thin sharp bones found in most fish, are usually round and soft enough to eat. They provide a nice crunchy contrast to the softer consistency of the fish. Mashing or blending canned salmon makes a handy spread for crackers or bread.

Caffeine and soft drinks

If you are accustomed to drinking lots of coffee, tea, or cola, you may wonder how the caffeine will affect your baby.

Excessive caffeine intake by the nursing mother may cause a reaction in her baby. The amount of caffeine in five or fewer five-ounce cups of coffee (less than 750 ml) will not cause a problem for most mothers and babies. You may be getting additional caffeine from tea or colas. Caffeine is also found in some over-the-counter medications. If you suspect that caffeine may be causing fussiness in your baby, cut down for a week or two and see if it helps. Since people do become addicted to caffeine, cutting it out abruptly may give you a headache for a day or so. Some mothers use herbal teas without caffeine and most brands of herbal tea are safe to use in moderation. However, certain herbs can be potent if taken in large amounts. In general, it's best to get most of your daily liquids in water, juice, or milk and limit your intake of coffee or tea.

Remember that in addition to caffeine, soft drinks contain lots of sugar and no food value. Sugarless soft drinks are not good either. Sugar substitutes, like aspartame and saccharine, may be easier on the teeth but could be hazardous to your health and they don't really satisfy your appetite. These artificial sweeteners should not be given to children. Remember—if you as a parent consume soft drinks daily, you can be sure your children will want to follow your example.

Supplements

Many people today report good results in preventing or eliminating certain deficiencies by taking vitamin or mineral supplements. Of course they are only supplements—they do not substitute for good food.

Your doctor may advise supplementary vitamins and minerals for you during pregnancy, particularly iron, to replenish the stores from which your baby is building up his own supply of iron to carry him through at least his first half year of life. During the time you are breastfeeding, your doctor may suggest that you continue taking them.

It is important for a mother who is on a vegan or macrobiotic diet that includes no animal protein to take a vitamin B12 supplement in order to avoid a vitamin B12 deficiency in her baby.

Weight Loss and Exercise

Mothers often wonder if it's possible to lose weight while breastfeeding. The answer is yes. In fact, breastfeeding makes it easier to shed the extra pounds put on during pregnancy. Those pounds were put there, after all, to store energy for producing milk. New mothers who do not breastfeed have to depend on diet and exercise for weight loss. Breastfeeding women have a head start, because the caloric demands of milk production are already using up extra energy. Studies have shown that breastfeeding mothers tend to lose more weight when their babies are three to six months old than mothers who consume fewer calories but are not breastfeeding. Of course, patterns of weight loss are highly individual and depend on diet and activity levels as well as whether you are breastfeeding.

According to Dr. Judith Roepke, a retired nutritionist and a member of LLLI's Health Advisory Council, lactation may be an ideal time to lose weight. Lactation seems to mobilize even fat accumulated before pregnancy. But it's important to go slowly. Dr. Roepke suggests that nursing mothers do nothing to consciously bring about weight loss during the first two months postpartum. Your body needs that time to recover from childbirth and to establish a good milk supply, and most breastfeeding mothers will lose a few pounds anyway while eating to appetite. If after two months you haven't lost any weight, you probably need to increase your activity level as well as decrease your caloric intake by cutting back on fats and sweets. Put the baby in a stroller or baby carrier and head out of doors for a two-mile walk five times a week. At the same time, eliminate just 100 calories from your daily diet (the equivalent of one tablespoon of butter or oil) and you can expect to lose two or three pounds in a month. Not a dramatic weight loss, but one that guarantees that you and your baby will both stay well nourished. And the exercise has benefits that go beyond pounds and inches.

Some questions have been raised about the effects of exercise on a mother's milk. One widely publicized study suggested that mothers should avoid nursing right after exercising because of changes in the composition of their milk. Other studies did not show this same effect; in fact, one study showed that breastfeeding mothers who exercised regularly had a higher milk volume than those who did not exercise.

After reviewing many studies of breastfeeding mothers who exercise, researchers concluded that moderate exercise during breastfeeding is safe and beneficial for most women.

Crash diets, fad diets, and quick weight loss present problems for nursing mothers. In the past there was concern that losing weight too quickly would release environmental contaminants into a nursing mother's blood and increase the levels in her milk. However, more recent research shows that this is not a risk. Exceptionally high protein/low-carbohydrate diets are potentially harmful for breastfeeding mothers because of substances released into the milk by the mother's altered metabolism. Any kind of drastic weight loss carries the risk of a drop in milk supply.

Many mothers find that weight loss takes care of itself while breastfeeding. Steering clear of sweets and "junk foods" (high-calorie foods with little nutritious value) and concentrating on good nutrition are often all it takes. Good nutrition will also help you combat the fatigue and emotional ups and downs that are an inevitable part of new motherhood.

PART FIVE

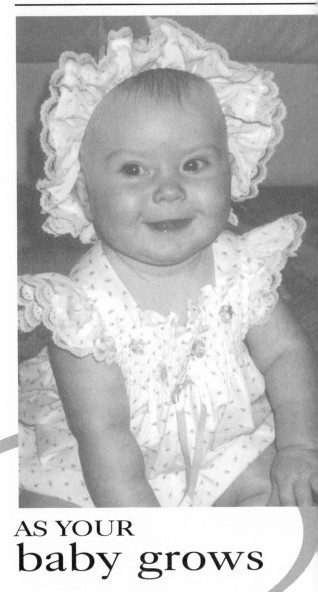

AS YOUR
baby grows

CHAPTER THIRTEEN

READY FOR
solids

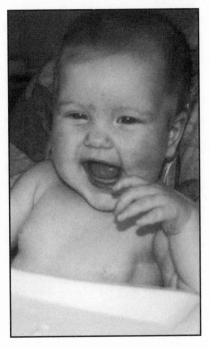

H and in hand with formula feeding of babies, a trend toward feeding solids earlier and earlier in infancy developed and took hold in the United States. A spirit of rivalry and competition arose among mothers (and sometimes doctors) to have the biggest baby who ate the most foods in the largest quantities at the earliest possible age. The baby food industry promoted and encouraged this trend. Mothers were led to believe that there was an advantage in giving early solids.

Today medical scientists all over the world have verified that human milk gives the best assurance of proper nourishment because it is nature's complete food for the baby. Young babies do best without the early addition of solids to their diet. Human milk is the perfect food for at least the first six months for the healthy, full-term infant, and there is usually no reason for adding any foods to the breastfed baby's diet before that time. In its 1997 recommendations, The American Academy of Pediatrics advocates only human milk for six months for the full-term breastfed infant.

There are at least two good reasons for waiting to start your breast-fed baby on other food. First, you want to maintain your milk supply, and the more solids the baby takes, the less milk he will want; the less he takes from the breast, the less milk there will be. Research has confirmed that babies who start solids early balance their energy intake by reducing the amount of mother's milk they consume. When solid foods replace human milk in a baby's diet, it decreases the protective anti-bodies the baby receives. Starting solids too early substitutes an inferior food for a superior food.

The second reason for waiting is that the younger the baby, the more likely it is that any foods other than mother's milk will cause food allergies. Most solid foods are poorly digested by a young baby, and may cause an unpleasant reaction in a two-month-old, but are readily assimilated by the same child if they are delayed until he is six months or older.

Until his immature digestive system develops to the point where it can utilize other foods without upsets, it is both kind and wise to give the baby the benefit of a few extra months of the food that is perfectly suited to meet his needs.

Some babies with a tendency to allergies will refuse solids even at seven or eight months. This could be nature's way of protecting that baby from foods that will cause him problems. Such babies can continue to do well on human milk alone until their systems are ready to tolerate other foods.

At some point around six or seven months, most babies start to teethe, and your baby's natural urge to chew and bite begins to develop. His mouth and tongue are ready for the new skills he will need, and his digestive system is probably ready to handle new foods. Your baby will let you know when he is ready; watch him, not the calendar.

Vitamin supplements

Vitamin supplements are not routinely recommended for a breastfed baby. If the nursing mother gets an adequate supply of vitamins from her diet, her milk will have an adequate supply of vitamins, in just the right proportions for her baby. Research continues to bear this out. Your physician may suggest that you continue taking prenatal vitamins while you are breastfeeding. As long as your baby is thriving on your milk alone, he has no need for additional vitamins, iron, fluoride, or other supplements in the early months.

The exception to this could be vitamin D. The amount of it in human milk is small. Sunlight is the normal source of vitamin D for

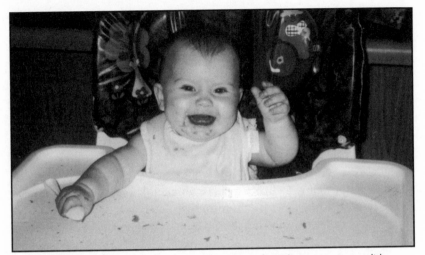

Watch your baby not the calendar for signs of readiness to start solids.

babies and adults. However, problems associated with overexposure to sunlight have caused various medical groups to advise limiting or avoiding exposure to sunlight in young babies and suggest instead that all babies be given a vitamin D supplement. More information on vitamin D is found in Chapter 18.

Baby's first foods

By the time babies are ready for solids, they are also ready and able to sit up with support and they just naturally want to put everything in their mouths. The simplest way to begin solids is to sit baby in his chair or, if he prefers, on your lap, and let him experiment with a tiny taste or so of his first food.

These first feedings of solid food usually go more smoothly if you nurse your baby first, to take the edge off his appetite. Otherwise he will be in no mood to try something new. With practice and patience on your part, he will catch on soon enough. These first few attempts are merely to introduce the idea of solids to him, not to fill him up. At first, use a small spoon and place just a small amount of food on it, about a teaspoon or less. If you have an independent baby who balks at spoon feeding, provide him with finger food, small bites of food he can pick up and put in his mouth by himself. Learning to grasp small finger food like cooked peas or beans will help him gain finger control and coordination. By the time he is one year old, he will probably be feeding himself with very little help from you.

A word of warning is in order here. Most babies have an excellent gag reflex and manage to get up anything that goes down the wrong way. But while your little one is learning to handle food all by himself, you don't want to leave him alone and walk away. Also be sure your baby is not given any foods to teethe on while he is lying down, as these could go too far back into his throat and cause him to choke.

Go Slowly at First

New foods should be introduced one at a time. This means a single food, not a mixed food like stew or soup, or even a mixed-grain cereal. The reason for this precaution is that although the baby of six or seven months is not nearly as likely to have an allergic reaction as a younger child, it is still possible. If you introduce foods one at a time and he develops a rash or a sore bottom, which are potential indications of allergy, you will know what the most likely cause is and can eliminate the food temporarily. Wait until baby is at least a year old before introducing foods that cause allergic reactions in other family members.

It is a good plan to allow a week between each new food introduced. There is no advantage to be gained by striving for the widest variety of foods in the shortest time possible. Rather it is good for the baby to be given the opportunity to experience each new food thoroughly before going on to another. Start with a teaspoon or so of a new food once the first day. Increase the amount little by little until by the end of a week he is getting as much as he wants two or three times a day. He will probably let you know when he has had enough by turning his head, clamping his mouth shut, spitting the food back out, or some other unmistakable gesture. Take his word for it. Don't start feeding problems by coaxing, pushing, or forcing. Give him only as much as he wants, not what you think he should have.

Babies have likes and dislikes about foods, as we all do. So if your baby turns away from any particular food, don't panic. Just skip it and try something else. Even if he has happily consumed a whole banana every day for a week, and suddenly he won't look at one, go along with him. He's not sick—just sick of bananas.

Once a food has been started, try to keep at least a bit of it on his menu once a week or so thereafter, to avoid the possibility of an allergic reaction if it is reintroduced after a lapse of time. This precaution should be kept up during the baby's first year.

Neatness doesn't count

Now is not the time to worry about neatness. A hungry baby is easily frustrated when he is suddenly attacked by a wet washcloth instead of another tasty bite of food. Squelch your tidy impulses for the time being. Your baby is just learning the basics of eating and isn't ready for lessons in manners yet. Put a big bib on him and move his chair off the rug or put a sheet of plastic under it. (A hungry dog is handy for cleaning up under the high chair!)

You will avoid some messes, though, and make the learning process easier for him, if you have only one thing at a time on his tray—one piece of the finger food, later one unbreakable dish with a small serving of one food, and (not at the same time) a small unbreakable cup with a tight-fitting lid and a spout. Keep servings small and let your baby ask for more.

What Foods to Choose

Most of us find it unnecessary to use commercial baby foods at all. They are relatively expensive, and some varieties contain undesirable fillers and preservatives. If you do use commercial baby food, read the labels to determine exactly what is in them. Though improvements have been made in recent years, for most babies, starting with table foods is easiest and best. If you understand good nutrition and your family's eating habits are pretty good, then the food from your table will be fine for your baby, too. This also makes the transition to family meals easier. (See Chapter 12, "Nutritional Know-How.")

In her excellent book about preparing nutritious food for little ones, WHOLE FOOD FOR BABIES AND TODDLERS, Margaret Kenda writes:

> The baby food you create yourself is stunningly superior [to commercial baby foods]. Besides huge advantages in nutrition, you can give your baby other advantages with your own baby food.... Your child will know how fresh foods taste. Your growing child will naturally prefer the best, most nutritious food....You will have given your daughter or son a lifetime advantage.

She goes on to explain that making your own baby food does not have to be complicated:

> You really don't need any special cooking equipment. Many beginner foods can be cooked along with food for adults, leaving out spices and other ingredients for which the baby is not ready. Many baby foods can be mashed with an implement as simple as a fork.

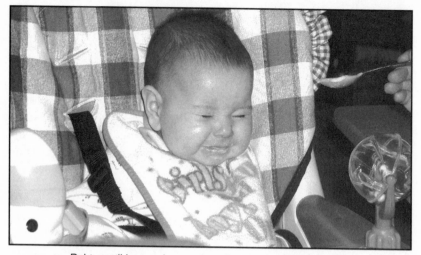

Babies will let you know when they are not ready to eat.

A blender, baby food grinder, or food processor can be used to make some table foods easier for baby to manage. However, mashing the food with a fork works nicely for most things you'll be giving him. If baby is six months or older when he's starting solids, he does not need foods pureed or liquified.

Suggested guide for introducing solids

Fresh, Mashed Banana. This is a good food to start with, since it is fresh and wholesome and contains more food value than cereals. Babies usually love the smooth consistency of a ripe banana. After you've given your baby a small taste the first time and gradually increased the amount, you can offer the baby a whole piece of banana to handle himself, thus quickly eliminating one mashed food as well as pleasing the baby who likes to feed himself, and mash it himself, too...between his fingers!

If your baby doesn't care for banana, sweet potato (yam) and avocado are good alternatives. It is preferable to bake the sweet potato whole to preserve the nutrients. Sweet potato has a fine flavor and maximum food value. Avocado has a smooth consistency and is high in vitamins and iron. You can slice off a piece and refrigerate the rest for another day. Most babies love it.

Meat. Meat is introduced early among solid foods because of its high iron and protein content. In vegetarian families, other foods high in protein may be substituted for meat. It is not difficult to reduce table meats to a consistency right for baby. Chopped beef, stew meats, or tender pieces of chicken can easily be cut up into small pieces or mashed with a fork. Better yet, scrape across a piece of raw meat with a knife. Tough connecting fibers will remain behind while the tender portions can be gently cooked for baby to eat.

When baby has had a week or so on one meat, try handing him a good-sized bone with no splinters or sharp corners, but with a few fragments of meat still on it. A chicken drumstick is good, and just about the right size for his grasp. (Be sure to remove the needle thin splint bone and gristle cap on the end.) Chances are he will chomp away on the bone with great relish, especially if he has the urge to chew and bite. He'll be developing muscle coordination in the process, too.

To make sure you have on hand the kind of meat your baby can handle, keep individual portions of cooked, chopped, or scraped beef or chicken, wrapped and frozen. When you have meat at the table that might be too difficult for the baby, you can quickly prepare a small portion of frozen meat for him.

Fish is another excellent protein food and quite easy for baby to eat, but it is a common source of allergy. If allergies are not common in your family, and your menu often includes fish, you can introduce it carefully to your baby. Watch out for bones. Check each piece between your fingers before giving it to baby. And wait until baby is older to introduce smoked and pickled fish or shellfish.

Whole-Grain Breads and Cereals. Finger-sized pieces of dried or toasted whole-grain bread are good chewing foods for your baby and handy to offer him, perhaps between meals or while you are preparing dinner. Whole-wheat bread is the type most commonly available, but other whole-grain breads are also good. If you regularly serve a cooked whole-grain cereal you might want to introduce this; but be sure there is no sugar or other sweetener added, and cook it with water, not milk. Avoid mixed-grain cereals until baby has been introduced to each one. Baby cereals do not have quite as much food value as your own freshly cooked whole-grain cereals because they are more highly processed. They are an additional expense as well.

Another nice thing about whole-grain toast (or a day-old heel of the loaf) is that it's good for spreading things on. A very thin layer of smooth peanut butter or almond butter, for instance, is a popular spread, once baby is old enough to handle it without choking. (Be cautious of peanut butter in families with a history of allergy.) Be sure to buy the natural spreads, without added sweeteners and preservatives. Later on, cheese and other homemade nutritious spreads can be used on the bread.

Fresh Fruits. Raw, peeled apple or pear can be grated, or scraped with the edge of a spoon, and put in a little mound on baby's high-chair tray. It won't be long before you can hand him a piece of peeled apple, ripe pear, or peach to munch on. Apricots, plums, and melons are good, too. If baby is eight months or older, other fresh fruits in season may be offered, but with caution. Some berries have seeds that babies are not old enough to handle well and some tend to cause allergic reactions, especially strawberries.

Frozen blueberries make wonderful finger food; baby will love the cold, crunchy taste, especially if he's teething. They do leave stains on baby's clothing so a large plastic bib may be useful. Citrus fruits and citrus juices can cause allergy, so wait with those until baby is about a year old. Tangerine segments are good to start with, but be sure to take all the seeds out.

Avoid canned fruits that contain sugar. They have less food value than fresh fruits, but unsweetened canned fruits are better than no fruit at all. Dried fruits such as raisins, dates, or figs should not be given at all in the first year, and later only on a limited basis. Although they are nutritious, they tend to stick between the teeth which can cause tooth decay.

Vegetables. Sweet potato and white potato are both good choices for baby. Don't add butter or margarine to baby's portion. He'll enjoy the natural flavor of the food without these enhancements.

Finely grated raw carrot can be mixed with grated apple or some of the other foods baby is getting. Cooked carrots are good, too. Other cooked vegetables may be offered from your table one at a time, just as you do with any new food. Some little ones enjoy frozen vegetables right from the package—especially frozen peas they can pick up and pop into their mouths one at a time. Wait until baby is about a year old before offering corn or tomatoes, as these are potential sources of allergy.

Don't be concerned if, in the beginning, you find little bits of vegetable, virtually unchanged, in the diaper. Even cooked vegetables are harder to digest than many other foods.

Raw vegetables have more food value than cooked vegetables, but most of them are too hard for a little one to chew and digest. Some raw vegetables—particularly carrots and celery—can be dangerous as small chunks can be inhaled rather than swallowed.

Eggs. Since eggs, especially the whites, seem to be a common cause of allergies, it's usually best to wait until the baby is about a year old before introducing them. At first the egg should be hard-boiled. Place the egg in water and bring to a full boil. Remove from heat, cover, and let stand for twenty minutes. Peel under cool water. Feed baby only the yolk at first, mashed and moistened to suit his preferences. Start with no more than a quarter-teaspoon and increase gradually, a quarter-teaspoon at a time. After baby has been eating eggs well for a month or so you can give him scrambled eggs. Babies usually love to eat them as a finger food. Or cook an egg in with his cereal for extra nutrition.

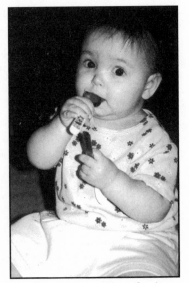

Some babies like to feed themselves right from the start.

Cow's Milk and Other Dairy Products. If there is a history of allergy in the family, or baby has already shown signs of it, avoid cow's milk entirely. The only milk your baby needs is yours. In some parts of the world, adults do not drink milk at all, but eat well otherwise, and the people are healthy and well-nourished.

Cottage cheese, yogurt, and natural cheeses can be introduced when baby is nine or ten months old. These dairy products provide calcium and other nutrients and they are much less likely to cause allergies than regular cow's milk.

Introducing the cup

At some point during baby's first year, you can start offering your baby water or juice from a cup once a day at mealtime or in between, whichever suits you best. There's no need to rush. A tip on getting the baby started with a cup comes from Betty Wagner: let him drink through a short straw. (The bendable kind works well.) The sucking comes easily to him, and it's neater too—no drips or dribbles. Or, try the kind of plastic cup that comes with a tight-fitting lid and a spout.

Baby's beverages should consist mainly of your milk, water, homemade soups (canned soups may contain a lot of salt and preservatives), and unsweetened fruit or vegetable juice. Dilute the juice with water so it is not so concentrated. Giving babies or toddlers too much fruit juice has been found to contribute to malnutrition by decreasing their appetite for wholesome foods. Limit fruit juice to four ounces or less per day. No soft drinks or colas please—these are heavy on sugar or sugar substitutes and sometimes caffeine, and are lacking in anything worthwhile. Soft drinks with artificial sweeteners such as aspartame or saccharine should also be avoided. There is still no substitute for a good drink of water.

What to avoid

You will notice that from the beginning we are suggesting you feed your baby wholesome, nutritious foods. We would strongly urge you to avoid processed foods that are full of sugar, salt, dyes, preservatives, and chemicals.

Once you have given your baby the best start by breastfeeding him, we are sure you'll want to continue along those lines when he starts to eat other foods. Your baby will do just fine without cookies, pretzels, teething biscuits, puddings, cakes, and ice cream. Let him first develop a taste for the natural sweetness of fresh fruits and the natural goodness of whole grains. Now is the best time to start developing habits of good nutrition that will last a lifetime.

Raw honey should also be avoided for babies under one year old because it may contain bacteria that causes infant botulism.

The whole process of starting your baby on solid foods may take from three to six months. Once he's eating a variety of foods without any signs of allergy or distress, you can be less concerned about mixing foods or introducing something new. As long as what you offer him is good, nourishing food, you can let his appetite be your guide as to what he wants to eat and when he wants to eat it.

As you are getting your little one well launched in the eating department, you'll want to learn as much as you can about good nutrition for your whole family. LLLI's cookbooks—WHOLE FOODS FOR THE WHOLE FAMILY, WHOLE FOODS FROM THE WHOLE WORLD, and WHOLE FOODS FOR BABIES AND TODDLERS—will give you good suggestions for keeping baby, and everyone else in the family, deliciously well-fed. For details, see the Appendix.

CHAPTER FOURTEEN

WEANING GRADUALLY,
with love

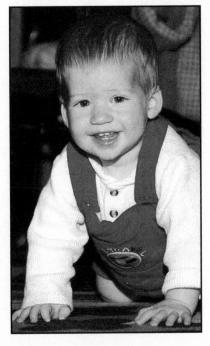

"When shall I wean my baby? How shall I go about it? How long will it take?" Some mothers begin to worry about weaning when their infant is only a few weeks old.

Why do mothers begin worrying about ending breastfeeding almost as soon as they've started? No doubt there are many reasons, but we suspect that not the least among them is the fact that society often expects babies to be weaned early. Mothers are uneasy about the thought that their babies might still be nursing after everyone expects them to be weaned from the breast.

We don't agree with society's attitudes about early weaning. We believe that ideally the breastfeeding relationship should continue until the baby outgrows the need.

One mother who had weaned because of criticism from others, had this to say about her decision: "I let pressure from people prematurely end one of the most meaningful experiences I have had with my son.... I wish I had it to do all over again now that I am more sure of myself."

More Than Milk

Your milk continues to provide special benefits for your baby as long as you nurse him. It doesn't lose its goodness with the passing of time. Research has shown that the immunological benefits of human milk that protect your baby from illness in the early months continue to offer significant protection as your baby gets older.

If we consider breastfeeding only as a means of nourishing the infant, then we can see why it might be feasible to bring nursing to an end as soon as the baby can handle a variety of solid foods and drink from a cup—perhaps even before his first birthday.

It is when we view the breastfeeding experience as a whole, when we understand that the baby has emotional needs which can easily be satisfied through the closeness of breastfeeding, that it is hard to understand why we must set a specific time for ending this important, intimate relationship. If we do not satisfy these needs when our children are small, they may be as undernourished emotionally as they would be physically if they were deprived of an important nutrient in their diet.

Emotional needs

The breastfeeding mother and her baby build a relationship based on their mutual needs, and the relationship changes gradually as the needs change. One of the most urgent needs of the tiny baby is food, and during this period of infancy the mother's physical need is to be relieved of the milk that fills her breasts for the sake of the baby. However, the mother and baby depend upon each other for many other things. The baby needs affection, and the mother enjoys responding to his need to be loved. The mother has a strong desire to be truly needed by this tiny one. But at some point, usually gradually, the baby's dependence on mother lessens. He begins to broaden his horizons, to try his wings. But nursing is still important, for it is a secure haven in a sometimes difficult world.

When the baby does not wean by a year or so, a mother may wonder if this means he is too dependent on her. She may fear that letting him continue to nurse will prevent him from growing toward independence. But weaning is a step toward growing up and, like walking or talking, a child takes these steps according to his own timetable. All children stop nursing sooner or later. Some have the need to continue the nursing relationship longer than others—but they do grow out of it eventually. And still they do not become overly dependent. We have been reassured on this point many times over because we have observed firsthand hundreds of babies who were considered "late weaners."

Independence, not dependence, is one outstanding trait they seem to have in common as they grow up.

In the American Academy of Pediatrics book, *New Mother's Guide to Breastfeeding*, editor Joan Meeks, MD, writes:

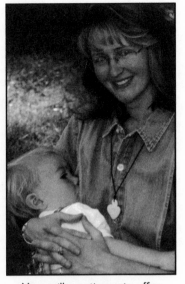

Your milk continues to offer significant benefits as your baby gets older.

> **Certainly there is no evidence that extended breastfeeding makes a child more dependent or harms him in any way. On the contrary, many parents proudly tell how independent, healthy, and exceptionally bright their long-term breastfed children become. As long as you are comfortable breastfeeding your toddler, there is no reason to stop.**

Dr. William Sears, author and pediatrician, confirms this with his observation: "Some of the most physically and emotionally healthy children in my practice are those who have been breastfed in terms of years."

Remember, too, that as he gets older your baby will not be nursing as often as he was at two weeks or six months. The toddler who is "still nursing" may only be enjoying a bedtime snack or a "pick-me-up" when he bumps his head or has caught a cold. Nursing is so comforting to him when he's ill and your milk continues to provide antibodies that help him recover sooner.

Still nursing?

Keep in mind that all children wean eventually. Young children have a tremendous desire to move on to the next stage of development. You are certainly not out to set a record for prolonged nursing. Nursing a toddler is not something you strive for, but it is part of a very special relationship between mother and child.

One mother, Susan Redge from Michigan, tells how she and her son grew into and out of this special relationship:

> **When my son was a newborn and he and I were at our first LLL meeting, the mother sitting next to me was nursing her**

two-year-old. I assumed that she came to get help with weaning. I was surprised to hear that instead she was there to
learn more about toddler nursing. I was sure I would never
need to learn about toddler nursing!

When my baby was about eight months old, my mother-
in-law couldn't understand why he didn't eat solid foods.
Although I had offered him solids, he didn't seem too interested and I knew he was thriving on "mother's best." I was
savoring our nursing time because I knew it couldn't last forever.

By the time he was a year old, my husband said "Don't
you think he ought to quit? After all, it's been a year." I was
ready for that and told him all about baby-led weaning and its
benefits to both mother and baby. "Why some even nurse
until three years old!" I said. "But, of course, our child will
certainly wean before then!"

By the time he was two, I couldn't imagine not nursing
him. I didn't think he would ever go to sleep without it. I was
pleased that out of our chaotic life I could take time to relax
and nurse knowing that I could close my eyes and the plants
would be safe, he wouldn't be cracking eggs on my living
room rug, or having a tantrum, or doing any of the other
things two-year-olds might do. I felt real sympathy for mothers of two-year-olds who did not nurse.

By that time, no one asked me about nursing anymore.
Most people assumed that he was weaned. I never dreamed
I'd be nursing this long! He nurses at night to go to sleep,
maybe once more in the wee hours, and usually once during
the day.

The most important thing I have learned from La Leche
League is to meet my child's needs. As a baby, he needed to
be held close and nursed often. As he has grown, his needs
have changed. He needs to know I am there for him and there
are still times when nothing else but nursing can calm him.
I've had the thought countless times that it is nursing that
soothes the savage beast. It has many times turned a kicking,
screaming, out-of-control toddler into a calm, smiling, confident and contented young man, bravely ready to face the
world.

Now he's been telling me that only babies nurse, and he
is a big boy. Sometimes he even falls asleep without being
nursed. I probably will not have a nursing toddler much

longer. I just hope I can continue to satisfy his needs as easily and with as much joy when breastfeeding is no longer a
part of our lives.

Natural weaning

"But when will he wean?" you ask, as your two-year-old holds up his
arms to be picked up and nursed again. Actually, he's been weaning
himself ever since his first bite of solid food. "To wean," says the
Concise Oxford Dictionary, is "to teach the sucking child to feed otherwise than from the breast." While many people see weaning as the end
of something—a taking away or deprivation—it's really a positive
thing, a beginning, a wider experience. It's a broadening of the child's
horizons, an expansion of his universe. It's moving slowly ahead one
careful step at a time. It's full of exciting but sometimes frightening
new experiences. It's another step in growing up.

In her warm and insightful book, MOTHERING YOUR NURSING
TODDLER, Norma Jane Bumgarner talks about the "unpredictable
course of natural weaning." She says there will come a time "at some
age" when "your child will not find nursing so absolutely essential to
her well-being. She may stop asking so often. Or she may be distracted
sometimes from nursing....You will very naturally and with hardly a
thought respond a little less quickly to her requests to nurse.... In
time—how much time no one can say—your child will abandon all but
a few favorite nursing times."

Norma Jane goes on to describe how some children will continue
to enjoy one or more of these special nursing times for a while, dropping them ever so slowly until eventually they are weaned. She concludes: "Every natural weaning is unique so that it is impossible to
guarantee anything about it except that it will happen."

In Diane Bengson's book, HOW WEANING HAPPENS, mothers
describe a wide assortment of weaning experiences that range from
early to late, abrupt to gradual, natural to planned. The book reassures
parents that weaning is a natural process that does not have to be
stressful for either mother or child.

Author Diane Bengson explains:

The age when weaning happens is influenced by many factors. Your life circumstances, your baby's needs and personality, your needs and feelings—all of these figure into your
baby's unique weaning timetable.

What If I Want to Wean My Baby?

Each of us must make decisions about breastfeeding and weaning in keeping with our family situations and personal circumstances. Perhaps you do not agree with the concept of natural weaning or you don't think it will work out for you. Before you decide that circumstances will make it necessary for you to wean your baby, think over all possible alternatives. Perhaps there are some compromises that could be made in order to allow your baby to nurse at least once or twice a day. Stop and think about whether weaning your baby will really improve matters. Norma Jane Bumgarner says, "Nursing makes the job of mothering easier, not harder." Remember that illness, medications, surgery, or returning to work do not necessarily mean you must wean before you and your baby are ready.

If at all possible, you'll want to take your time with weaning and proceed slowly. We talk about weaning as something to be done "gradually and with love." You'll need to step up the loving attention you give your baby in other ways during the time that you cut back on nursing him.

Basically, weaning is accomplished by substituting other kinds of food and loving care at the times you would usually be nursing. You'll want to eliminate just one nursing at a time, distracting your little one with a cup of juice or water, a story, or a walk around the block at the time he would usually nurse. Wait a few days to allow him to get used to this change and to avoid feeling uncomfortable yourself from over-full breasts, and then tackle another nursing time. This may take up to two weeks or more depending on how many times a day your baby has been nursing. It is not a good idea to rush things. Weaning is a big change for both of you and it takes time to adjust.

Since weaning involves substituting other kinds of food for the nutrition your baby has been receiving from your milk, you'll want to carefully plan how to do this. If you decide to wean when your baby is under a year old, you'll want to talk to your doctor about giving him a bottle and ask the doctor what to put in it. If you are weaning from breast to bottle, you'll be substituting a bottle for some of the times you used to nurse the baby. Remember that your baby was also nursing for comfort and will probably not need as many bottles per day as the number of times he was nursing per day. You'll need to double up on cuddling, rocking, hugs, and kisses throughout the day to make up for this. Instead of holding your little one in the familiar nursing position, bring his face close to yours and hold him cheek to cheek as you rock or comfort him.

With an older baby or toddler who is eating well and drinking from a cup, you'll want to keep tasty things to nibble on within easy reach.

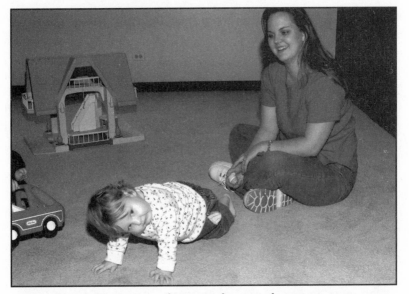

Your little one will need lots of attention from you if you are trying to wean.

By frequently offering him drinks of water or, occasionally unsweetened juice, during the day, his thirst will also be quenched, often before he even realizes he's thirsty and asks to nurse. Chunks of fresh fruit are good, too—oranges, melons, or peaches. You'll want to be careful to offer foods that are high in protein and nutritious in other ways at his regular meals because he will no longer be receiving the nutrients from your milk.

Go out of your way to make the time at which you are omitting the nursing warm and happy. Your baby's father can be a tremendous help at this time, by taking the baby out for a stroll or putting him to bed at night, and getting up with him if he wakes during the night.

Your toddler may be enthralled by your sudden interest in going for walks, visiting the playground, or doing puzzles. You may need to avoid the situations in which he is accustomed to nursing, such as in a favorite rocker or climbing into bed with you in the morning.

You may need to be flexible, too. If your little one reacts strongly to the idea of not nursing at naptime or bedtime or whenever, you may decide to let him continue with that one nursing for a while. Weaning doesn't have to be an "all or nothing" situation.

This method of weaning "gradually and with love" can be a lot of work. But abrupt weaning can be physically and emotionally traumatic and is never a good idea for you or your baby. By substituting lots of "other-mothering" you can help your little one come through the weaning process with his confidence and trust in you still intact. He may have a hard time understanding why he can no longer nurse, but at least he'll be reassured that his mother has not deserted him. She's still there with lots of love and understanding.

One mother from Missouri, Maggie Bryan, tells how the course of weaning took place with her son:

> While attending La Leche League meetings with my constant companion, Sean, I learned with great surprise about baby-led weaning and witnessed the wonderful closeness of mothers and nursing toddlers. The months slipped by; I was confident that he would eventually decide to stop nursing at his own pace, in his own time.
>
> Imagine my dismay when I found myself becoming increasingly impatient with his continued nursing. I yearned to have a night free of bedtime nursing, to enjoy my bodily privacy once again, and a small thing, to read a few pages of the morning newspaper uninterrupted. It seemed to me that sometimes Sean was using nursing to trap my attention.
>
> Whether or not my perceptions were accurate, my feelings were definitely a reality and had to be dealt with. So, with some trepidation, I decided to try to reduce the number of Sean's nursings and see if my impatience would lessen.
>
> I began to ask him to wait a minute until I was finished with the morning paper, and, to my surprise, I found that he could cooperate for about five minutes. I found that delay also worked well in public situations. I found life with a nursing toddler becoming easier to manage. Sean nursed mainly at naptime, bedtime, and occasionally once at night.
>
> As time passed, Sean began to give up naps and then stopped asking to nurse at night. On the rare occasions when he awakened, his Daddy held him close for a snuggle while he went back to sleep. Then to my astonishment Sean began to prefer to get up and have a bowl of cereal rather than stay in bed and nurse in the morning!
>
> All of a sudden, it seemed, Sean was weaned! But actually the process had taken about six months. Sometimes I led, and sometimes Sean led. But his father and I only encouraged new behavior that he was ready and willing to learn. In this gentle way, I feel weaning was a maturing experience for both Sean and me.
>
> Although our experience was not exactly the way I had imagined weaning would be, it did happen gradually and with love.

Toddler Nursing

Our culture today has geared us to thinking that all babies should be off the breast at an early age. But this is far from the custom that prevailed in centuries past. In biblical days weaning at age three was often mentioned, and still today in many parts of the world children wean themselves at ages up to three, four, or even older. The late Niles Newton, PhD, pointed out that in most periods of history and in most parts of the world babies have been breastfed for two to four years. She also observed that the changes in breastfeeding customs do not seem to have come alone, but in conjunction with a whole body of customs related to child rearing.

Since cultural expectations about weaning vary, anthropologist Katherine Dettwyler decided to do research into the weaning ages of primates and other mammals to determine a "natural" weaning age for humans. She examined criteria such as length of gestation, age of eruption of permanent teeth, relationship of offspring to adult body size and made comparisons to average age of weaning in each species. Using these criteria, she determined that a "natural" weaning age for humans might be between three and seven years. Knowing this may not influence the decision you make about weaning your baby, but it can be reassuring if you and your baby are satisfied to follow a natural weaning and others are critical of this decision.

Benefits of toddler nursing

Fulfilling your child's individual needs is the key. From the moment he is born, a mother strives to respond to the needs of her child. As the child grows, if he continues to express a need to nurse, it is a natural response for a mother to continue to meet this need.

If your toddler continues to enjoy nursing, you may find there are many advantages that continue to go along with toddler nursing. It is so easy to help an overtired or fussy child calm down and often fall asleep through nursing. If he hurts himself there is no better way to soothe him. Because nursing eases frustration, many families find that it helps turn the "terrible twos" into the "terrific twos," minimizing the usual competitive behavior of the two-year-old. Sometimes behavior that is normal for a toddler is blamed on breastfeeding if the child is still nursing. Behavior such as clinging and demanding normally occurs at this age, whether the child has weaned or not.

Traveling with a child is much easier when he is still nursing. Even though you are away from home, your little one can be kept happy with the familiar comfort of your breast.

Your milk continues to provide immunities, vitamins, and enzymes for as long as your child continues to nurse. In one study, mothers reported fewer instances of illness requiring medical care in toddlers sixteen to thirty months of age who were still breastfeeding. If your child does become ill, nursing will be a comfort to him. If he has an upset stomach, he may be unable to keep anything down but mother's milk.

You will probably find it convenient to encourage your child to use a special word for nursing. Choose carefully so that the word can contribute to discreet toddler nursing. One family uses "num num"; another calls nursing "mama." When the child shouts out, "I want mama!" in a restaurant, no one even turns around.

There will be occasions when it would be very inconvenient to nurse a toddler. If your two-month-old infant had begun to scream in a long check-out line at the supermarket, you might have pushed the basket to one side and gone out to the car for a few minutes to feed him. When he is older and has demonstrated the ability to wait and understand the concept of time, you may offer him a nutritious snack and ask him to wait until you get to the car to nurse. If you are about to visit someone you know would be extremely upset to see your child nurse, you might encourage him to nurse before you go, in the hope that he would then not need to nurse during the visit.

Nursing too much?

Many little nursing persons nurse only occasionally, such as to fall asleep or for comfort when they hurt themselves. Sometimes however, a small child nurses much more avidly. If you feel your little one wants to nurse "too much" for his age, take a close look at what is happening in his—or your—life right now. Make sure he has lots and lots of other kinds of attention from you, and provide him with a nutritious snack or story before he asks to nurse. You can talk with him, sing, read, play games, or explore the outdoors together. Let him be a part of the jobs you do. He can wash pan lids while you do the dishes; he can carry socks to the clothes washer and push the vacuum cleaner around.

Is he away from you more than is comfortable for him? Are you home with him but busy with other projects? Are you spending lots of time on the phone or at the computer? Are you going through a time of emotional upset? Moving? Is he making great strides in some other area of growth? Does he have an ear infection, allergies, or other illness? You can probably add your own ideas of things that might cause a child to want the extra reassurance of increased nursing.

When your child asks to nurse, if you are unsure that he really needs to nurse, you may choose to offer him a sliced apple and a story instead of nursing. If the child is happy with this, fine, but if he asks repeatedly or cries to nurse, this would indicate that he feels a real need. You can respect the laws of inner growth and individuality, nursing him with the confidence that he will grow away from this kind of closeness at his own pace.

In HOW WEANING HAPPENS, Diane Bengson discusses the signs that a child may not be ready to wean:

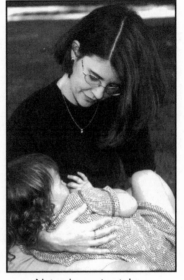

> A child not able to accept substitutes for nursing is telling you she isn't ready to wean.... Seeming distressed and listless is often another sign of not being ready.

Natural weaning takes place according to a child's individual needs.

It may be that the process is moving along too fast for the child. Diane Bengson goes on to say:

> Sometimes a child is upset by the pace of weaning. Even if your child seems ready to wean, it is important to give her time to get used to the idea.... If you suspect that weaning is happening too quickly, the obvious answer is to let your child nurse more often.... Your child may need more time to become comfortable with substitutes for nursing, such as alternate ways to go to sleep or other ways to be reassured of your love and attention.

Some little ones continue to want to nurse several times a night as well as during the day. When your little one wakes up during the night, pick him up, cuddle him, take him into bed with you, and nurse him if he wants it. Then, if he's willing, put him back into his own bed. However, he may sleep better and wake less often if you keep him in bed with you. There are a number of reasons why toddlers want to nurse often at night. He could be teething, which is a common cause for little ones to fret. Perhaps he's hungry or thirsty during the night and needs a nutritious bedtime snack. Or it could be that he's been so busy all day he hasn't had his share of hugging and cuddling and just needs time to be close to you.

What do you do when there's nothing to do?

Sometimes a mother needs to evaluate the nursing relationship she has with her toddler and consider whether things are really going well. In some situations, nursing can become the easy way out, substituting for other kinds of attention the toddler really needs.

An older baby or toddler may want to nurse simply because he has nothing more interesting to do, or because it is the only way to get mother's attention. As your little one is growing out of the infant stage, his need for mother does not really lessen. It changes, certainly, and mothering a toddler requires a great deal of ingenuity and even physical dexterity. His whole being is growing. His mind as well as his body needs stimulation. He needs conversation and a companion to explore and experience all the new and exciting things his broadening horizons have brought into focus.

No one can better share these things with him than you, his very own teacher, guide, protector, and special person. No one knows his "language" as well as you do, nor understands so well his interests and needs. You know best when he's hungry and needs a snack to tide him over until dinnertime. You know when he's over-tired and needs to wind down in your arms.

One mother tells this story about how she realized her daughter needed more kinds of loving attention besides just nursing. Freda Main from Arizona writes:

A month ago Celeste was a two-and-a-half-year-old nursing child who had become increasingly demanding of me. She seemed discontented and often angry at everything and everyone including herself and me. This is not unusual, I know, for a child whose baby sister had come into the family five months earlier. I had always assumed Celeste would eventually stop nursing when she was ready, with no part played by me.

One day the light dawned. I had been thinking, "This child does nothing but nurse!" Then I realized this was precisely the case. I had not stopped thinking that nursing met all of Celeste's needs—as indeed it had for a long time. I had not observed until then that I was not giving Celeste the attention she deserved at times when she was not nursing.

For me nursing had become so easy and effortless that I had fallen into the trap of not growing in my relationship with my daughter. What had always worked so well before was not meeting her needs now.

I began to change my complacent ways. I began faithfully spending time with Celeste each day and giving her my undivided attention. We did many things together: making playdough, collecting Popsicle sticks and gluing them together, and reading many stories. I would sit and hold her and hug her and kiss her even without "nursies." We talked. When my five-month-old slept, I spent the time with Celeste instead of crossing off items from my list of things to be done. We started having regular mealtimes, reading bedtime stories, and following daily routines. I started to be conscientious about eye contact and really made an effort to do less talking and more listening.

To my amazement, in a matter of days the little girl whose nursing I had once seen no end to, was hardly nursing at all. I was becoming more attuned to what she really needed and was giving more of myself to meet her needs.

It was hard for me to change. In weaning myself, Celeste weaned also. Now I no longer think of baby-led weaning as "mother doing nothing." As in everything else, experience is the best teacher.

Night waking goes on

Even if your baby begins sleeping almost all night when he's a few months old, that may not be the end of your nighttime parenting role. Toddlers often wake up at night for a variety of reasons. Many one-year-olds have erratic eating habits and may wake up really hungry during the night. If you think that this could be the reason your toddler is waking at night, be sure there are nutritious foods available to him frequently during the day and offer him a good bedtime snack. Perhaps he is thirsty. Offer your toddler water often, especially in warm weather.

The older baby or toddler who wakes a number of times at night may be bothered by teething. Even though there doesn't seem to be much of a problem during the day, his gums may hurt more at night when he isn't distracted by a busy daytime world. Have you ever had a mild toothache that started throbbing madly just as you were dropping off to sleep? A toddler cannot express what he is feeling in words, but since frequent waking during the night is so common in children during their second year, teething might have something to do with it.

Fatigue or aching muscles might cause a busy and very active toddler to be wakeful. There are other possibilities. Is he getting enough fresh air and exercise? Was there tension during the day caused by such things as long shopping trips or visiting? A frightening experience? A scary show on television? Were there enough hugs and kisses? Too many restrictions? If your answers to these questions satisfy you, and your toddler is still waking at night, blame it on whatever you like and remember that it will pass. Whatever the reason, nursing seems to offer special comfort in satisfying nighttime needs.

Dental Caries

When multiple cavities appear in the mouth of a nursing toddler, parents may find themselves on the receiving end of a stern lecture from the dentist about the hazards of nighttime nursing. As decisions are made about repairing the child's teeth and preventing further decay, the dentist may urge a mother to wean her toddler, at least at night. But what if this child is not ready to give up bedtime and middle-of-the-night nursings, let alone wean completely?

Fortunately, weaning is not necessary, either as a prerequisite for fixing cavities or as a preventive measure to guard against future decay. There is no strong scientific evidence to support the theory that nighttime breastfeeding causes rampant dental caries in older babies and toddlers. Meanwhile, there are many factors other than breastfeeding that are known to influence tooth decay in toddlers and young children. Many mothers have found ways to work with their dentist on improving their toddler's dental hygiene while continuing to meet his emotional needs through breastfeeding. Occasionally, this may involve switching to a dentist who is more supportive of toddler nursing, or at least more flexible about working with families who believe that breastfeeding plays an important role in meeting the needs of small children.

Studies of large populations of breastfed and formula-fed babies do not show a link between long-term breastfeeding and higher levels of dental caries. Researchers have pointed out several ways in which human milk may actually prevent cavities, when compared with infant formula. For example, human milk does not lower the pH level of the mouth as artificial baby milk does. Lower pH levels allow the bacteria that cause decay to thrive; various immune factors in human milk may inhibit the growth of these bacteria. Formula may damage tooth enamel, making it vulnerable to decay. Human milk actually deposits calcium and phosphorus in the teeth, making them stronger.

Researchers have found that human milk on its own, with no other sugars available in the mouth for bacteria to feed on, does not cause teeth to decay. This makes a lot of sense—as dentist Brian Palmer has said, "It would be evolutionary suicide for human milk to cause decay."

Some dentists believe that milk pooling in the mouth as baby nurses is a significant cause of dental caries. Those who are more knowledgeable about the mechanics of breastfeeding disagree, pointing out that sucking at mother's breast delivers milk to the back of baby's mouth, bypassing the front teeth. And since sucking stimulates swallowing, human milk leaves the mouth quickly, unlike formula or juice, which may drip from the bottle nipple into the front of a sleeping baby's mouth. Mothers who are warned that nursing at night may harm their child's teeth should keep in mind that the vast majority of toddlers who breastfeed to fall asleep and breastfeed during the night do not experience dental caries. Often a child with serious tooth decay problems has siblings who nursed at night and whose teeth are fine.

Of course, there is reason for concern when a toddler has a mouthful of cavities. Parents want explanations. Some children are genetically predisposed to be vulnerable to tooth decay. The mother's prenatal diet and stress level may affect tooth formation in the womb, as do antibiotics taken during pregnancy. Certainly the child's diet beyond mother's milk is a contributing factor. Foods that bathe the teeth in sugar cause cavities. Preventing tooth decay is one of many good reasons for feeding your family nutritious whole foods and avoiding sugar-laden treats and soft drinks. Even large amounts of fruit juice can cause tooth decay.

Pediatric dentists recommend that you begin cleaning your child's teeth as soon as the first one appears, especially if the child is already eating foods other than human milk. When tooth decay is a problem, the dentist may suggest cleaning baby's teeth with a soft cloth after every nursing, at least during the day. A few sips of water after nursing can also help to clean the teeth. One mother, whose son had extensive cavities, found that gently taking him off the breast when he finished nursing during the night, and encouraging him to roll to his back, ensured that the last mouthful of milk was swallowed as he drifted off to sleep.

Renee Cox, a mother from Michigan, tells the story of her toddler's experience with tooth decay and what she did to prevent further problems:

My daughter, Katherine, who is four now, had numerous cavities and even has one crown, so I was sure to bring William

in for his first checkup as soon as his first few teeth appeared at about one year. At that point I heard the bad news: four cavities in the top front four teeth.

William's having so many cavities was somewhat surprising. William had very few sweets and very little juice (mostly water, instead). He did nurse on demand and William slept in our bed and nursed through the night.

With a clear understanding that William was going to continue to nurse on demand day and night, my dentist suggested a routine in which we would try to keep his teeth immaculately clean, wipe them with a cloth after every breastfeeding, brush his teeth three to four times a day, and apply a small amount of topical fluoride (being sure to wipe off the excess fluoride). This was a solution that would allow us to continue breastfeeding as much as we needed to and have healthy teeth for William as well.

So we started on this experimental program—wake up, brush his teeth, apply topical fluoride, nurse throughout the day, keep a dry cloth handy, wipe his teeth after every nursing (which he didn't like), go to sleep, nurse at night. I must confess that I did not wake up at night to wipe his teeth with a dry cloth. One of the reasons William is in bed with us is so he can nurse and I don't even have to wake up.

We continued this routine for three months, had a checkup and no cavities. Then we had another three-month checkup and no cavities. Six months with no cavities! Everyone in the dental office was happy for us and even William managed a smile. I was pleased to know that continued nighttime nursing had not caused further decay.

William still protests through every brushing, but at 21 months old he still nurses on demand, is cavity-free, and oh, he has the sweetest smile.

Repairing a mouthful of cavities in a young child may require the use of general anesthesia. Or the doctor may give the child medication that leaves him conscious but very relaxed during the procedure. The child may not be allowed to eat, drink, or nurse for several hours beforehand, because of the medications. Ann Davis of Ohio went through this experience with both of her daughters:

When my daughter was two years old, we discovered caries in two of her teeth. Because the cavities were in molars, which wouldn't come out until around age 12, we agreed that they needed repair. After interviewing several dentists, we found one who told us he could perform the needed work in his office using nitrous oxide and a calming medication. I was able to give the medication to my daughter before leaving for the dental office, which put her in a very agreeable mood. The repair work was completed in just under 30 minutes, to my astonishment, and since the medication was still in effect, she was fine! The dentist did restrict my presence in the treatment room, but I was allowed to escort her to the chair and get her settled. All things considered, I was happy with the outcome.

My next experience with dental caries was more difficult, mainly because our second daughter had more extensive damage at an earlier age. At 17 months, I noticed spots on her teeth, which were confirmed as caries in eight teeth, some with multiple caries. Again, we agreed that repair was necessary. However, because more work needed to be done, our dentist recommended general anesthesia at the local children's hospital.

In both instances, I provided my dentist with literature to support my being allowed to nurse my daughters until just a few hours before the surgery. My dentist was wary, but agreeable. Our first daughter had her work done at an early morning appointment, which made for some difficult nighttime hours, but we coped. Learning from that, we scheduled our second daughter's surgery for around noon. She nursed when she woke up, and then I was able to distract her from nursing by playing with her. This was easier for both of us to cope with than restricting nursing in the middle of the night.

Pregnant and Nursing?

If you find that you are pregnant, there is no sudden need to wean. Your child may wean himself early in the pregnancy when a few little ones notice a taste change in the milk, or he may stop nursing around the fourth month when some women notice a reduction in the milk supply. He may even wean toward the end of pregnancy when the milk changes to colostrum, or after the birth because of the separation if you are in the hospital for several days or because the increase in your milk supply does not suit his taste. If he seems to have a strong desire to nurse in spite of the changes that occur during pregnancy, feel free to continue if you wish.

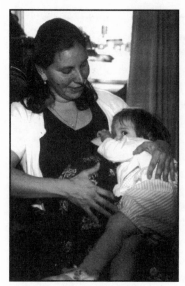

Pregnancy is not a reason to wean abruptly.

In a study of 503 La Leche League members who became pregnant while still nursing, researchers found that 69 percent of their babies weaned at some time during the pregnancy. Of course, there was no way to know how many of these little ones would have weaned if their mothers had not been pregnant.

You may have some concerns about continuing to nurse while you are pregnant. If you are eating a well-balanced diet including a variety of nutritious foods there should be no cause to worry about either baby being harmed. Some mothers may worry that nursing through pregnancy will cause a miscarriage. There are valid reasons to doubt that this would occur and many mothers who have previously miscarried have not done so while nursing a toddler.

In her book, ADVENTURES IN TANDEM NURSING: BREASTFEEDING DURING PREGNANCY AND BEYOND, Hilary Flower reviews current research on the effects of nipple stimulation on the pregnant uterus and concludes that there are safeguards in place during a normal pregnancy that block the effects of nipple stimulation on the uterus until the pregnancy is full term. But what about a situation where the pregnancy is at risk and the mother has been experiencing contractions? Should she wean her toddler?

Hilary Flower goes on to say:

How do you make the best decision? Remember that weaning will not guarantee that the pregnancy will be saved nor will continuing to breastfeed necessarily result in the loss of the fetus. Ultimately a mother must make the decision that best fits her situation as she understands it. Sometimes the answer is weaning...and sometimes the answer is to stay the course.

During your pregnancy, you may find that you are just not happy about continuing to nurse your toddler. In this case, we suggest you consider following the recommendations that are given for weaning "gradually and with love." It is up to you to make the decisions that will work best in your own family.

Again, to quote Hilary Flower:

A mother facing a weaning dilemma must often make a bold decision, one she considers far from ideal. A mother making this difficult choice needs to draw deep into her reserves for honesty and compassion in evaluating her own needs and the needs of her child.... In the end it is a leap of faith.

Tandem Nursing

Continuing to nurse throughout your pregnancy often leads right into a situation called "nursing siblings who are not twins" or more simply, "tandem nursing." Mothers find there are advantages as well as disadvantages to being in this situation.

It can be reassuring to the older child to continue nursing. Sharing these special times with his new sibling can help to avoid feelings of jealousy. You may worry, however, that your new baby will be somewhat deprived of milk or of the intimate one-to-one relationship with just you. Some mothers are surprised by the intensity of their feelings toward protecting the newborn which can cause resentment when their toddler wants to nurse. You may want to restrict your toddler's nursing to only certain times of the day, or establish a rule that he only nurses after the new baby is finished. Most mothers, however, find these things work out and the new baby gets plenty of milk without any problem. It helps to talk with other mothers who have gone through this experience.

One mother, Brenda May from California, tells how nursing two worked out in her family:

When I became pregnant with our fourth child, my son Jon was a very active toddler who still enjoyed his frequent nursings. I soon realized he was not ready to wean himself, and I did not feel it was necessary to encourage him.

By the sixth month of my pregnancy, my lap seemed to completely disappear. This made our nursings somewhat awkward, but with the help of a pillow under his head, Jon continued. As my birthing time grew nearer, my milk supply decreased, and I thought Jon might decide to wean. However, he still continued, seemingly content with whatever he received at the breast.

On the morning of what was to be our fourth child's birthday, Jon and I lay in bed together nursing. It helped me to relax, as my labor had already begun. Six hours later, Jacob Allen was born at home with his family all sharing the experience. That day we began tandem nursing. Jon was twenty-one months old.

For the next three weeks, we spent most of our days nursing. Jon had increased his nursings, and Jake was nursing every hour or so. Soon after, my toddler went back to his regular routine but clearly enjoyed the abundant supply of milk now available.

I didn't know anyone who had tandem nursed; no one in our LLL Group had done it. So I felt unsure at times, but I just trusted my mothering instincts that told me what I was doing was right for myself and my children.

A mother from New Zealand, Juana Atkins from Auckland, tells how breastfeeding her children helped them to establish a strong bond with each other:

When Willow was born, I was not surprised to see how eagerly two-year-old Cadell returned to breastfeeding even though he had been close to weaning before her birth. The bonding between them seemed instant. They held hands and looked into each others' eyes as they fed.

Occasionally, after apparently being completely weaned, a toddler might suddenly ask to nurse again. (This sometimes happens when the new baby arrives.) This request may or may not result in the toddler returning to the breast. A mother from Ohio, Mary Beard, recalls:

After Julian was born, Elliott asked once if he could nurse. I said, "Yes," and he said, "Oh," and walked away. Apparently he only wanted to make sure he could. Once he was reassured, we never heard anything more about it.

And another mother, Mandy Clifton, from Ohaupo, New Zealand, had a similar experience:

After Daisy was fully weaned, a chance remark from a friend of mine asking whether Daisy was still breastfeeding caused Daisy to say to me, "I miss having milk from you." Since I was nearing the end of my pregnancy, I told Daisy I would let her nurse again once the baby was a few weeks old and she

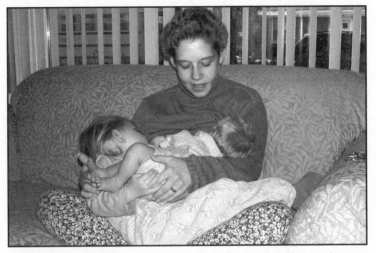

Sometimes a toddler continues to nurse after the new baby is born.

agreed to this plan. When the time came and I offered to breastfeed Daisy, her eyes lit up and she climbed into my lap. However, when she tried to latch on, she discovered she had forgotten how to do it! She was so surprised she didn't even get upset!

If your toddler asks to nurse and he reacts with enthusiasm and delight at the discovery of this bounty, you can relax and let him nurse if you are comfortable doing so. Most mothers who are nursing a toddler along with a new baby have ambivalent feelings about it. Yet they realize that many little ones still need lots of reassurance and continuing to nurse along with their new sibling is one way to provide this.

In ADVENTURES IN TANDEM NURSING, Hilary Flower suggests that a mother consider whether or not she is willing to tandem nurse before she allows her child to resume nursing:

> **Some mothers already know they aren't up for tandem nursing. If you decide that offering the breast is not your best option, you will do well to figure out why your child wants to nurse again, and address that specific need as actively as you can in other ways.**

Jan Wilcke of Kansas writes about her experience:

> **When Ardith was twenty-eight months old, Carrie was born and I weaned Ardith. The weaning would have been too**

abrupt by itself without the added burden of a new sister contending for mommy's affection. Ardith seemed more tense, and I was unhappy about the situation. So, after two months, Ardith began nursing again.

For about six months after that, Ardith nursed twice a day. She now nurses once every few weeks. I believe this occasional nursing is important to her in a different way than it is for Carrie. Her need to nurse occurs quite often when she's had a bad morning, and we're both "nearing the end of our rope." It's as if she's asking, "Do you love me as much as Carrie? Do you love me enough to let me nurse?" I think tandem nursing, while difficult at times, is a wonderful way to reassure a toddler when a new sibling arrives. And a warm lap with some mommy's milk is a safe retreat for the child when the demands of his enlarging world are too much for him.

Several books mentioned in this chapter include information based on the experiences of other mothers as well as advice from experts. MOTHERING YOUR NURSING TODDLER by Norma Jane Bumgarner, has been an LLL classic for more than 20 years. Revised and updated in 2000, it is an excellent resource for mothers who are nursing toddlers, considering weaning, nursing while pregnant, or tandem nursing. Another book recently published by La Leche League International is HOW WEANING HAPPENS, written by another LLL Leader, Diane Bengson. The newest book addressing issues related to weaning and toddler nursing along with nursing during pregnancy and nursing a toddler along with a new baby is ADVENTURES IN TANDEM NURSING: BREASTFEEDING DURING PREGNANCY AND BEYOND, written by Hilary Flower. You can order copies of these books from La Leche League International or your local LLL Group. They are also available in bookstores and through our LLLI Web site at www.lalecheleague.org. See the Appendix for further details.

CHAPTER FIFTEEN

DISCIPLINE IS
loving guidance

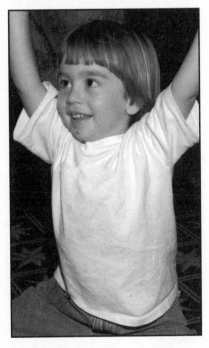

As parents, our goal is to have the wisdom to guide our child's growth so that he can become an independent, mature, loving person, with his talents and abilities developed to their fullest.

Our first job is to meet his physical and emotional needs as fully as we can, so that a secure foundation is laid for his advance to maturity. Through breastfeeding we are getting him off to the right start. The breastfeeding relationship itself makes us more sensitive to his needs, so we are quicker and surer in devising ways of meeting them. As a child grows, his needs change. We must progressively let go of him as he assumes the direction of his own life. This process will not be complete until he is fully grown, but it starts in babyhood. This book, therefore, would be incomplete if we did not look into the beginnings of independence.

Before your baby enters the toddler years, it is important for you and your husband to share your feelings and ideas about discipline with each other as you develop your own style of parenting.

Setting the Stage

Discipline is an integral part of everything we do for and with our children. Having developed a philosophy of mothering our babies and toddlers through breastfeeding and weaning, we are now ready to go on to develop other aspects of mothering our young child. "If you have been doing a good job of mothering, you are already doing a good job of disciplining," says Dr. Hugh Riordan, psychiatrist and LLL father.

A need for guidance

As the baby-child grows, he will need guidance, instruction, and sometimes correction to learn the ways of our world. If the foundation of secure love was laid when he was a baby, and if he sees his parents as kind, polite, and considerate people, he will try to imitate them, because he wants to act in ways that will please them (most of the time). We still have to respect his growth patterns and not ask of him more than he is capable of giving at his stage of development, but we can and should give some direction to his inexperience. How to do this is where the difficulty often lies. Before we can successfully begin to discipline our little ones we must have a clear idea of why we are doing what we are doing and how we should go about doing it. There should be no sharp break in our ways of guiding our child's development. From infancy on, children need loving guidance which reflects acceptance of their capabilities and sensitivity to their feelings.

Elizabeth Hormann, an experienced mother and La Leche League Leader, wrote this about toddlers' needs:

> We would like to think that children learn the civilizing virtues—caring, compassion, consideration—simply by our good example, but most children need a little more than that. A clear definition of acceptable behavior, our expectation that they can meet that standard, and periodic guidance when they stray—all of these are necessary. Sometimes we have to thwart our wee ones....We have to be alert so that they don't hurt other people or their possessions; we need to know the difference between the normal behavior of toddlers and small children and behavior that becomes disruptive and out of hand. It is not easy to guide a small child when she clearly wants to go in another direction, but she needs us to do that for her.
>
> It is not really so very different from what we did when they were babies. We looked to their needs, met them, and tuned out the critics who said we were spoiling them or baby-

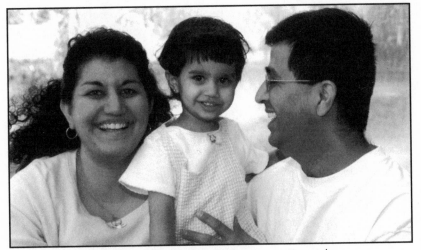

Parents need to develop their own parenting style.

ing them or ignoring our own needs too much. We were confident we knew our babies and ourselves best—and for the most part, we did. That hasn't changed. We still know our children better than anyone else does. Because we know them and love them dearly, we are better equipped than anyone else to guide them through the complex steps of growing up, of learning the rules, of developing character.

Guiding our children—lovingly—is an important part of caring for them and helping them be loving and lovable to people within our families and beyond. Next to breastfeeding, it is the best gift we can give a small child; and like breastfeeding, the benefits last a lifetime.

Discipline and Punishment

Discipline is a much maligned word, often associated with punishment and deprivation. Yet discipline actually refers to the guidance which we as parents lovingly give our children to help them do the right things for the right reasons—to help them grow into secure, happy, and loving persons able to step out into the world with confidence in their own ability to succeed in whatever they set out to do.

In *The Discipline Book* by William and Martha Sears, the authors explain their approach to discipline based on their professional knowledge and their personal experience raising eight children:

Discipline is grounded on a healthy relationship between parent and child. To know how to discipline your child you must first know your child.

They go on to explain:

Wise disciplinarians spend time and energy keeping one step ahead of their child and setting conditions that promote good behavior, leaving the child fewer opportunities to misbehave. Wise disciplinarians:

- stay connected to their children

- develop a mutual sensitivity between parent and child

- spend more time promoting desirable behavior, so they need less corrective discipline

- have a working understanding of age-appropriate behavior

- use humor to promote cooperation in the child

- are able to get behind the eyes of their child and redirect behavior.

In discussing the role of punishment in discipline, the Sears' believe that it must be used wisely:

The child who is punished too much (or too severely) behaves more out of fear of punishment or the punisher than for the satisfaction of behaving right.

William G. White, MD, an experienced family practice doctor and father, offers the following observation:

The goal of parenting is not to produce good children, but good adults. The "good child" is marked by docility, the good adult by character.... The word "discipline" comes from the word "disciple." ... Discipline, therefore, is not punishment. Children are not Pavlov's dogs, to be programmed with rewards and punishments. They are human beings, persons of infinite worth and dignity. They deserve not only to be treated as persons, but to know that we regard them as persons, that we value them, their intellects, their wills, their feelings, their desires, their needs, their judgments as much as we would have them value ours.

What about spanking?

Outwitting a determined toddler is a challenge. His pranks and explorations are to him just innocent fun but they may be dangerous or destructive. It's our job to teach him and set limits for him. But we have found that in the long run, spanking a defiant toddler only leads to tears, resentment, and an uncontrollable (and understandable) urge to hit a baby brother or sister. Our children learn by examples they see, and parents are the ones they most desire to imitate. So we must ask ourselves what kind of example we want to set for them. Punishing young children by spanking and slapping reflects the impatience and frustration of the parent. It is not the kind of behavior we want our children to imitate. Spanking does not help a child learn self-discipline.

In their book, *The Irreducible Needs of Children,* T. Berry Brazelton, MD, and Stanley I. Greenspan, MD, emphasize:

> Physical punishment, such as hitting or spanking, is no longer an acceptable alternative to discipline. Discipline means teaching, not punishment. Physical punishment is not respectful and is bound to undermine the child's self-image.

As psychologist Eda LeShan writes in her book, *When Your Child Drives You Crazy*:

> Is spanking a helpful, constructive form of discipline? No, it is not. Unequivocally! It may relieve our anger and clear the air when the atmosphere has gotten pretty tense and wound up, but it does not teach any constructive lessons about human relations, and after all, that's what discipline is all about: the way in which we try to teach our children to live in a civilized fashion with themselves and others....
>
> Even when we think we are being rational about spanking, we're still not teaching any terribly valuable lessons. We say, for example, "I have to give you a spanking in order to make you remember how dangerous it is to run across the road." The lesson there is: "Here I am, a grown-up—a college graduate, even—and the only resource I have at my disposal to teach you the dangers of traffic is physical violence!" What a discouraging picture of human potential!

Of course, there are other things parents do that can be harmful to a child. Physical punishment is only one aspect. Parents can under-

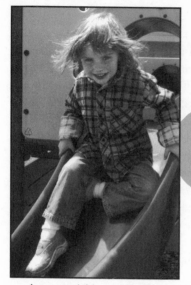

A young child needs lots of opportunities to have fun.

mine a child's self-esteem in other ways, too. Nancy Samalin, author of *Loving Your Child Is Not Enough*, explains:

Children take criticism from a parent very personally. They feel attacked by someone whose admiration they crave.... Children need appreciation and praise, not indifference and criticism.

No child ever has too much self-esteem. If you take every opportunity to point out what children do well, praise them descriptively for it, and express appreciation, your child will become more cooperative, competent, and confident.

Normal Toddler Traits

Parents sometimes find it difficult to make the changeover from the total giving that a baby needs to the more active role of meeting the needs of a toddler. Over the years many of us had to unlearn some of the attitudes about discipline we had been raised with. We learned to relax a little, laugh a lot, and be incredibly quick on our feet.

A large part of mothering a toddler is helping him through the transition from babyhood, when his every wish was a real need, to later on, when he becomes an outward-looking youngster just starting to become aware of the needs of others. In the process he needs help in learning that not all of his wants are needs, and in fact, some of them, if granted, would most surely not be good for him at all. As the infant becomes a toddler, parents need to begin to set limits.

While most people tend to respect the growth pattern of the infant, the eighteen-month-old or two-year-old is another story. When little fingers reach for electrical outlets, coins go into mouths, and lamps are toppled over, parents face a new challenge. Of course, we can't permit utter chaos in our home, or unrestricted freedom. But we need to recognize that another stage of growth is taking place. The toddler is discovering the world around him, as he wants to touch, feel, and take apart everything he sees. He is an inquisitive two-year-old private eye, investigating everything. This is normal behavior for his age; punishing him is entirely out of place and will only frustrate him. That doesn't mean that you should do nothing at all. What's needed here is distraction and firm but gentle steering in another direction.

Not all children are alike; with some it is only necessary to caution them a few times about a forbidden object. If a child can learn to respect a few taboos without being nagged or scolded and without frustration on his part, then this method is fine. Usually it is wiser to remove dangerous or breakable objects from sight.

If your explorer discovers a "forbidden" object, one good way to satisfy his curiosity is to sit down with him and let him touch, feel, and even hold it himself. Show him how the electric hair dryer works, and explain in simple language, with lots of gestures, that we must be careful because it can be dangerous, break, or come apart. Give him plenty of time to explore it with your guidance. Than change the subject, distract him, and put the forbidden article away—out of sight or reach or, better yet, both. (Remember that toddlers are great climbers.)

An ounce of prevention

The time-honored adage, "An ounce of prevention is worth a pound of cure" can be most important in avoiding upsets with our busy little toddler. "It makes good practical sense," says Nancy Stanton of Florida, "to baby-proof your house as much as possible, because otherwise you'll spend your entire day battling with your child. It's hard enough to protect your child against the things you have no direct control over (such as cars on the street), so, especially if you have several preschoolers, keep your home environment as simple as possible."

Nancy continues: "With very active toddlers, extreme measures are sometimes necessary to preserve your sanity. Someday you can put the knobs back on your kitchen cabinets. Most likely you have already given up at least one lower cupboard to your toddler anyway. Be sure to fill it with real utensils—pots and pans, plastic bowls, large spoons, and spatulas."

Dangerous situations

In the case of a really dangerous situation such as chewing on an electric cord or running out in the street, mother should allow herself the full emotional expression of her fears; the child will gradually adopt these justifiable fears of real dangers and avoid them. A sudden shriek of alarm, accompanied by some fast footwork gets the message across pretty well when your little one reaches for the electric plug or runs toward the street.

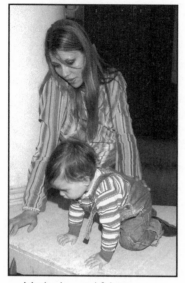

Mother's watchful presence keeps a little one safe.

In any case, always keep an eye on your toddler, for his own safety. Pediatric experts who have carefully studied accident patterns in the very young child state that it is only when a child has reached the age of approximately three that you can begin to teach him how to protect himself. Until that age he can only be protected by the watchful eye of his caretakers, and it's up to you to make sure the eyes are there.

In their book, *The Irreducible Needs of Children*, T. Berry Brazelton, MD, and Stanley I. Greenspan, MD, say that:

During infancy, toddlerhood, and preschool years, children should always be in the sight of caregivers.

Look to the cause

When your little one is crabby and uncooperative, there may be a variety of reasons. Is he tired? Bored? Hungry? Over-stimulated? Sometimes figuring out the cause of misbehavior is a good way to avoid future problems.

Little children (like grown-ups) are often at their worst if they are over-tired or hungry. Nancy Stanton observes: "Toddlers usually need some extra sleep in the daytime, but they don't want to miss anything. If your child is really tired, stop everything—close the drapes, turn off the TV, don't do anything yourself—put a pillow on the floor and both of you lie down."

Or maybe his behavior is a signal to mother, telling her it's time to stop talking on the telephone, visiting with the neighbors, or working on the computer, or whatever it is she is doing that takes her away from her little one, mentally if not physically. It's time to get back down on his level and notice him.

Say what you mean

"Come in the house right now, Kate," you call for the fifth time. Kate, still ignoring your summons, goes right on playing. Do you really want her to come in "right now" or don't you care? If you don't care, then don't call her until you do. Then, call her once. Wait a couple of minutes and call again. If she doesn't respond, go out, scoop her up, and carry her cheerfully and speedily into the house. She will soon learn that you mean what you say.

"To a young child, a call to stop playing and come in for lunch may be asking too much," says Edwina Froehlich, one of LLL's co-Founders. "Try going out there ten minutes in advance with a nutritious snack you know he'll like, and when that's finished start the getting-in process."

Limit television time

Television programs can be a tremendous influence on young children's behavior. You need to monitor the kinds of programs your children watch as well as how much time they spend watching TV. A young child needs to learn from a variety of activities and interactions. Television does not offer the opportunity for these types of learning. What children do learn from TV may not be in keeping with your family's values. Preschoolers often cannot distinguish fantasy from reality and programs depicting violence can be particularly upsetting and frightening for them.

But often, it's not so much what's happening on the television screen that causes the biggest problem—it's what's not happening that matters most. Too much television interferes with active communication among family members.

There are, of course, educational programs directed toward young children which you may find of value. As a parent, you have the responsibility to make informed judgments. Even so, you need to be aware of the hazards of commercials. A child can be enticed into wanting expensive toys and non-nutritious food products simply because he is bombarded with advertising campaigns.

Some mothers prefer to allow their children to watch videos for a limited amount of time, instead of tuning in to a children's TV station that plays continuously. Videos have another advantage over regular television shows because there are no commercials.

In 1999, the American Academy of Pediatrics issued a controversial statement that said no child under two should be allowed to watch TV at all. The AAP was concerned that TV watching is too passive and keeps toddlers from enjoying healthier activities that are important for their development. In their book, *The Successful Child*, Dr. William and Martha Sears explore the topic of children's TV watching. They say:

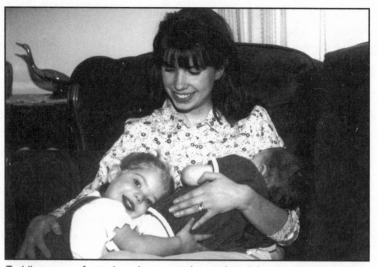

Toddlers are safest when they are right nearby while you nurse the baby.

> **During the first two years, especially, babies and toddlers need direct interaction with caregivers to develop to their full potential.**

They also discuss the increase in aggressive behavior seen in children who have been exposed to violence on TV and in video games. They conclude:

> **As with many issues in child rearing, decisions about television watching require a balanced approach.**

Temper tantrums

On the subject of toddlers and tantrums, Edwina Froehlich recalls her own experiences:

> **Temper tantrums can be devastating to both mother and child. Having had to cope with two children who had tantrums, I did learn a little. I followed the usual suggestions with the first boy—a spank on the bottom made him scream harder, of course; trying to firmly take him to his room was hard on my shins; a stern reprimand couldn't be heard over his screaming. Ignoring him was the best of the lot, since at least it didn't add to the child's hysteria. Still, this neither solved anything, nor prevented future tantrums. As I became better informed about our nutritional needs, I became aware**

that the timing of the tantrums often coincided with periods of hunger. They seldom occurred immediately after a meal. Once in progress, you can't stop a full-blown tantrum by offering food, but understanding the cause at least enables you to cope better. Better still, it can perhaps show you the way to help prevent or at least lessen future tantrums.

When our youngest was about two-and-a-half, a friend had come for lunch, and Peter had his first tantrum! I went over and sat on the floor beside him and reached over to pat him gently. At first he literally threw my hand back at me. So I just sat by him and waited, whispering, "I love you Petey." Soon, he rolled himself over to me, burying his face in my lap sobbing. When the storm was over he had forgotten what started it and we trotted immediately to the kitchen. While I was relieved to know that I had been able to calm him, I girded myself for repeat performances. To my surprise, he had only two or three more tantrums, and they were mild and quickly over.

If your child has tantrums often, try to determine if there is a pattern. Do the tantrums occur at the same time each day? Only with certain people? What seems to be the source of the frustration? Can you possibly remove the source? Do what you can to avoid the frustrating situations that cause him to explode.

If your child does have a tantrum, he'll calm down sooner if you remain calm and nonthreatening. As soon as the child will permit it, touch him gently and try to help him recover. When the sobbing has stopped you can offer him a nutritious snack if you suspect he is hungry, but be sure it is not a sweet, or he may react with another tantrum soon afterward.

The tantrum a child throws in public is no harder on him than if he were at home, but it is agonizing for the parent. Onlookers are quick to show their disapproval of your "naughty" child. Embarrassing though it is, the basic approach to handling the tantrum is the same— the parent cannot react in anger, but must remain calm and speak in quiet, soothing tones. Both mother and child are in a state of distress in this situation, but the child is the more helpless of the two. He cannot just turn off his rage on command. If it is at all possible, pick the child up and move to a more secluded spot where he will bother fewer people. Any attempt to reason with him in this highly emotional state will be wasted. It may be that the only thing you can do is stand by quietly and wait it out.

The biting child

What about the child who bites or hits? This seems to be a rather common problem, and a difficult one, especially when other children are around. Norma Jane Bumgarner, from Oklahoma once told this story:

> About two years ago (at an LLL meeting), my beautiful, superbly mothered, absolutely perfect toddler was bitten by somebody's rotten, neglected, little monster—or so it appeared to me at the time. As I comforted my baby I shot reproachful glances in the direction of the little culprit's mother, making no attempt to hide the feelings we all have when somebody hurts our child.
>
> As proof that there is justice in the world, our next child turned out to be not only a biter, but the most determined, dangerous biter I have ever seen. This is one of the most difficult things I have ever dealt with in my life, and it was made even harder for me by those few mothers who reacted the way I did two years ago.

Naturally, when we realize this is going to be a problem with our youngster, it behooves us to be ever watchful and intervene by removing him from the scene with great dispatch and firmness. Speed is of the essence. Yelling, spanking, or biting the child back doesn't solve the problem. Diane Kramer of New Mexico writes, "Young children are usually very oral in reaction. They use their mouths to feel, to love, to test, and to argue, and it takes time and maturity for them to realize that not all these reactions are acceptable. Meanwhile, love them, cuddle them, help them through their frustrations, and recognize that this too shall pass."

If your child seems to resort to biting when confronted with groups of children, you may need to avoid these situations for a while. Help him learn to get along with just one other child at a time, with careful vigilance as he does so.

The sandman cometh not

In some families, bedtime is a source of frustration, with everyone ending up exhausted and exasperated before finally getting to sleep. Planning a course of action ahead of time may help to avoid disaster! While it may not matter whether or not your preschooler goes to bed at a predetermined time every night since he doesn't have to get up early the next morning, some bedtime regularity is a good idea.

Don't set bedtime too early though, or he just won't be sleepy. Children can only sleep a certain number of hours, and if your child goes to bed at seven, he may be up bright-eyed at five in the morning. You can't have it both ways.

When bedtime comes, make it a cozy, quiet time, with no rush or hurry. A warm bath with time to play in the tub, a nutritious snack such as an apple, with tooth brushing afterwards, and a quiet story while you snuggle together under the covers, all lead to a relaxed little person, ready and willing to go to sleep. He may want you to stay with him for a while, and of course, you should. It's scary all by himself.

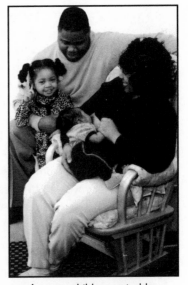

As your children get older, parenting becomes less intense but it is always challenging.

A Look Ahead

As your children get older, discipline becomes even more of a challenge. Children will keep pressuring you, testing the limits, on into their teens. If they know that you are and always have been firm and consistent and loving, and that you trust them, it will be easier.

As you set limits for your older child you may find that at times he may be really angry with you, but he'll get over it soon as long as he knows that you really love him. Show him you love him by your actions, even when you have to say "no." As Dr. Ross Campbell reminds us: "The first fact we must understand in order to have a well-disciplined child is that making a child feel loved is the most important part of good discipline."

Whatever happens, remember that each child is an individual, and you can't have hard and fast rules that will be appropriate for all children. In this matter of discipline, what works for one child or one family may not work for onother. Decide what works for your family. If you have the intimate understanding of your little one that the breastfeeding relationship fosters, and if you are clear in your mind about the real nature of discipline, you can safely follow your own instincts as parents. "It's not our job as parents simply to take care of our children, but to help them learn how to take care of themselves," says Norma Jane Bumgarner.

When your child is born, you devote yourself to meeting all of his needs; you nurse him when he is hungry and hold him close as long as he needs and likes it. As he grows, he wants less snuggling and more sociability; you prop him up in the midst of the family from time to time. As the days and weeks and months go by, he becomes more independent in other ways; he starts eating solid foods and does not nurse so long or so often. Soon he picks up bits of food to bring them to his mouth himself. And one day, he is feeding himself, handling a spoon with dignity and aplomb, albeit with occasional spectacular messes. Now he is drinking from a cup, and as the months speed by, taking no more than a friendly nightcap from the breast. You are still there when he needs you. Secure in knowing that he can retreat for a bit into babyhood if he wants to, he ventures further and further into childhood, and finally (all too soon, it seems in retrospect), he isn't a baby anymore. Before you know it, he will be on his way to school, with a cheerful wave good-bye as off he goes.

The years go by, and though parenting does get somewhat less intense, it is always challenging and interesting. Our children will never stop needing us in one way or another, thank goodness! But we have to learn when to stand back and when to offer our help. And someday, your little boy will be standing over his own wife as she happily nurses their baby, or your daughter, looking so like her mother at that age, will be proudly nursing hers. All the work and worry, the time and the endless patience, will have paid off. It was all very much worthwhile.

With your understanding guidance, your child will grow from dependence to independence gradually, and always with the love that is his birthright and the great need of our world.

PART SIX

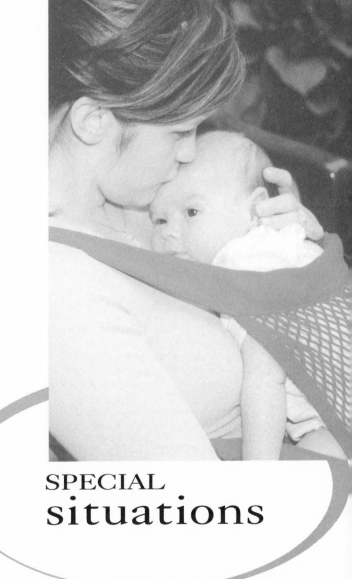

SPECIAL
situations

PROBLEMS AT THE
beginning

For some mothers and babies, breastfeeding may get off to a slow start because of unexpected challenges, such as a cesarean birth or problems with jaundice. These kinds of difficulties should not keep you from breastfeeding your baby. With information, support, and a determined attitude, you can work things out and go on to enjoy many happy hours of feeding your baby at the breast. The extra effort pays off. Your baby will benefit from the good nutrition and immunological protection available in human milk, and both of you will treasure the closeness and convenience of just sitting down to breastfeed.

Breastfeeding after a Cesarean Birth

Of course you can breastfeed your baby after a cesarean birth. You will probably get off to a somewhat slower start, however, as a cesarean section is major abdominal surgery, and it will take time to recover. If you know you are going to be having a cesarean, you'll want to find out in advance as much as possible about cesarean births. But whether you are reading this before or after having a cesarean birth, you can be confident that you and your baby can still enjoy a happy breastfeeding experience.

271

Be sure to discuss the choice of anesthetics with your doctor ahead of time, if possible. While a general anesthetic may be the easiest to administer and may be necessary in an emergency situation, it will make you unconscious for the birth and drowsy for some time afterwards. Your baby may also be sleepy at first. This may postpone your first contact with the baby you have waited so long to hold and nurse. A regional (spinal or epidural) anesthetic allows you to be conscious so you can hold and nurse your baby soon after he is born.

It is important to breastfeed your baby as soon as possible not only because of the importance of early contact and bonding, but also because breastfeeding helps the uterus to contract and return to its normal size more quickly. This also aids healing.

Breastfeeding can begin on the delivery table in the operating room, although you will need help in positioning and holding the baby. Because you will still have an IV in one arm, and the other arm may be strapped down while the doctors finish stitching the incision, it will be difficult for you to maneuver the baby. The baby's father or a nurse can help you place the baby tummy down on your chest to nurse, moving him gently toward your nipple.

If you are breastfeeding for the first time in the recovery room, position baby so he can reach your nipple easily. You may have to lie flat on your back due to the anesthesia, so make sure he is well supported and close enough to you to easily latch on. You should be fairly comfortable, if the anesthesia is still in effect. Again, feel free to ask for assistance in positioning the baby.

The early days

Rooming-in is a wonderful way to get to know your baby and get nursing off to a good start. Some hospitals do not allow rooming-in for cesarean mothers for the first twenty-four hours, but most are becoming more flexible about this. Mothers find it comforting to have their babies with them all the time. Plan on having your baby's father, another family member, or a friend with you to help with the baby.

For the first few days after giving birth your abdomen will be sore and tender. Most medications that are given for pain will not affect your baby through your milk, so do not feel that you must endure discomfort. You and your baby will get off to a better start if you are comfortable.

Babies born by cesarean may be more lethargic than those born without the aftereffects of anesthetics. It may take a few days for these effects to wear off, and your baby may temporarily have a weak sucking reflex. Pay special attention to the baby's sucking patterns and

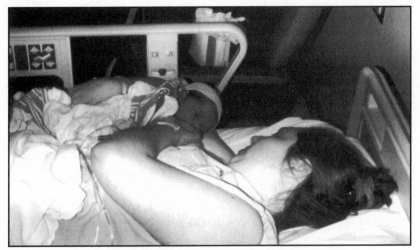

Nursing early and often is important after a cesarean birth.

how he latches on to your breast. It is especially important to avoid the use of artificial nipples that can interfere with the baby's efforts to learn how to breastfeed effectively. If baby is showing any signs of difficulty in latching on or sucking effectively, check to see if the hospital has a lactation consultant on staff who can assist you. Or contact your La Leche League Leader for further help.

Positioning while lying down

It may be easiest to nurse while lying down for the first day or so. You and your baby can nap together, enabling you to spend more time with him without becoming fatigued.

With the bed in a flat position, have a helper raise the side rails of your bed and place extra pillows behind your back for additional support. Carefully roll to one side while grasping the side rail and relaxing your abdominal muscles. Move slowly to avoid any strain. Cover your abdomen with a folded towel or rolled-up blanket to protect you from baby's kicking. Flex your legs and place a pillow between them for more support and less strain on your stomach muscles. Lean back into the pillows behind your back.

Ask your helper or a nurse to place the baby on his side facing you so you are positioned chest to chest. Baby's head may need to rest on your arm or a rolled-up blanket to bring his mouth up to the level of your nipple. In this position, the baby should be able to latch on well.

It is important to nurse on both breasts at each feeding in the early days, which means you will have to roll over. Turn your hips a little at a time with your knees bent and your feet positioned flat on the bed. Move slowly, being careful not to pull suddenly on your incision. Again, use the side rails to help. Reposition the pillows and have a nurse help you ease the baby onto the other breast.

Once your incision is less tender, you can roll over in bed by yourself while holding the baby on your chest. Use the technique described above while securely grasping the baby.

Positioning while sitting up

It is wise to use several different nursing positions in the early days in order to speed your recovery. Some women prefer to nurse while sitting up in bed or in a chair.

Place the head of your bed upright while elevating your legs slightly. Flex your legs from time to time to help circulation. Prop a pillow (or rolled-up blanket) under the arm that will support the baby's head and place baby on a pillow over your incision. This not only raises him to your nipple, but also protects your sore abdomen. Hold baby very close, with his whole body facing yours, resting his head on your arm for support. This allows your free hand to support your breast.

Football hold or clutch position

This is a good way to avoid direct pressure on your incision as baby is lying beside you, not on your lap. While sitting in an upright position, tuck a pillow under one arm. Place baby's head close to your breast, facing toward you, with his body tucked under your arm. His body should be bent at the hips, with his bottom against the back of the chair or bed you are leaning against. Support the back of his neck with your hand. Be sure he is up at the level of your nipple so you are not straining forward to reach him.

When you get home

Because you have had major abdominal surgery, as well as having given birth, you will need plenty of rest when you go home. Put the baby in a cradle next to your bed or right in bed with you so you don't have to get up and down. With plenty of diapers, a pitcher of juice or water, and a snack, you'll be set for several hours. You'll both get lots of rest while getting to know one another.

If at all possible, find someone to come and help out with cooking and household tasks while you rest in bed. Ask friends to bring meals, entertain toddlers, or do laundry.

Some women have trouble adjusting to a cesarean birth when they had envisioned themselves giving birth vaginally. Major surgery, especially when unexpected, can be upsetting when other plans had been made for the birth experience. Mothers who have had cesarean births may want to get in touch with a support group for opportunities to share their common problems and experiences. Many mothers who have previously had cesarean deliveries have been able to deliver subsequent babies vaginally. For further information, see the Appendix. La Leche League can also help you through your local Leader, who can provide suggestions, support, and more information about breastfeeding and mothering after a cesarean birth.

Ann Hague, a mother from Georgia, writes:

> **After a cesarean, a mother and baby may have to be more patient and persistent, but the rewards are well worth it. My surgery healed nicely, and my baby and I are experiencing a beautiful relationship through breastfeeding. A cesarean birth can be an apprehensive time, but it should not rob you of the remarkably loving experience of breastfeeding.**

What If Your Baby Is Jaundiced?

Your baby may be only hours old, but more likely he is two or three days old. You notice that the whites of his eyes as well as his skin have a yellow cast. Or maybe he looks as though he's been to the tropics and acquired a golden tan. The doctor informs you that the baby is jaundiced and may refer to the bilirubin level in the baby's blood.

Jaundice is common in babies during the first weeks after birth and tends to occur more often in breastfed babies. In almost all cases, it is harmless and no treatment is necessary. The jaundice disappears, and the baby is none the worse for the experience. You can continue to nurse your baby, and both of you can be assured of receiving breastfeeding's ongoing benefits. In fact, nursing your baby soon after he is born and frequently thereafter is an excellent way to keep jaundice from becoming a problem. Even when treatment is necessary, there are a number of ways to avoid any separation between mother and baby. Knowing more about jaundice will help you understand what is happening so that you don't have to feel anxious about your baby's welfare. Understanding jaundice will also help you communicate more effectively with health care providers.

Normal or physiologic jaundice

Jaundice in the newborn is a common and usually harmless condition. More than half of all newborns appear jaundiced in the days after birth to a mild or moderate degree with no ill effects. In most cases the jaundice will disappear by itself in two to three weeks.

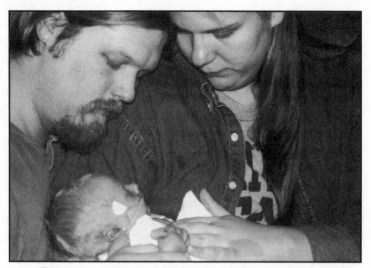

Parents are understandably frightened when their newborn
has a serious health problem.

Normal newborn jaundice is called "physiologic jaundice." This
means the jaundice occurs as part of a normal physiologic process.
Jaundice itself refers to an excess of bilirubin being temporarily stored
in the baby's blood and tissues. The bilirubin is an orange-yellow pig-
ment which gives the baby's skin the yellowish cast that is characteristic of jaundice. Bilirubin comes from the normal process of breaking
down extra red blood cells, part of baby's adjustment to life outside
the womb.

In the normal course of events, new blood cells are continually
being produced and old ones broken down. Newborns have an excess
of red blood cells because the oxygen supply in utero is limited and
the baby needs the extra red blood cells to carry oxygen. After birth,
the baby's lungs supply plenty of oxygen and the extra cells are no
longer needed.

The breakdown of these old cells releases iron and bilirubin, a
residual product of the process. The iron is stored in the liver and
other tissues to be used later in the manufacture of new blood cells.
Bilirubin must be disposed of by the liver. When a newborn's immature
liver cannot eliminate the bilirubin as fast as it is produced, the excess
is stored in the tissues and the result is jaundice. To determine if
treatment is needed, the bilirubin level is measured, using a special
meter held against baby's skin or with a blood test. If the baby has an
abnormally high level of bilirubin, or if levels are rising rapidly, these
tests may be repeated several times a day in the first week in order to
monitor the changes in the bilirubin level.

Physiologic jaundice usually appears on the second to fourth day in normal, full-term babies. In most cases, it gradually disappears by itself, although this may take several weeks in some babies. Normal jaundice is not a disease; it is a harmless condition that has no aftereffects. In fact, because physiologic jaundice appears more often in breastfed babies, some experts believe that higher bilirubin levels may be nature's norm for newborns; they actually may have a beneficial effect.

Jaundice starting on the first day

Pathologic or abnormal jaundice is often visible at birth or within the first 24 hours, and the bilirubin level may rise quite rapidly. Medical treatment is usually necessary in cases of pathologic jaundice, but breastfeeding can continue during treatment and often helps to reduce the jaundice. Pathologic jaundice in a newborn is most commonly caused by Rh or ABO blood incompatibilities. While Rh incompatibility is becoming relatively rare, ABO incompatibility, a much milder condition, is still quite common. Your doctor will know whether he needs to watch for either of these conditions by checking your blood type before your baby is born. Other causes of pathologic jaundice include infection, metabolic problems, or gastrointestinal obstruction.

The reason for concern about very high bilirubin levels is that bilirubin can damage brain cells. A level of 20mg/dl or above is considered to be a high level in the first forty-eight hours; after that 25 mg/dl or above is considered a high level in an otherwise healthy, full-term baby. Problems can occur at lower levels in premies. Kernicterus, the medical term for the brain damage that can be caused by excessively high concentrations of bilirubin, is quite rare, and is of greater concern in the premature or sick baby with pathologic jaundice.

Why jaundice causes problems for newborns

When parents are told that their baby's bilirubin level is elevated, that the baby needs more blood tests, or that their baby's jaundice needs treatment, they may become very worried. Their precious newborn, who was fine yesterday, suddenly seems to have a frightening and complicated condition. Parents may have lots of questions, and the answers may be confusing.

Some mothers may even be told that their baby's jaundice is caused by human milk. At one time it was thought that high bilirubin levels that persisted past the first few days in breastfed babies were a special kind of jaundice called "breast milk jaundice." Many physicians suggested feeding the baby formula for 24 to 48 hours as the best way to bring down bilirubin levels. Unfortunately, even if this weaning was meant to be "temporary," for many mothers it was the beginning of the end of breastfeeding. Mothers of jaundiced babies, in general, tend to wean earlier—not because jaundice interferes with breastfeeding, but because the treatment often does.

It is important for parents to remember that complications or damage from high bilirubin levels are very rare. Decisions about treatment will depend on how old the baby is, whether there are other health problems, and how quickly bilirubin levels are rising. Parents have input into treatment decisions, and you should let your doctor know how important it is to you to continue breastfeeding and not be separated from your baby. Your feelings will influence your doctor's recommendation. While some physicians may still recommend a day or two without breastfeeding to bring down the bilirubin level, many have come to recognize that this advice is not in the best interest of either mother or baby. Guidelines from the American Academy of Pediatrics on newborn jaundice emphasize that parents should participate in treatment decisions, and these guidelines suggest several treatment options that include continuing to breastfeed.

In fact, frequent breastfeeding will help lower bilirubin levels and should be considered an important part of the treatment plan. Continued monitoring of the baby's condition along with efforts to encourage the baby to nurse often and effectively may be all that is needed to bring down the bilirubin levels.

Babies with jaundice may sleep more than other newborns, so mother may have to wake the baby for some feedings. Babies with jaundice should be breastfed ten to twelve times in a twenty-four period. Mother may need to encourage the baby to nurse actively for longer periods of time, using breast compression (described on page 315) or any other technique that prevents baby from falling asleep after just a few minutes of sucking. Babies born more than two weeks before their due date are more likely both to be jaundiced and to have difficulty with breastfeeding in the early days. These babies need lots of gentle encouragement.

Phototherapy as treatment

If your doctor feels that your baby's jaundice requires treatment, he or she will probably prescribe phototherapy. "Bili-lights" are used to speed up the elimination of bilirubin. The baby is placed under the lights, wearing only a diaper, with protective patches covering his eyes.

This treatment is designed to keep the bilirubin from approaching critical levels at which, in extreme cases, an exchange transfusion may be necessary.

Generally speaking, the earlier and more rapid the rise in the bilirubin level, the sooner phototherapy will be started. It might be started at 18 mg/dl in a full-term baby who is two to three days old, or at 20 mg/dl in a baby more than three days old. Sick or premature infants who are jaundiced present special problems, and medical treatment is often necessary at lower bilirubin levels.

If it becomes necessary to treat the jaundice, breastfeeding can and should continue while the baby receives phototherapy. Frequent breastfeeding is still important in helping the baby get rid of excess bilirubin. You'll want to be sure he nurses even more frequently than usually recommmended for a newborn—approximately every two hours, or ten to twelve times per day. This will also help him avoid dehydration.

Light therapy does not have to be continuous to be effective. When you nurse your baby, remove his eye patches, cuddle him close, and look into his eyes. Holding and stroking him even when he is under the lights will be reassuring for both of you.

In some cases, you may be able to have your baby and the bililights moved into your hospital room. You'll feel better with your baby close by, and frequent nursings will be that much easier. Light therapy can also be done at home with a rented light unit, so that baby does not have to remain in the hospital after mother is discharged. Another option is the Wallaby unit, a fiberoptic blanket that wraps around the baby's trunk. The baby doesn't need eye patches and mother can hold the baby and breastfeed without interrupting the treatment. (See Appendix for information on the Wallaby unit.) Further blood tests will be needed to monitor the baby's bilirubin level, and you may need to return to the hospital for these.

"Flushing out" jaundice

At one time, it was thought that giving a baby bottles of water would help to "flush out" the jaundice. But research has shown that water supplements given to newborns in the first few days do not help to reduce jaundice. In fact, one study showed that the more water the baby received the higher the level of bilirubin reported.

Bottles of water may reduce the amount of nursing the baby does and cause nipple confusion. Anything that makes the baby less interested in the breast or interferes with nursing at least ten to twelve times per day can increase jaundice in the breastfed baby. Since bilirubin is eliminated in the baby's stools, frequent nursing is one of the best ways to help the baby get rid of the excess bilirubin.

Hypoglycemia in Newborns

Newborns are often tested to determine their blood glucose levels and parents are sometimes told that their baby has hypoglycemia—or low blood sugar—and needs to be treated with a glucose supplement. Babies at greater risk for hypoglycemia include those who are premature or postmature, those who are small or large for gestational age, and those who have been deprived of oxygen. Hypoglycemia can also indicate infection or a metabolic disorder.

The most common cause of hypoglycemia is delayed or inadequate feedings. A baby who is put to the breast soon after birth and kept near the mother so he can nurse freely will be much less likely to show signs of hypoglycemia. In adults, treatment for low blood sugar includes small, frequent, high protein meals which is exactly what the baby receives when he nurses often. For most babies at risk for hypoglycemia, frequent feedings at the breast (10 to 12 feedings in 24 hours) will stabilize glucose levels.

Giving glucose water feedings instead of nursing causes a sudden rise in blood glucose levels and then a sudden drop. Glucose water feedings in the early days have also been associated with greater weight loss and higher bilirubin levels. A baby who is receiving feedings of sugar water is receiving little nutritional value but he is filling his tummy so he will nurse less often and less effectively.

In some hospitals, glucose feedings are given to all babies whose birth weight falls above or below certain standards. It's a good idea to discuss this with your health care provider before the baby is born and request that routine glucose supplements not be given. If a blood test indicates a glucose supplement is necessary, artificial nipples can be avoided by giving the glucose by spoon, cup, or eyedropper. Sometimes the glucose is given by IV. Nursing at least ten to twelve times per day is the best way to stabilize a baby's glucose levels.

If Your Baby Is Premature

Premature babies come in many sizes. Some may weigh two pounds or less; other premies may be fully developed and weigh close to five pounds. Some will be able to nurse soon after birth, while others will have to be kept warm and protected in an isolette and will not be ready to nurse at the breast for several weeks. If your baby is very small, he may have to stay in the hospital for a month or more and may at first be fed through a tube. Whatever the situation, your milk is very important to your baby. Giving your baby your milk is also important for you. Pumping milk for your baby is something only you can do, and it will help you overcome the worry and fear you feel about his condition. Kathie Patten of South Dakota writes:

> It was a good feeling knowing that I was able to do something for my baby. Giving birth prematurely had left me with subtle feelings of guilt. Even though I could not give our baby the warm, loving feelings of motherly touch and sounds, I knew I was the only one who could provide him with superior nourishment.

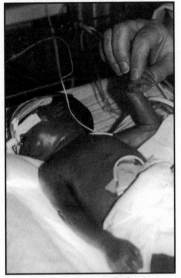

Pumping your milk for a tiny premie is the one thing only you can do.

Later on, when baby is ready to nurse at the breast, breastfeeding helps make up for the separation you and your baby have experienced. Rebecca Strasser from Tennessee was happy that she persevered in her efforts to breastfeed her son, Jonathan, who was born twelve weeks early weighing just under three pounds. She explains, "Nursing Jonathan has soothed the pain of our early separation.... I am forever grateful to all who encouraged me to persevere so that I could know the precious joy of nursing him."

Human milk is best

Human milk is the best possible nourishment for premature infants, just as it is for full-term babies. Human milk is easy for your baby to digest; premature babies use the fats and proteins in human milk more efficiently than those in formulas. Studies have shown that human milk enhances brain development in premies; one study that compared children who had been born prematurely and were fed human milk with those who were given formula showed higher IQ scores at ages 7 1/2 to 8 in the human milk group. Babies who receive human milk in hospital nurseries have fewer infections than formula-fed infants and are at lower risk for necrotizing enterocolitis, a serious bowel problem that may develop in tiny premies. Milk from mothers who deliver prematurely contains greater amounts of antibodies and of some important nutrients than does the milk of mothers delivering at term. It has been found that some of these differences are evident for as long as six months. When you provide your own milk for your baby you are making a critical contribution to his care. Medical technology cannot duplicate mother's milk, the perfect food for your baby.

A very tiny premie, born more than two months before his due date, may require a vitamin and mineral supplement in addition to mother's milk. If your doctor finds your baby needs this type of supplement, don't think that something is wrong with your milk. It's just that such very tiny premature babies may need more of certain nutrients to grow and develop properly. Your milk still provides the basis of the special nutrition your premature baby needs, plus the immunological protection that can't be found in formula.

If your premie is unable to nurse directly from the breast at first, you'll want to start pumping or expressing your milk as soon as possible. Frequent pumping in the first several weeks after birth helps to ensure that your body will be able to make enough milk for your baby in the months to come. You should pump about as often as a newborn would nurse—eight or more times a day. Use a hospital-quality electric pump that can pump both breasts at the same time. This type of pump has been shown to be the most effective at maintaining a mother's milk supply when a baby cannot nurse directly at the breast. Your health insurance should cover the cost. (This may require a note from your doctor or your baby's doctor.)

Colostrum, the first milk you pump, is especially important for your baby because of the immunities it provides. If the colostrum you pump cannot be given to your baby right away, ask that it be frozen and saved for your baby's first tube feedings. As soon as your baby is able to take anything by mouth (or nasogastric tube), your milk is the best food for him.

In the first weeks, if you are pumping frequently, you may be producing far more milk than your baby can take. This is not a problem. Stimulating a bountiful milk supply in the early weeks lets your body know that it should continue to produce milk. The supply may decrease somewhat as time goes on. Your body doesn't respond to a pump the way it would to a cuddly baby. Thinking about your baby, looking at his picture, and calling the hospital for a report on his progress will help you pump more milk. Many mothers find that they are able to get more milk if they pump at the hospital, at baby's bedside, or right after holding their baby skin-to-skin in kangaroo care. (More information on pumping and storing your milk can be found in Chapter 7.)

Ideally, your milk should be stored in a refrigerator and fed to your baby within five to eight days of collection without any kind of processing. Heating the milk to high temperatures destroys many of its

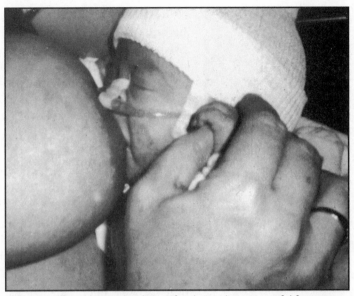

Studies have shown that breastfeeding is less stressful for a tiny premie than feeding from a bottle.

protective qualities. If your milk cannot be fed to your baby within five to eight days, it should be frozen.

The hospital may provide you with containers for collecting your milk. If not, any sterilized container may be used. Be sure your hands are scrupulously clean when you pump your milk. However, your daily shower is enough to keep your nipples clean, and it is not necessary (or even desirable) to clean them with soap, since nature has provided its own cleansing secretions.

The appearance of your milk will change over time. Colostrum may be clear or golden in color. As colostrum changes to milk, it will look richer and creamier and be white or golden-white. After a few weeks, mature milk will look thinner and bluish-white. You will notice that the fat globules may separate from the rest of the milk as it stands. The fat content of the milk may vary, depending on how long you have pumped, the number of let-downs, and the time interval between pumping sessions. All of these variations are perfectly normal; don't let them worry you.

Your need for support

It is a real asset when the doctors and nurses caring for your infant encourage and support you in your efforts to provide human milk for your baby. These professionals whom you see every day can help build your confidence in your ability to breastfeed and mother your baby. Sometimes the health professionals caring for premies are not fully

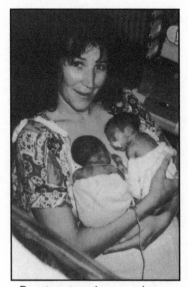

Premie twins who are only two days old are held close to their mother in "kangaroo care."

aware of how to help with breastfeeding, and it may be difficult for them to assist you. Knowing that many other mothers have nursed premature babies is bound to increase your self-confidence. A supportive La Leche League Leader or board certified lactation consultant can help at times like these.

Be persistent about keeping in touch with the hospital and doctor regarding the baby's progress. Most professionals are very understanding about parents' need to know what is happening to their baby. They will also encourage you to come in and give your baby as much personal care and attention as possible. Even when the baby is in an isolette, he needs human contact, and you need to be with him, too. Linda O'Brien of Arkansas tells of traveling forty-five miles to be with her son in an intensive care nursery:

No one seemed to understand the need I had for Jeff or the need I knew he had for me. At every turn I had people ordering me to rest—"Go home," they said, "Sleep! We can take care of your son." At times I felt maybe they were right and I tried. However, once home I could only weep. So I returned to the hospital, prepared to stay. Jeff was crying when I arrived but responded to my voice and stroking. It was very evident that he knew his mother even though he was only two days old.

Kangaroo care

Kangaroo care is becoming more widely accepted in neonatal nurseries as doctors and nurses are learning more about the benefits for both parents and babies. In kangaroo care the premature infant is placed skin-to-skin on mother's chest under a loose-fitting shirt, gown, or blanket that covers them both. Research has shown that this contact has almost magical effects on premies' physiology. Heart and breathing rates become more regular. Premies make eye contact with mother, explore her nipple, and maybe attempt a few tentative sucks. After a few minutes of quiet alertness, many babies will fall into a deep and peaceful sleep while held on mother's chest. Kangaroo care helps mothers feel more confident and more connected to their babies. After spending time with their babies skin-to-skin, mothers often find their pumping efforts produce more milk.

Ask your baby's nurses if kangaroo care is possible for your baby. Some hospitals allow even very tiny babies to enjoy skin-to-skin contact with their mothers. Fathers can participate in kangaroo care, too.

The first time baby nurses

Depending on his size and gestational age it may be days or weeks before your baby is finally ready to suck. Whenever possible, baby's first feedings from a nipple should take place at the breast rather than from an artificial nipple on a bottle. Research has shown it is easier for a baby to coordinate sucking, swallowing, and breathing during breast-feeding than during bottle-feeding, and therefore breastfeeding is less stressful than bottle-feeding. Some doctors suggest that when mother is not available to feed baby at the breast, he should be fed with a cup or by tube, in order to avoid nipple confusion.

Getting a premature baby to latch on and nurse for the first time often requires patience and persistence. Give yourself plenty of time. Ask for a comfortable chair, preferably in a private area, and lots of pillows. Ask for assistance from the hospital's lactation consultant or from a nursery nurse who has lots of experience with breastfed babies. Your baby may not be able to suck well for more than a few seconds at a time in these early feedings. Think of them as practice sessions. In fact a mother who has a plentiful milk supply may need to pump her milk first, so that her premie is not overwhelmed with too much milk the first time he nurses.

In these early breastfeeding sessions, your baby may latch right on and start nursing, or he may experiment briefly with sucking or just lick the nipple. Often these first nursings are made up of more loving and learning than actual nursing. Both of you are benefiting from the close contact. If your baby seems to be getting tired or stressed, take a break and just hold him skin-to-skin for a while. Premature babies tire easily, so these first nursing sessions will be short.

The usual positions for feeding a large, healthy infant may not work well for the small premature infant. This baby needs more support. If, for example, you are nursing on the right breast, use your left hand to support baby's neck and shoulders. Your left arm extends along the length of the baby's body which is supported with pillows in your lap. Use your right hand to support your breast with thumb on one side and fingers on the other in a U-hold. You will have a good view of what is going on and good control over your baby's movements. Be sure that your back and arms are well supported with pillows, and try to relax your back and shoulders. Reassure your baby with calm, gentle handling.

Some premies have difficulty latching on to mother's breast and drawing the nipple in, all the way to the back of the mouth. For some, it will be easier to latch on and obtain milk from the breast if the mother uses a silicone nipple shield. Mothers of premies may need to continue to use the nipple shield for several weeks. The nurses or the hospital lactation consultant will be able to help you obtain a nipple shield and learn to use it.

The nurses may want to monitor your baby's condition closely during these first feedings at the breast. After your baby has learned to latch on and actually suck for a few minutes at a feeding, he may be weighed before and after feedings on a very precise electronic scale to determine how much milk he has taken. Be sure to congratulate yourself for every single gram! Focus on the positive and use the scale results to help yourself learn what effective breastfeeding looks and feels like.

La Leche League's book BREASTFEEDING YOUR PREMATURE BABY contains detailed information on pumping for a premie and on making the transition to feeding at the breast. For more information see the Appendix.

Taking your baby home

The long-awaited day will finally come when you can take your tiny baby home from the hospital. You may find yourself feeling somewhat unsure of your ability to care for your baby, since up until now his life has been so dependent on nurses and complex medical equipment.

Be assured that your loving arms, careful attention, and warm milk are what he needs most at this point. Premature babies have a lot of loving and nursing to catch up on, and they need all the time and closeness you can offer. Sleep with your baby, carry him in your arms or in a baby carrier or sling, let him feel the nearness of you in every way. This will help you get to know him better, so that you will be able to tell when he is hungry or when he needs rest. Give him lots of skin-to-skin contact, with only his diaper between you and him. Keep your breast readily available to him. But be careful not to overstimulate him. Premies also need peace, quiet, and lots of rest.

If he has been on supplements (either formula or pumped human milk), ask your doctor for guidelines on how much supplement to give until your baby makes the transition to total breastfeeding. It's normal during these first days at home to be concerned about whether your baby is getting enough milk at each feeding. For some mothers, renting an electronic scale, like the ones used in the hospital, and weighing the baby before and after feedings may ease these worries and make it easier to gradually discontinue the supplements. As breastfeeding becomes established, the mother may weigh the baby only once a day until she feels fully confident that he will grow and thrive on her milk alone. You can also tell that your baby is getting enough milk by counting the number of wet and soiled diapers. As usual, five to six wet diapers and three to five bowel movements per day are good indications that he's getting plenty of milk.

If it is necessary to continue supplementing your premature baby, you can pump your milk after he nurses to have extra high-fat hindmilk to use as a supplement. Continuing to pump will keep up your milk supply until your baby learns to suck effectively. If baby is getting regular supplements of human milk or formula, you may want to try using a nursing supplementer at the breast. Check the information in Chapter 7 for tips on increasing your milk supply.

With lots of closeness and loving care your premature baby will grow and thrive. Is it worth the trouble to keep up your milk supply in order to breastfeed your premie? Jo-Anne Montgomery of Manitoba, Canada thinks so. Her daughter, Shannon, was born nine weeks early. She says, "Nursing my baby daughter has been and still is one of the greatest pleasures of my life. I encourage any mother who wants to nurse her premature baby not to give up."

A Baby with Special Needs

The baby born with a disability or medical problem needs breastfeeding even more than a healthy baby does. The baby with special needs benefits particularly from the stimulation, attention, and reassurance that are a natural part of nursing at the breast. Baby's mother benefits, too, since breastfeeding helps her to focus on her baby as a baby first and foremost. If your baby has a health problem that complicates nursing, remember that breastfeeding is nearly always possible and is important for both baby and you. If your baby has a problem, contact your local La Leche League Leader or LLLI for information and help with breastfeeding.

The Baby with Down Syndrome

For the baby with Down Syndrome, a loving home environment with maximum interaction between baby and the rest of the family will help to develop his capabilities to the fullest.

Breastfeeding communicates your love and affection to your baby in a very special way. It is something "normal" you can do with your baby even as you are coping with all the emotions that accompany the birth of a disabled child. Breastfeeding is especially important for Down Syndrome babies because they may be more susceptible to respiratory and ear infections and breastfeeding offers some protection against these problems.

The baby with Down Syndrome responds readily to love and returns it enthusiastically to those around him. He is often a delight to the whole family. Lucille Clancy says this about her son, "My heart said 'I love him,' my head said 'I wish it didn't have to be this way,' but soon Chad's big, happy smile thanked me a million times for the extra love I had given him."

A baby with Down Syndrome is often sleepy during the first few weeks and may have a poor sucking reflex, so extra help and patience with breastfeeding are in order. Be calm and patient as he learns to latch on, suck, and swallow. You may need to pump after feedings in the early days to stimulate your milk supply. If your baby needs supplements at first, you can offer this high-calorie hindmilk in a cup, eye dropper, feeding syringe, or nursing supplementer. Breastfeeding may get off to a slow start, but babies with Down Syndrome will eventually learn how to nurse. Don't be discouraged if you encounter problems. The rewards of nursing your baby are well worth the extra effort. With your loving help your baby will catch on.

A Baby with a Cleft Lip or Palate

A cleft lip or cleft palate will make breastfeeding more challenging. However, babies with a cleft lip can usually suck effectively at the breast, even before they have corrective surgery. A cleft palate presents much greater obstacles to breastfeeding.

A baby with a cleft lip may need assistance in forming a good seal on the breast while sucking. Some mothers use their thumb to close the gap left by the opening in the baby's lip. Other mothers find that the breast naturally fills in the space. Lots of practice on a soft, relatively empty breast in the first day or two after birth will help your baby learn how to latch on and suck well before your milk comes in.

Lip-repair surgery is often performed while the baby is still quite young and receiving all his nourishment from the breast. Talk to your baby's doctors about your desire to continue breastfeeding your baby before and after surgery. Guidelines from the American Society of Anesthesiologists state that infants may receive human milk up to four hours before general anesthesia, and many surgeons allow infants to breastfeed as soon as the baby is awake after cleft lip surgery. The idea that babies can breastfeed immediately after cleft lip repair has become more widely accepted in recent years, and articles on this subject have been published in medical journals. Still, some doctors may be reluctant to change their usual procedures, so be prepared to seek a second opinion, if necessary.

Tammy Shaw from Illinois persuaded her doctor to allow her son, Peter, to nurse immediately after his lip-repair surgery. She writes:

> My husband and I showed Dr. Johnson the information about nursing. He enthusiastically agreed to allow me to breastfeed soon after surgery. He understood my wish to nurse Peter right away. He assured me that if any stitches pulled out after nursing, it would not harm Peter in any way to have him quickly replace a stitch. He agreed it was important that Peter be comforted. After surgery when Dr. Johnson appeared and saw that Peter was nursing happily, he commented that it was nice to see him calm and not crying so soon after surgery.

Another mother, Valerie Hawkes-Howat from Massachusetts, went to a great deal of effort to find a doctor who was willing to allow her son to nurse immediately after lip-repair surgery. But she was glad that she did. Valerie writes about Willie's first nursing after his surgery:

> When Willie was brought down from surgery, his bright eyes looked up at me and his little mouth opened into a wide, sleepy smile. I could have wept with relief. The only bandage on his face was a trio of narrow "steri-strips" across the upper lip. The nurse helped me take him into my arms and get him settled in my lap without disturbing the IV in his foot. I snuggled him and he began to root at my breast, so I immediately began to nurse him. He showed only profound pleasure to be back at my breast again—no signs of discomfort whatsoever. I noted the way his upper lip lay over the top of my areola, completely free of stress. There was no swelling or bruising around the sutures.

A cleft palate presents multiple obstacles to effective sucking. Whether or not breastfeeding will be possible for your baby depends a great deal on the size and location of the cleft. Many babies with a cleft palate cannot create enough suction to hold the breast in their mouth. They may not be able to compress the areola between the tongue and the roof of the mouth. Milk may flow from the breast into baby's nasal cavity, causing choking and sputtering. These feeding problems are not unique to breastfeeding. Bottle-feeding a baby with a cleft palate can also be challenging and time-consuming.

Experimenting with different positions and techniques will help you determine if breastfeeding is possible for your baby with a cleft palate. You will want to seek assistance from a board certified lactation consultant, in addition to the other health professionals who are caring for your baby. Some babies feed more effectively with a palatal obturator, a device that fits in baby's mouth and covers the cleft.

Because your baby may not be able to suck very well, you will need to use an electric breast pump to build up your milk supply. The milk you pump can be given to your baby as a supplement. Even if your baby is not able to nurse directly at the breast, continuing to pump your milk will provide him with the important nutritional and immunological benefits of human milk.

Cystic Fibrosis and Other Metabolic Conditions

Babies with cystic fibrosis, celiac disease, or other malabsorption problems benefit from being breastfed. In fact, the point at which symptoms appear is often delayed in babies who are breastfed. Human milk helps protect these babies from respiratory infection and promotes more normal growth.

Kathleen Winterer's son, Ben, gained weight steadily on human milk despite cystic fibrosis; Ben was much healthier because he was breastfed:

At the time of Ben's hospitalization we were told we could expect one or two bouts with pneumonia his first year, and I am very happy to say Ben just turned two last month and hasn't had any yet. Of course, I like to think that my milk helped him through that first crucial year.

Metabolic disorders

In the United States, almost all newborns are tested routinely for PKU (phenylketonuria), a rare metabolic disorder that interferes with normal brain development if left untreated. Babies with PKU are unable to digest the amino acid phenylalinine, although they still need small amounts of this nutrient to grow normally. Human milk contains less phenylalinine than cow's milk formula, so doctors have found that a baby with PKU can continue to receive some of his daily nutrition at the breast while also being given supplements of a special formula.

One study found that babies who had been breastfed before their PKU diagnosis scored an average of 14 points higher on IQ tests during elementary school than those who had been formula-fed from birth. False positives can occur on PKU tests, so it's important to know that breastfeeding can continue while re-testing is done to confirm the diagnosis.

Galactosemia is another rare metabolic disorder. Babies with galactosemia are unable to digest lactose, the main carbohydrate in human milk. Babies with galactosemia cannot be breastfed and must be fed lactose-free formula.

When a Baby Dies

The death of a baby, whether through miscarriage, stillbirth, shortly after birth, or later through illness or accident, is an experience most of us shudder to think about. Sadly, the lives of many families are touched by such tragedies. Parents who suffer this terrible loss are usually shocked and grieved to find themselves also coping with the fact that the mother's body doesn't immediately realize what has happened; milk will begin, or continue, to be made.

A mother whose infant dies at birth or shortly after or who miscarries in the second trimester of pregnancy or later, is often discharged early from the hospital. So the process of the milk coming in will take place at home. It helps to be prepared for what will happen, but often mothers are shocked to experience engorgement—hard, painful swollen breasts. Mothers whose baby dies when the milk supply is well established will also experience engorgement, and will need to seek relief. Check into the treatments suggested for engorgement in Chapter 4.

Women are often afraid to relieve their discomfort by expressing milk for fear of encouraging their breasts to make more milk. However, expressing enough milk to relieve discomfort is probably the most useful thing to do. A hot shower or a hot bath is a good preliminary to

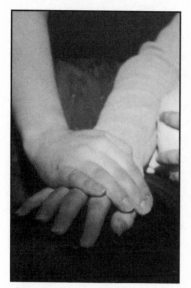

Having a friend to listen helps a mother deal with grief.

expressing some milk. Not only will the warmth enable you to handle your painful breasts, but the warm water often helps the milk to be released. At first, you may need to express a small amount of milk several times a day, and at night too, if you wake in discomfort. The point of expressing a little milk is first to alleviate discomfort, and secondly to prevent undue accumulation of milk in the ducts, which could lead to a breast infection. You may also find it helpful to wear a firm bra for support and comfort. One size larger than usual may be necessary for a few days.

When the milk supply is already fully established, some mothers report that expressing milk and donating it to a local milk bank helps them feel they are doing something positive to help another baby. If you choose to do this, you will be able to cut back gradually and decrease your milk supply more comfortably.

Many mothers are taken aback by the way the let-down reflex can be triggered just by thinking about the baby. Comforting hugs from friends may also make the milk let down. Wearing absorbent nursing pads, loose and patterned clothing, even taking a change of clothing with you on outings can help.

Whatever your feelings are, accept them as normal. Grief can continue for a very long time indeed. Remembering the baby's birthday and the anniversary of the funeral, sharing photographs, naming the baby, even if he was stillborn, can help. Couples need to support each other and understand that grief may affect husband and wife in different ways, at different times. Often there is a lot of help provided initially, but after a few weeks people may expect parents to "get over it." This is a vulnerable time for bereaved parents, who may find grief welling up repeatedly. Dr. Penny Stanway, a British physician whose third baby was stillborn, says: "Most women find that they want to go over the circumstances of their baby's death time and time again with whoever will listen. A mother will have to have time to incorporate her loss, and the best way of doing this is by repetition of the event in her mind or by talking, as if to stamp on her mind what has happened."

How can friends help?

Support from friends, family, and involved health professionals is vital. Celia Waterhouse, from Great Britain, whose baby Leo died at three months, offers this suggestion to friends. "Say simply how sad you are to hear about it. Your saying so will not make the mother any sadder for being reminded of her baby—as if she could ever forget! Even if nothing further is said between you, your acknowledgment of her sorrow will have helped."

Certainly practical help will also be welcome—help with meals, laundry, or the older children—but having friends willing to talk, cry, and listen is a comfort in itself.

Support groups for parents who have lost a child offer a chance to share feelings and experiences with other parents. See the Appendix.

CHAPTER SEVENTEEN

WHEN EXTRA CARE IS
needed

B reastfeeding often requires patience and commitment, but mothers have continued breast-feeding in almost every situation imaginable. They have discovered that when the circumstances surrounding breastfeeding are less than ideal, the special benefits of breastfeeding become even more important.

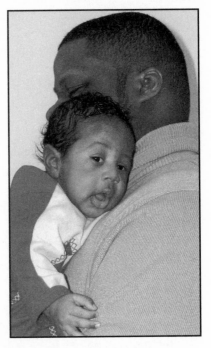

New babies and mothers struggling with problems appreciate the emotional closeness and reassurance of their unique breast-feeding relationship. Breastfeeding helps them get to know one another despite the complications. In addition, human milk's nutritional and immunological benefits are especially important for the baby at risk.

Circumstances that might legitimately prevent you from nursing your baby are rare. Be confident that your milk is the best possible nourishment for your baby. If he can have any liquid or food by mouth, the best choice is human milk. Not only is human milk safe for the sick baby, it is one of the best medicines for him. Doctors have often commented on how quickly a breastfed baby seems to recover.

If you or your baby become ill, make it clear to your doctor or health care provider that you want to continue breastfeeding your baby and ask for his or her cooperation in bringing this about. Your positive attitude toward breastfeeding is a most important factor and one your doctor will take into consideration. Your insistence on continuing to breastfeed whenever possible during a period of medical treatment may make a difference in the type of treatment the doctor suggests. If your doctor is unwilling or unable to take positive steps to keep your baby nursing, you have a right to seek other medical advice and assistance. Your baby's welfare comes first.

In the case of an unusual breastfeeding situation, your doctor can contact La Leche League International's Center for Breastfeeding Information (CBI) for additional information. Please encourage him or her to do so. See the Appendix for further information about the CBI.

You will appreciate the support of your local La Leche League Leader. She may be able to put you in touch with another mother who has breastfed in a situation similar to yours. Don't hesitate to call on her for help. You may also find helpful information about your special situation on La Leche League's Web site (www.lalecheleague.org) or in other books published by La Leche League International.

Multiple Births— Multiple Blessings

Can a mother breastfeed twins? Of course she can. In fact mothers who breastfeed their twins find that the benefits of breastfeeding are multiplied when they have two babies to love. In her book, MOTHERING MULTIPLES, Karen Gromada, a La Leche League Leader and mother of twins herself, writes about the benefits of breastfeeding twins:

> The advantages of breastfeeding one baby are even more important and intense for multiples. How nice to save twice the money and twice the preparation time. And it is twice as nice to curl up at night for feedings in bed, rather than awaken to crying babies who must wait for you to warm their meals.... One advantage is particularly important.... Breastfeeding ensures maximum skin contact with each baby.

Plenty of milk

All of the doubly blessed mothers agree that having enough milk is no problem. The tried and true maxim for breastfeeding holds for multiples as well as for one baby—the more you nurse, the more your milk supply builds up. A mother in Illinois, Lee Mueller, had twins who

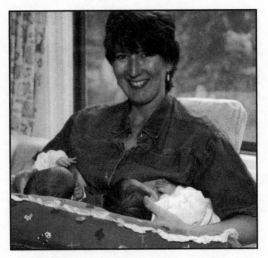

Nursing twins brings special rewards.

each weighed eight pounds at birth, yet she found no need to resort to supplementary formula or to start solids earlier than usual. A Wisconsin mother of twins, Judy Latka, commented, "I've taken breastfeeding so much for granted that it surprises me when people are amazed that the twins are nursing. That part is easy—it's the extra set of loving arms that I need." Judy was aware of the importance of nursing the babies soon and often, and she adds, "I had discussed my desires many times with my doctors, and it was well worth the effort. My hospital stay was brief. We went home when the babies were twenty-eight hours old."

Because twins sometimes come in smaller packages, they need the protection of mother's milk even more than single babies. Twins and other multiples are more likely to be born early and as a result, they are more likely to spend time in the hospital's special care nursery. Your milk will help them grow and stay healthy. If you cannot nurse one or both babies right from the start, plan to use an electric breast pump to express your milk and establish the supply.

Plan ahead

In planning for two or more (and we hope you have prior notice so you can plan), take the hints for easy housekeeping and relaxed mothering and multiply them to fit your needs. Cut your housework to a minimum. Your babies need the same loving attention that every baby deserves, and a tired mother is hard pressed to give this. Plan on getting help with the housework for at least the first few months. Your partner can take over more than his usual share of the chores, or you

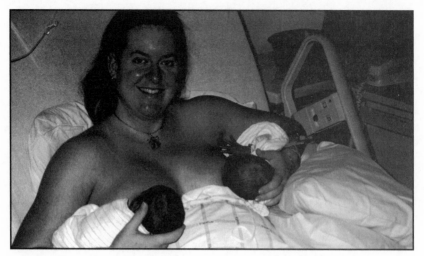

Breastfeeding ensures maximum skin contact with each baby.

can ask friends and family to help out. Hiring a mother's helper is a
good investment, if you can afford it. Your spare minutes should be
spent resting and relaxing, not catching up on laundry.

Feeding two babies

Whether to nurse the babies together or separately is one of those
things that mothers work out in their own way to suit themselves and
their babies. La Leche League Leader Carolyn Johnson of Illinois
described her method of satisfying two hungry babies:

> When time was a factor, I nursed the twins together, sitting in
> a rocker, with Jill on Judy's lap. Otherwise, I found it much
> easier to nurse the babies separately. I would awaken one
> about half an hour before the other was "due" to get up so as
> to avoid nursing them together. Of course, I alternated so
> that one twin wouldn't always have "first pickings."
>
> If one was still hungry after nursing on one side, I would
> offer the other breast. Then the next one would begin on the
> breast last nursed by the other. Usually, the last to be nursed
> would be the first to wake up hungry. There were times when
> they would want to nurse again after only one-and-a-half to
> two hours, and this served to increase my milk supply to
> meet their demands. Usually it would take two days of very
> frequent nursing and they would again be satisfied with a
> less demanding schedule.

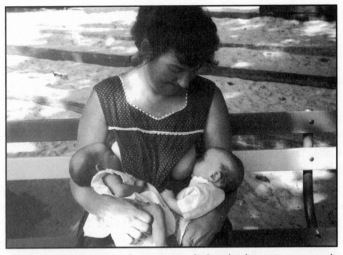

Twins can be positioned to nurse with their bodies criss-crossed.

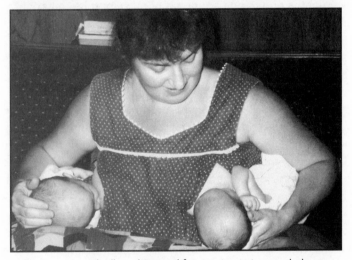

Using a special pillow designed for nursing twins can help you
position both babies in the football hold.

I always made sure the twins were nursed at least every
three hours and would awaken them if necessary. At night
I didn't watch the clock, but kept them alongside our bed in a
bassinet and buggy, and all I had to do was scoop the hungry
one into bed, doze and nurse until the other one awakened,
and then switch. This was a marvelous system for me
because it gave me the sleep I needed. I also didn't change
them at night unless they had soaked through everything.
They never got diaper rash and didn't seem to mind not being
changed at night.

A question that was uppermost in Paula Johnson's mind as a new mother of twins was how to feed both babies when they decided to nurse at the same time. This Missouri mother tells of her experience:

The first try was hilarious! If you're holding a baby in each arm, what do you do when a newborn loses the nipple? Wish for a third hand, that's what! I soon discovered pillows, and we've got the system down pat now. For a couple of frantic weeks, they refused to nurse at the same time. But with practice and the aid of pillows we finally discovered a lying-down position that is comfortable for all three of us. The nicest part is that now I can doze off while nursing, whereas before I sat upright until both were finished. That made for short nights! Looking back now, I realize I did little else but nurse the babies in those first couple of weeks. But now here we are at five months and things are going fairly smoothly—most of the time!

Patti Lemberg from Texas, found several different ways to nurse both babies at once:

When they were tiny, each rested in the crook of an arm, bottom at my hand, legs extended along my thigh. If one wriggled out of place I caught the back of the diaper and pulled him back. In fact, I still use this position if they both want to rock and nurse at the same time. Another good position is sitting on the couch with both heads in my lap and bodies extended under my arms onto the couch. This one is great because both hands are free to hold a book and sip a beverage. When they are still tiny it's best to put a pillow under each for height and comfort. These days, we prefer to nurse lying down on their bed (a mattress on the floor), with David on the left in the standard nursing position for lying down and Alan on the right across my chest. That may sound awkward, but any position that is comfortable to all is fine. You need to work with the furniture and pillows until you find what's best for you.

Almost all mothers who nurse more than one baby comment on their hearty appetite and increased thirst. Some make a practice of eating an extra meal before going to bed. Regarding the work of managing more than one baby, one mother of twins commented, "The

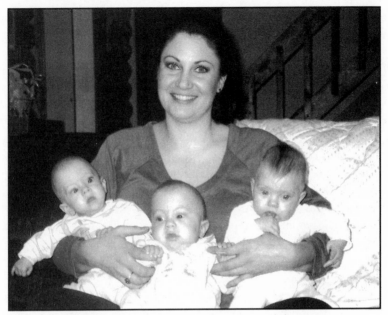

Breastfeeding triplets is quite an accomplishment!

rewards are great, but during the first three months you won't have time to think about them." Marge Saphier suggests that mothers of twins make time in their busy lives for La Leche League. She comments, "Although I am a La Leche League Leader myself, I cannot tell you how much I needed and appreciated the support the other mothers gave me."

With more than one baby, your attention is focused on the babies in a special way. Just watching them—noticing their differences, their different growth patterns, their inherent temperamental leanings—is an ever-interesting, ever-changing spectacle. It can give you insight and knowledge that add greatly to your competence as a mother, as well as to your enjoyment of your babies. As one twin mother puts it, "I'm afraid having one baby will be rather dull after watching two bloom and grow!"

Nursing more than two

If nursing twins sounds like an amazing accomplishment, it may astonish you to know that mothers have also been able to fully breastfeed triplets, and even quadruplets! Supplements may be needed at first, but once the babies are breastfeeding well, a healthy milk supply is usually no problem.

One mother of triplets pumped her milk for many weeks while her premature babies were in the hospital. After all three babies came home, she had no trouble nursing the two boys, but her daughter had become nipple confused and continued to prefer the bottle.

The mother was so determined to provide the benefits of human milk for all three babies that she continued to pump her milk for her daughter while fully breastfeeding the two boys.

With three or four babies to feed and care for, mothers often find it helpful to keep track of feedings as well as wet and soiled diapers to be sure each baby is nursing often enough and getting plenty to eat.

If you are expecting multiples (or have them already), you'll find additional information on breastfeeding and caring for more than one baby in Karen Gromada's book MOTHERING MULTIPLES, BREASTFEEDING AND CARING FOR TWINS OR MORE! Revised in 1999, this book is available from La Leche League Groups or La Leche League International. See the Appendix for details.

Relactation and Induced Lactation

In the usual course of events, a mother's body prepares for lactation during pregnancy, and the birth of the baby signals the mother's breasts to begin producing milk. With the baby's eager sucking, the milk continues to be produced. If the baby is not put to the breast after birth, or if breastfeeding ceases soon afterward, the milk "dries up." Relactation is the process by which a mother is able to re-establish her milk supply several weeks or months after lactation has stopped. It requires patience and determination, but it can be done. The baby's sucking will stimulate milk production. In fact, some mothers have been able to establish a milk supply for an adopted baby without the impetus of pregnancy and birth. This is called induced lactation.

Often mothers who have attempted relactation have been those whose babies could not tolerate any artificial formula.

One mother, Kimberly Fradejas from Florida, was understandably concerned when her daughter, Brandy, didn't seem able to tolerate any of the formulas they had tried. When the baby was three weeks old, they took her to see a nurse practitioner at the clinic. Kimberly tells what happened next:

> I asked if it was too late for me to breastfeed. The nurse said it might not be too late. She showed me how to guide the baby to the breast, and Brandy took right to it. She nursed for the first time right there in the office. I never will forget the look on her cute little face. It was as if that was what she had

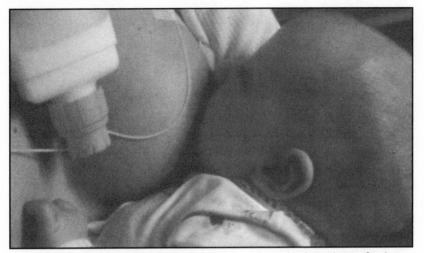

Using a nursing supplementer can allow an adopted baby to breastfeed.

wanted and needed all along. The nurse then advised me to let Brandy nurse first whenever she was hungry, then to supplement her afterward with a small amount of formula. As my milk supply increased, I decreased the amount of formula Brandy was taking until she no longer needed a supplement.

The nurse arranged for me to talk with a La Leche League Leader, who gave me information on increasing my milk supply and books on breastfeeding. Since I knew nothing about nursing a baby, she invited me to come to La Leche League meetings where I could meet other nursing mothers.

Brandy is four-and-a-half months old now and weighs nearly twenty pounds. She is a very healthy and happy baby. I am proud to be doing the best I can for her. My only regret is that I didn't begin nursing her the minute she was born.

Nursing adopted babies

The first few adoptive mothers who were in touch with LLL were nursing their toddlers when they adopted their new babies. By putting the young baby to their breast often, they were able to increase their milk supply to meet some or all of the infant's needs.

But even mothers who have never been pregnant have been able to establish at least a partial milk supply by putting the baby to the breast, expressing milk with a pump, or both. In most cases, adoptive mothers are not able to bring in a full milk supply. Their babies receive supplements of infant formula along with human milk from mother. Supplements can be given at the breast using a nursing supplementer, so that these mothers and babies can enjoy the closeness of full-time breastfeeding.

Jo Young, from England, who had never been pregnant, was able to bring in her milk for her adopted son, Peter. She began when he was three weeks old and explains it this way:

> With great effort and sacrifice from a small handful of people I succeeded in my effort to induce lactation, and incredibly, Peter was completely nourished and sustained at my breast by the time he was three-and-a-half months old. He remained solely breastfed from then until he began to experiment with solids at about six months. During the early months when he was basically dependent on formula, Peter looked rather fragile and unwell, suffering from constant colds. I am convinced that the human milk he has had is responsible for the marvelous changes in his looks. His skin has cleared and he is now a large, bouncy, blooming, typical breastfed baby.
>
> I can never hope to convey totally the depth of my gratitude to the friends who helped us. I think they realize the wealth of the gift they have given Peter and me.

The closeness and intimacy of the breastfeeding relationship is what matters most to adoptive mothers regardless of how much milk they produce. From Arizona, Anne Sanger writes:

> It seems like such a short time since we took Lisa from the adoption agency into our family. She was four days old then and seemed so small. Now she is a happy, beautiful one-year-old.
>
> I was able to nurse Lisa with the help of a nursing supplementer. I did a lot of preparation prior to her arrival. When Lisa was ten months old and eating a variety of other foods in addition to breastfeeding, we were able to discontinue using the supplementer. We are still a happy nursing couple.
>
> It is difficult for me to explain what it means to me to be able to nurse Lisa. I wanted to give her the gift of love and the wonderful way of communicating that the nursing relationship opens to mothers.
>
> Breastfeeding my adopted child was not the easiest thing I ever did in my life, but it has been one of the most rewarding. We feel very fortunate to be the parents of such a happy child.

The basic technique

The basic technique for relactation or induced lactation is to encourage the baby to nurse as often as possible. This is how you stimulate the breasts to produce milk. Adoptive mothers can often begin establishing a milk supply before they have their babies. It helps, of course, to know when you'll get the baby. Use a pump or hand-express for three to five minutes on each breast several times a day, gradually increasing the number of times per day. If this is kept up faithfully, the breast will begin to produce milk—usually in two to six weeks. It may be only a few drops at first, but this will increase once your baby starts to nurse.

Certain herbs and medications are sometimes used to stimulate lactation or to boost a mother's milk supply. Substances that stimulate the body to produce milk are called galactagogues. Your La Leche League Leader or a board certified lactation consultant can provide more information about their use. Taking medication to stimulate or increase milk production will require a prescription from your doctor.

If it is possible for you to hold and nurse your baby in the first hours or days after birth, by all means arrange to do so. One of the most difficult aspects of relactation is getting the baby interested in sucking at the breast if he has been used to bottles and artificial nipples for several weeks or months. This requires a great deal of patience and determination. The mother who is attempting to relactate needs a generous amount of support and encouragement. For a time she will be working almost around the clock, feeding her baby as often as she can. Of course, the more often the baby nurses, the more milk there will be waiting for him the next time. It's a good idea to be in touch with a La Leche League Leader who can provide further information.

You will need to continue giving the baby some formula. Nurse the baby first, for as long as he is willing, before you offer the supplement. Many mothers avoid bottles and artificial nipples completely and use a spoon, cup, small flexible bowl, or feeding syringe to give supplements. If a nursing supplementer is used, the baby can receive his supplement as he nurses at the breast. (See the Appendix.) A baby who is having a great deal of difficulty making the transition from artificial nipple to mother's breast may benefit from the use of a nipple shield, which will feel more like a bottle nipple in his mouth. A nipple shield can be used in combination with the nursing supplementer.

If you are putting the baby to the breast as often as possible and giving the supplement only during or after a feeding, you may be able to gradually cut back on the total amount of supplement you give the baby as your milk supply increases. If you write down the amount of supplement he takes each day, and you see the total decreasing slowly, you'll know your milk supply is increasing. You'll need to watch the baby's wet diapers and bowel movements to be sure he is still getting plenty to eat.

While you are establishing a milk supply, it is very important to keep in touch with the baby's doctor and check the baby's weight on a weekly basis to be sure he continues to gain weight.

Many adoptive mothers are able to gradually discontinue using supplements as their babies near their first birthday and are taking large amounts of solid foods. Their babies continue to nurse at the breast both for the milk that's there and for comfort.

Further information from mothers who have nursed adopted babies including details on establishing a milk supply, having realistic expectations, and keeping your perspective about the situation can be found in other publications available from your local La Leche League Group or LLLI. The LLLI Web site also has stories from mothers who have done this. See the Appendix for details.

If Your Baby Gets Sick

Most of the time your breastfed baby will be happy and healthy. You will be pleased and proud to know that your milk is contributing to his good health. Because of the immunological protection received through mother's milk, a breastfed baby is less likely to become ill when colds and flu are going around. Even when a nursing mother is ill, it is best for her baby to keep on breastfeeding. The baby has already been exposed to the germs causing the illness, and human milk will help protect the baby. In fact, the nursing mother produces antibodies on demand to the specific germs that challenge her baby.

But what if your baby does develop an illness, such as a cold or ear infection, vomiting or diarrhea, or something more serious? No matter how serious your baby's illness is, he can almost always continue breastfeeding. If a baby can take anything by mouth, your milk is the best food for him except in the situation of a baby with a metabolic disorder. Human milk provides perfect nutrition that is easily digested and also provides antibodies to help him fight infection. And the comfort provided by breastfeeding is also important in recovering from an illness.

Colds and ear infections

Studies have shown that breastfed babies are less likely to have respiratory infections and ear infections. But that doesn't mean your baby won't ever experience these problems. A baby with a cold, sore throat, or ear infection may find it difficult to nurse. These suggestions may help:

- Carry the baby in an upright position, perhaps using a sling or baby carrier, for a short time before trying to nurse him. This may help to drain the mucus from his nose.
- Nurse the baby in a semi-upright position. This may help with an ear infection as lying down to nurse puts pressure on baby's ears.
- Use a cool-mist vaporizer in the room where baby sleeps and where you'll be nursing him.
- Clear baby's nose with a soft rubber suction bulb before feedings.

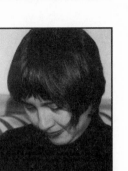

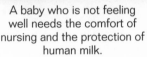

A baby who is not feeling well needs the comfort of nursing and the protection of human milk.

If baby is still too uncomfortable to nurse, pump or express your milk and offer it to him in a spoon, cup, or eyedropper. Of course, you will want to be in touch with your doctor if baby has a fever or is refusing to nurse for more than a few hours.

Diarrhea or Vomiting

If your baby is otherwise well and thriving, it really doesn't matter how loose his bowel movements are. Not all loose, frequent stools constitute diarrhea. In the breastfed infant it is quite normal for baby to have very loose, runny bowel movements. Many breastfed babies, especially in the early weeks, have as many as six or eight stools a day; some will soil a diaper every time they nurse. Later on, when they are more than six weeks old, they may have only one bowel movement a day or one a week or even less often. If a baby has infrequent bowel movements, they are usually quite profuse. All this is well within the realm of normal. Even the occasional green, watery stool in an otherwise healthy baby is nothing to worry about.

If a baby with diarrhea or vomiting is not running a fever, it is wise to consider other possibilities before assuming that the baby is ill. Antibiotics can cause diarrhea, as can vitamin supplements. Sometimes antibiotics or vitamin, iron, or other supplements taken by a nursing mother can cause digestive problems in her baby. An occasional bottle of formula could result in diarrhea or vomiting in a sensitive baby. Another possibility is that the baby is sensitive to a new food that has been introduced. In some cases, a food eaten by the nursing mother may affect her baby, causing an upset stomach or diarrhea.

If a baby is having twelve to sixteen stools a day, or if the stools have an offensive odor or contain flecks of blood, the baby most likely has a gastrointestinal infection. For the breastfeeding baby, the rule of thumb is that if the baby can take anything by mouth, he should continue to receive human milk. Human milk is digested so quickly that some nutrients and fluid will be absorbed even if it seems as if most of the feeding comes right back up. Usually baby's symptoms will improve in three to five days, if not sooner.

Diarrhea occasionally causes more serious problems in babies and young children. When the lining of the intestine is inflamed and irritated by an infection, it tends to leak fluids and pass nutrients through the body too rapidly. The loss of water and minerals can lead to dehydration and eventually to shock. Signs of dehydration include listlessness, lethargy, dry mouth, less than the usual amount of tears, minimal urine output, and fever. You should call your doctor if you suspect your sick baby is becoming dehydrated. You can help prevent dehydration by making sure that your baby gets plenty of fluids. The best way to do this in a breastfed baby is to offer small, frequent nursings.

As long as the baby is having at least two wet diapers per day during his illness, he is not in danger of dehydration. In more serious cases of diarrhea, the doctor may want you to give the baby supplementary feedings of an oral rehydration solution, to restore the lost fluid and minerals to his system. Even if an oral rehydration solution is recommended, breastfeeding can and should continue. Human milk continues to be a valuable source of both fluid and nutrients during gastrointestinal illnesses, and the antibodies in the milk will help to fight the infection.

Health professionals may advise mothers of formula-fed babies and toddlers who drink cow's milk to avoid giving their child any milk products until the vomiting or diarrhea clears up. This "no milk" advice applies only to cow's milk, not to human milk, which contains substances that reduce inflammation and fight infections in baby's tummy. Research has shown that babies who continue to breastfeed recover more quickly from bouts of diarrhea.

Mothers with breastfeeding babies or toddlers know that abrupt weaning, even if it is only temporary, can make life miserable for both mother and baby. When the familiar source of solace is taken away, a sick baby becomes even more frustrated and upset. Meanwhile mother's breasts become fuller and more uncomfortable.

For the baby who's vomiting, it will be best to take him off solid foods until he is no longer throwing up. If his stomach is very upset, it might help to hand-express most of your milk and let him nurse for comfort on a fairly empty breast. If he gets only a small amount of milk each nursing (while nursing fairly often), the baby may be less likely to lose it all again. Staying at the breast and sucking for comfort will also help to keep the milk in his tummy. After a few hours of tolerating these smaller feedings, the baby can begin to take more milk at each nursing. If even the smaller feedings repeatedly come back up and this continues for several hours, you should call your doctor and watch for signs of dehydration.

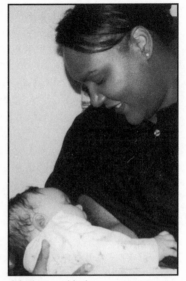

Mother and baby can continue to benefit from breastfeeding even if one or the other is ill.

For the baby who is six months or older, or the toddler who is begging for something because he is thirsty, perhaps a few ice chips or water from a teaspoon will satisfy him for a while. Freeze some of the milk you are expressing to keep yourself comfortable and use frozen mother's milk to quench his thirst. The advantage of ice is that it goes down slowly and is an interesting distraction. If you can hold him off with something like that, fine. If not, let him nurse on the emptied breast but don't give him anything else. In any case, weaning is not necessary or advisable.

Human milk is the best food there is for the sick baby, and as long as he can take anything by mouth it should be your milk. When a nursing baby is sick, the comfort he receives at the breast may be the most important benefit of all.

Lactose intolerance

Occasionally, when a baby has very frequent, loose stools it may be suggested that he has something called "temporary lactose intolerance," and you may be told to take the baby off the breast. This may happen after an intestinal illness or treatment with antibiotics. The lining of the stomach may be irritated, or the friendly bacteria that live in baby's intestines may need time to recover from the infection or the antibiotic. It may take some time before baby's bowel movements return to their previous consistency. There is no need to substitute lactose-free formula for human milk. True lactose intolerance is virtually unknown in babies and young children under weaning age.

Dr. William Sears, in his book, SAFE AND HEALTHY, calls this "nuisance diarrhea." The best thing to do in such situations is to take baby off everything by mouth except your milk. Give the baby plenty of opportunities to nurse, but be sure to allow him to "finish the first breast first," so that he gets plenty of the hindmilk that contains higher amounts of fat and less lactose. With a toddler whose diet normally includes solid foods and other liquids in addition to mother's milk, you may want to avoid giving him foods that are difficult to digest. Offer bananas, rice, unsweetened applesauce, lean meat, or strips of whole wheat toast, along with frequent nursing and water in a cup. As the effects of the illness or the medication wear off, the stools will return to normal, although it may take two to four weeks before the baby's usual bowel pattern returns. In the meantime, because of the special closeness and comfort he derives from the breastfeeding relationship, as well as the physical benefits of your milk, he will recover much faster.

Gastroesophageal reflux

If your baby spits up after feedings, or even vomits frequently, he may be suspected of having gastroesophageal reflux (GER), a condition in which the acidic contents of the stomach flow back into the esophagus, causing pain and irritation. Some babies with GER do not spit up at all but develop other symptoms. If your baby is suspected of having this condition, be assured that breastfeeding can and should continue. Breastfed babies with GER have been found to have fewer and less severe episodes of reflux than formula-fed babies. The digestibility of human milk is definitely an advantage.

Ways to manage breastfeeding include feeding the baby in an upright position and keeping the baby upright in a carrier or sling after feedings. Some physicians suggest short, frequent feedings, believing that lower volumes of milk are less likely to come back up than larger amounts. Feeding from just one breast at each feeding may be helpful for some mothers and babies. Pediatrican and breastfeeding expert Jack Newman, MD, recommends that the baby with reflux be encouraged to suck at the breast as long as possible with each feeding. Sucking produces waves of muscle contractions in the esophagus that move food toward the stomach. Continuing to suck for comfort, even after the breast is relatively empty, may prevent baby's meal from coming back up.

Further information about GER can be found in the pamphlet "Breastfeeding the Baby with Reflux," available from La Leche League International. Also see the Appendix for information about a group called PAGER, which is made up of parents and professionals who offer information on this topic.

Surgery on a breastfed baby

If your breastfed baby requires surgery, you will want to minimize the amount of time the baby will need to fast prior to receiving anesthesia. You can discuss this with the surgeon and the anesthesiologist ahead of time. The "nothing by mouth" period is shorter for breastfed babies than for formula-fed babies, since human milk is digested more quickly. Current guidelines from the American Society of Anesthesiologists state that breastfed babies should be allowed to nurse up to four hours before surgery. Some hospitals and doctors are comfortable with fasting times of two to three hours for breastfed infants. You'll need to find ways to distract the baby during the time he is not allowed to nurse. After surgery, many mothers are able to be with their baby in the recovery room and nurse the baby as soon as he awakens. Breastfeeding can be comforting at this time for both mother and baby. Again, as soon as baby can have anything by mouth, human milk is the first choice.

Slow Weight Gain

When babies do not seem to be breastfeeding well and are not gaining weight on mother's milk alone, everyone becomes concerned. The mother may feel frightened and inadequate. The doctor stresses that something needs to be done, but he or she may not know how to help mother and baby breastfeed more effectively. Slow weight gain in an otherwise healthy breastfed baby calls for a close look at baby, mother, and the nursing routine.

How do you know if there is reason to be concerned about your baby's weight gain or the way he is breastfeeding? Here are some indications that baby may not be getting enough milk at the breast:

- If baby has not regained his birth weight by two weeks of age.

- If there are too few wet diapers or scanty bowel movements. After mother's milk has "come in," a breastfed baby should have five to six wet diapers and three to five bowel movements daily. (Older babies may have bowel movements less frequently.)

- If baby's weight gain is below the average of six ounces a week in the first three months. (A weight gain of less than six ounces per week may be acceptable for some babies.)

- If the baby is nursing fewer than eight to twelve times a day.

- If the baby is not waking to nurse at night.

Most of the time, difficulties with breastfeeding can be readily resolved, but in all cases of slow weight gain, the baby should be under the care of a doctor. Your doctor can make sure that your baby does not have any other health problems that may be keeping him from gaining weight. As you work to improve your baby's breastfeeding, frequent weight checks at the doctor's office will reassure you that your baby is healthy and will help you measure your progress.

Some babies who are gaining weight slowly, or not at all, at the breast will need supplemental feedings for a time. These can be given in ways that will not interfere with baby's learning better breastfeeding skills. (See descriptions of alternative feeding methods on page 318.) Mothers of slow-gaining babies may need to pump their breasts to protect their milk supply. If milk is not removed from a mother's breasts frequently throughout the day in the first weeks of lactation, milk production will slow down and it will be more difficult to build up the milk supply later.

Helping baby breastfeed better

Review the section in Chapter 7 called "Is Baby Getting Enough?" It covers basic information on how to help your baby breastfeed effectively, so that he will get more milk from your breasts and gain weight more quickly. Then consider the following points.

More time at the breast. If a baby is not gaining well, the first question is how often is the baby being breastfed? Not nursing often enough is probably the most common cause of slow weight gain. Human milk is quickly digested, and frequent nursings are easier for the baby and provide him with a steady supply of nutrients. If slow weight gain is a problem, it's important that the baby nurse at least every two hours, with perhaps one longer stretch of three to four hours at night if baby is asleep. If a feeding begins at eight o'clock, put the baby to the breast again at ten, regardless of how long the eight o'clock nursing lasted. Plan to nurse the baby ten to twelve times in each twenty-four-hour period while you are trying to improve baby's weight gain.

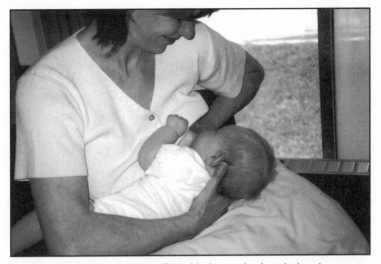

In the crossover or cross cradle hold, the mother's right hand supports the baby's neck and shoulders and her left hand supports the breast when baby nurses on the left side. Using the "U" hold on the breast may be more comfortable than the "C" hold used here because mother's arm would be close to her side. This position is often used to get baby started at the breast when he is having trouble latching on.

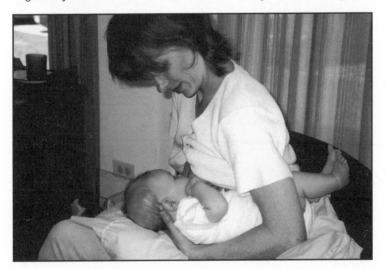

In the football hold, the mother has a good view of how her baby is latching on.

The slow gainer may be a placid baby, a quiet infant who regularly sleeps for four or five hours at a time. If your baby is one who sleeps a lot, you may be thinking, "Such a good baby." But don't be lulled by such placidness. This little sleeper may not gain weight well because he just isn't nursing as much as he should be. Keep a careful check on the number of wet and soiled diapers. After the first few days, you should be getting at least five or six wet diapers and three to five bowel movements per day. As baby gets older, he may only have a bowel movement every three or four days, or sometimes even less often, but in these cases, the amount will be substantial.

With a sleeper, mother takes the initiative and actively encourages her baby to nurse more often. You have to become a clock-watcher. For a time, you are the gentle prod encouraging your baby to nurse. Handling baby and nursing him often helps to rouse him. He needs this stimulation as much as he needs your good milk. It all works together to get him going.

To wake a sleepy baby who needs to eat more often, strip him down to a diaper and hold him, skin-to-skin, next to you. (If you are chilly, throw a blanket loosely around the two of you.) Rub his back or feet. Talk or sing to him. If baby is still too drowsy to nurse, try sitting him in your lap with his chin in your hand and bend him forward at the hips. Or gently bring him from a horizontal to a vertical position with one hand supporting his head. Or try walking your fingers up and down his spine.

If your baby tends to drift off into sleepy, ineffective sucking after only a few minutes at the breast, you will need to encourage him to keep nursing. The breast compression technique described below is an effective way to do this. Verbal encouragement helps too. One mother of a sleepy baby said that every time her baby opened his eyes during a nursing, she'd say loudly, "Yes! Good! You can do it!" Each time he responded to her words by nursing well for another minute or so. Whether it was mother's pep talks or her all-around attentive mothering we can't say, but baby's thinness was soon replaced by dimpled elbows and chunky legs.

Latched on well? Some babies spend a considerable amount of time at the breast, but still lag in the weight department. The question then is—how well is the baby sucking? Is he latching on to the breast well? He should be getting a large portion of the areola, the dark area surrounding the nipple, into his mouth. The baby who sucks in a fluttery manner on the end of the nipple will get the milk that has already collected in the breast, but he will not take in the additional milk that comes when he draws the nipple far back into his mouth and sucks vigorously. He isn't getting as much milk as he should, nor is it the richest milk, with the highest fat content. If you have sore nipples, this may be an indication that your baby is not latching on correctly.

If you suspect that your baby is not latched on well or is not sucking well, look carefully at how he is nursing. A baby who is sucking well will swallow often once your milk lets down. You will see his whole jaw move when he sucks and you will notice a "wiggle" at his temples, by his ears. You may be able to hear him swallow, or you will notice a slight pause in his breathing when his mouth is open wide which indicates he is swallowing milk. Babies who are breastfeeding effectively will suck actively and swallow milk for ten minutes or more at a feeding.

Getting baby latched on better will help him suck more effectively and get more milk in less time. Check over the section in Chapter 4 called "Breastfeeding in Slow Motion." Be sure baby is positioned at the breast with his whole body facing you, so he does not have to turn his head in order to reach your nipple. Be sure that baby opens his mouth wide as he latches on and that he gets a good-sized mouthful of breast, so that the nipple is positioned far back in his mouth. Baby should latch onto the breast chin first, so that his lower jaw is positioned well back from the nipple.

Some babies find it easier to latch onto the breast effectively when the mother uses a silicone nipple shield over her own nipple. The nipple shield may only need to be used for a few feedings or the baby may need to use it for several weeks. At one time it was thought that the use of a nipple shield interfered with a mother's milk supply. This is no longer considered to be true. Still, if a baby is already gaining slowly, a mother may want to use a breast pump or hand expression after feedings for a while to be sure that her breasts are being stimulated enough. This milk can be fed to the baby if he needs to be supplemented.

You may want to try using the football-hold position or the cross-cradle or transitional hold in order to support his head and have a better view of baby's position and sucking techniques. With the football hold, be sure his body is bent at the hips and he does not arch his back.

Breast compression. Some babies do not gain well because they tend to fall asleep at the breast or they prefer to "nibble" or suck very gently, mainly for comfort. Breast compression is a technique suggested by Dr. Jack Newman that helps to keep the milk flowing. Babies respond to the flow of milk by continuing to suck vigorously, and this enables them to obtain more of the higher-fat milk in the breast. Breast compression is used at the point in the feeding when baby's sucking slows down and he is no longer taking the deep sucks that indicate that he is getting milk. For some babies, this may be after only a few minutes of nursing.

When baby's sucking slows or stops, hold your breast with your thumb on one side and your four fingers on the other. Bring the thumb and fingers together, compressing the breast firmly, but not so hard that it hurts. Compressing the breast will move milk down toward the nipple and the baby will react to the milk flow with active sucking and swallowing.

Keep up the pressure on the breast until baby goes back to "nibbling" instead of sucking actively. Then release the pressure. Some babies may resume active sucking when you release the compression on the breast, as the milk that backed up in the breast behind your hand flows down toward the nipple. Others will not resume sucking until you compress the breast again. Reposition your hand slightly so that you apply pressure to a new part of the breast with each compression.

Continue the breast compressions until they no longer stimulate active sucking. Then switch the baby to the other breast and repeat the process. If needed, you can repeat the breast compression process on both breasts several times in each feeding, as long as the baby responds with active sucking. You might want to experiment with different techniques for compressing the breast to find what works best for you and your baby.

Getting enough hindmilk. While it's a good idea to offer baby both breasts at each feeding, switching sides too soon may prevent baby from getting the high-fat hindmilk he needs. The fat content of the milk in the breast increases the longer a baby nurses. If you switch him to the other breast too soon, he will not get the milk with the higher fat content that helps him grow and leaves his tummy feeling satisfied.

This situation is called a "foremilk-hindmilk" imbalance or an overabundant milk supply. The mother seems to have a good supply of milk but her baby is gaining slowly. He may be nursing often, but he is fussy, very gassy, and has loose greenish stools. He seems to be getting too much milk and may even spit up after feedings. This baby may be filling up on the thinner foremilk from both breasts and not getting enough of the rich hindmilk that comes later in a feeding.

A mother whose baby shows these symptoms can use the breast compression technique described above to encourage her baby to nurse actively for a longer time on the first breast. When baby is finally satisfied at the first breast and pulls away, she can offer the second breast. Some babies may be willing to latch on and nurse some more; others will wait for the next feeding. One interesting study showed that babies who nurse on both breasts at a feeding take in a higher volume of milk, while babies who nurse on only one breast at a feeding have a higher fat intake.

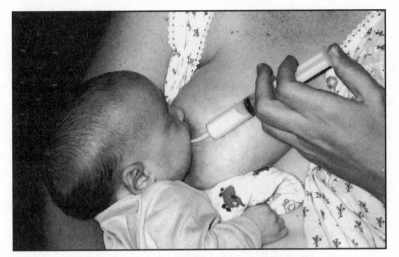

A feeding syringe can be used to give the baby a
supplement at the breast.

Nipple confusion. Using a pacifier or supplemental bottles of water, formula, or juice can cause nipple confusion and interfere with baby's ability to suck effectively at the breast. Just one bottle is enough to confuse some babies, especially in the early weeks. A baby uses totally different techniques to remove milk from your breast than he uses to drink from a bottle. You'll want to be wary of bottles or pacifiers if your baby is gaining slowly as nipple confusion can interfere with a baby's ability to latch on well and suck effectively. If a slow gaining baby needs to be supplemented, alternate feeding methods can be used in order to avoid artificial nipples.

If problems persist

Some breastfeeding problems do not respond readily to the suggestions above. If your baby has gotten into the habit of taking only the end of your nipple or if he nurses "all the time" but is mostly sleeping or just "mouthing" the nipple, not actively sucking and swallowing, he is probably not getting much milk from the breast. Babies who stay at the breast only for a very short time or who refuse the breast entirely also will not get enough milk. If your baby's latch-on and sucking skills do not improve after a day or two of working with him, you will need to seek hands-on help from a La Leche League Leader or a board certified lactation consultant who has experience in this area. You, your helper, and your doctor can then work together to keep your baby growing well as he is learning to breastfeed better. Even babies who get off to a very slow start can eventually be nourished entirely at the breast, though they may need supplementary feedings at first.

A skilled helper can observe a feeding, evaluate your baby's breast-feeding skills, and show you ways to teach your baby to breastfeed more effectively. She can also help you make a plan for giving supplements and pumping your breasts during the time baby is learning how to nurse.

Mothers of babies who are not sucking well need to pump their breasts to protect their milk supply. If milk is not removed from a mother's breasts frequently throughout the day in the first weeks of lactation, milk production will slow down, and it will be more difficult to build up the milk supply later. Pumping prevents this, and the milk you pump can be given to your baby.

Giving supplements

Babies who are gaining weight very slowly (or not at all) at the breast will need supplemental feedings for a time. Supplements do not have to be given with a bottle. In fact, using artificial nipples can make it harder for the baby to learn how to breastfeed effectively. As an alternative to bottles, consider using a cup, eyedropper, feeding syringe, spoon, or bowl. All of these work well when baby needs supplements temporarily, while you work on improving the breastfeeding situation.

To give the baby supplementary feedings with a cup or bowl, choose a small cup, for example, a shot glass or a small flexible plastic cup. Fill it about half full. Be sure the baby is awake and alert and swaddle him in a blanket so that his hands don't get in the way. Hold him upright in your lap. Rest the cup gently on his lower lip and tip it so that a small amount of milk touches his lips. Do not pour milk into his mouth. Leave the cup in position as he swallows, then offer another sip. Let the baby set the pace.

Feeding with a spoon, an eyedropper, or a syringe is similar to cup feeding. Hold the baby in an upright position. Proceed slowly and patiently, and pay careful attention to baby's own feeding rhythm.

Supplements can also be given at the breast using a specially designed nursing supplementer. The baby receives the supplement through a tube while he nurses. This avoids any nipple confusion from artificial nipples and continues to provide the sucking stimulation that your breasts need in order to produce more milk.

First choice for supplementing the breastfed baby is the mother's own milk which she hand-expresses or pumps. If the baby is not breastfeeding effectively, the mother needs to pump so that her breasts will go on producing lots of milk. Regular pumping ensures that the mother will have plenty of milk for her baby as his suck improves. Pumping after feedings will yield milk with high fat levels, which is a particularly good supplement for slow-gaining babies.

Human milk from a milk bank would be the next best supplement after the mother's own milk. However, this may not be readily available. If your baby needs supplements of infant formula, ask your doctor what to use and how to prepare it.

Pumping and giving supplements can be very time-consuming, but it's important to remember that you will be doing

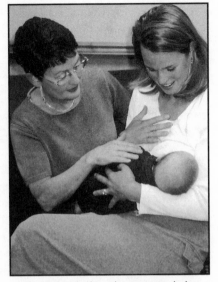

A mother with a slow-gaining baby may need help from someone who is knowledgeable about breastfeeding.

this for a relatively short time. Your investment of time and energy now will be rewarded with better health for your baby along with a long and satisfying breastfeeding relationship.

Checklist for mothers

If your baby is slow to put on weight, you'll want to take good care of yourself so that you have the energy and confidence you need to build up your milk supply and help your baby learn to breastfeed more effectively. Are you doing too much and not getting enough rest? One pediatrician's prescription for slow gainers is to put mother and baby to bed together for a few days. Try to reduce outside stress in your life. Ask friends and family to bring you meals and run your errands. Make your baby your main concern for the time being.

Making sure that milk is removed from your breasts regularly—either by your baby's effective breastfeeding or with a good quality pump—will ensure that your body continues to produce milk for your baby. Taking care of your own needs will help you stay healthy and deal with the stresses of being a new mother. Are you eating well? Think now—what did you have for breakfast today? Was lunch "on the run"? Are you drinking enough water or juice? Your liquid intake can include some coffee and tea, but keep in mind that caffeine will not help you feel any calmer and it will make it harder for you to nap when the opportunity presents itself. Excessive amounts of beverages containing caffeine have been known to adversely affect the weight gain of some babies. The same is true of smoking, especially if the mother is a heavy smoker.

Hormonal contraceptives, especially those that contain estrogen, have been found to affect a mother's milk supply. Could it be that you are anemic or have an underactive thyroid? Both of these conditions can affect a mother's milk supply if they are left untreated. Check with your doctor about these possibilities.

The doctor's advice

Your doctor will want to see your baby regularly for weight checks until everyone is assured that he is breastfeeding effectively and growing well. Tell your doctor what you are doing to help your baby breastfeed better and gain weight more quickly. If supplements are needed, discuss your preference for pumping or hand-expressing between feedings and supplementing with your own milk. If you cannot pump enough milk to meet your baby's needs, your doctor can advise you about supplementing with infant formula.

Over the past two decades, the medical profession has become more knowledgeable about breastfeeding, but most physicians will not have the in-depth knowledge of breastfeeding techniques needed to help a mother with a baby who is not sucking effectively. Your doctor should be able to refer you to a lactation consultant or another expert who can help you. If your baby's doctor is not helpful in your efforts to continue giving your baby human milk, you may want to seek another opinion from a more supportive physician in your community.

A slow gaining baby may be having difficulty sucking well because of a birth injury or other physical discomfort. This is something your doctor will need to check. A baby with a short frenulum (tongue-tie) may also have difficulty sucking effectively and his mother may have sore nipples. A short frenulum can be clipped in a doctor's or dentist's office with no stitches or anesthetic. This procedure often brings immediate improvement in baby's sucking ability.

Some babies who are not sucking effectively respond well to chiropractic adjustment, massage therapy, or other gentle, non-invasive treatments by practitioners who are accustomed to treating infants.

There are some situations in which the use of herbal or prescription medications can help to increase a mother's milk supply. Prescription medications would need to be recommended by a doctor or other health care professional.

In some very few cases a mother may not be able to increase her milk supply to fully meet her baby's needs. This could be caused by a variety of reasons—previous breast surgery, a hormonal problem, or inadequate breast development. Whatever the cause, a mother can continue to offer the breast while the baby receives whatever supplements are needed. She does not have to give up breastfeeding entirely.

Babies are meant to grow and thrive and everyone is happy when they do. If your baby is not gaining well, there may be reason for concern, but be assured that your milk is still the perfect food for him. Once he gets enough to eat, his glowing health and fat cheeks will be a source of pride and satisfaction for you in the months and years ahead.

Slow weight gain in an older breastfed baby

From four to six months, a breastfed baby's weight gain usually slows to four to five ounces (113 to 142 grams) per week. Increases in length, head, and chest circumference are also signs of growth. Alertness and good skin tone also indicate that baby is getting enough to eat. From six to twelve months, a healthy breastfed baby may gain only two to four ounces (57 to 113 grams) per week.

Studies comparing growth in breastfed and formula-fed babies show that there are differences between the two groups. After three months of age, breastfed babies gain more slowly than artificially fed infants. While changes in length and head circumference are similar, the breastfed babies, on average, are leaner at one year of age. The growth charts used by most doctors are based on formula-fed infants, and may not be accurate for breastfed babies.

Why do some babies grow more slowly than others? There may be one simple explanation or a combination of reasons. Could a minor illness be causing the problem? Often, a baby who is not feeling well does not nurse well. Of course, the baby's doctor will check him over thoroughly to be assured that illness is not the cause of the problem. And if the baby is sick, nursing is of even more value. An all-out effort to maintain breastfeeding, along with appropriate treatment for the illness, will speed recovery.

Sometimes slow weight gain in a baby who had been growing well can be attributed to a change in the breastfeeding pattern. The baby may be nursing less often as mother gets back into a busy routine. Some babies become so curious about the world around them that it's hard for them to settle in and nurse for very long. Making an effort to breastfeed more often and for a longer time may be all that is needed to get baby's weight gain back on track.

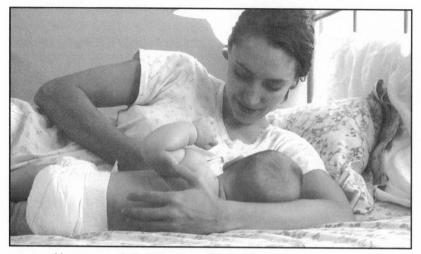

Nursing your baby lying down gives you a chance to rest when
you are not feeling well.

What If Mother Is Ill?

"How can I take care of my baby if I get sick?" This is a common question of anxious mothers. Of course, caring for an active, healthy baby is
a demanding job at any time, but when mother is ill it can be of real
concern. It is reassuring to know that nursing your baby makes caring
for him so much easier. For minor illnesses, such as a cold or the flu,
you needn't even consider interrupting breastfeeding. The germs are
not transmitted through your milk, and the baby has no doubt been
exposed to the illness for at least as long as you have, and certainly was
exposed to it before you knew you had it.

Your milk can actually protect your baby from getting sick when
you have a cold or the flu. A nursing mother produces antibodies to the
specific germs her baby has been exposed to. These antibodies are
transmitted to the baby through her milk. Continuing to breastfeed
also helps you get the extra rest you need when you aren't feeling well.
Sudden weaning would not be good for either you or your baby.

If your illness is more serious—for example, if you are being
treated for hepatitis or tuberculosis—doctors on our Health Advisory
Council still advise continued breastfeeding. Breastfeeding requires a
minimum of effort for you, giving you the most rest. In addition, your
milk helps to keep your baby healthy and happy.

If you become seriously ill and your doctor suggests weaning the
baby, explain how important breastfeeding is to both of you. If your
doctor still insists that weaning is necessary, you may find that talking
to your baby's doctor or seeking a second opinion helps you sort out
your options and find a way to avoid weaning your baby. It would be a

good idea to discuss your situation with your local La Leche League Leader as she may know of other doctors who are more supportive of breastfeeding.

Hospitalization

Consider all options before being admitted to the hospital. It is much better if you can remain at home during your illness. Get help with the necessary housework, laundry, meals, and caring for the older children. Tuck your little one in bed with you, where he will be close by all the time and able to nurse whenever he wants.

If a serious illness or an accident requires hospitalization, you will want to make arrangements to have your baby kept with you, or at least brought to you. Nursing mothers have found all kinds of ingenious ways to avoid being separated from their babies during hospital stays. Discuss your needs and those of your baby with your husband and your doctor. Your condition, the hospital's facilities, and your baby's age and usual nursing pattern will all influence the situation.

More and more patients are now being sent home from the hospital on the same day that they have surgery. If this is possible in your case, you can then return home to rest and nurse your baby without any prolonged separation. Procedures such as dental work can nearly always be carried out without interruption of breastfeeding. When the potential surgery is elective, it may be possible to postpone the procedure until the baby is older.

If you must stay in the hospital overnight or for several days, your husband or a friend or relative can bring the baby in to visit you and nurse. Some hospitals may be willing to admit the baby and allow him to room-in with you, though they may require that someone stay in the room with you to help care for the baby.

Be flexible and polite as you talk over your requests with the doctors and hospital. If you are willing to cooperate with hospital personnel, they will usually be cooperative, too. Let them see how much it means to you to keep your baby with you.

Major surgery

Even when a mother is required to have major surgery, arrangements can often be made to allow her to continue breastfeeding. If some feedings must be missed, you can plan on using a breast pump so your breasts will not become engorged. Ask that your need to pump your breasts is included in your medical chart. The hospital may be able to provide you with a breast pump, and nurses can assist you if you are unable to manage the pump on your own.

There is no need to avoid nursing your baby, or using milk that you have pumped, because of general anesthesia. You can breastfeed your baby or pump your milk as soon as you are awake after the surgery. The medications used for general or local anesthesia will not be harmful to your baby.

In some cases where a few days of separation are unavoidable, your little one will more than likely be willing and eager to return to nursing once you're back together. Marilyn Mastro of Florida needed to have a hysterectomy when her daughter, Frances, was a year old and still nursing. She tells her story:

> The surgery was successful. There were no postoperative complications, and my husband was allowed to bring the girls in to see me four days later. Frances was allowed to nurse (with a pillow under her to protect my stitches) for the first time in four-and-a-half days. I had used a breast pump to relieve the engorgement and to keep up my milk supply. Pete said that after that short period of nursing, Franny slept better than she had during any of the other nights while I was away.
>
> My doctor discharged me the next day and I came home and resumed breastfeeding and mothering my family. I had presumed that "complete hysterectomy" would mean the end of the joys of nursing, and this thought was very depressing and frightening. As my daughter suckled my milk supply back to her satisfaction I realized how important motherhood and nursing had become to me. I'm glad my doctor hadn't convinced me to wean Franny completely because I need her closeness now almost as much as she needs me.

Medications and Other Substances

Be sure to check with your doctor before taking any medication while you are breastfeeding, even drugs that are available without a prescription. Usually the amount of the drug found in mother's milk is so small that it won't affect the baby at all, but you still want to avoid unnecessary drugs for your own sake while you are nursing your baby.

If any doctor is prescribing medication for you, be sure he or she is aware that you are breastfeeding your baby and knows how important it is for you to continue. There are three questions to consider when a breastfeeding mother needs medication: Will the drug harm the nursing baby? Do the risks related to the drug outweigh the risks of weaning to infant formula? What alternative treatments are available?

When prescribing a medication for a nursing mother, some physicians routinely insist on weaning as a precaution. In reality, few drugs have been proven to be harmful to the nursing infant. A physician who advises weaning just as a precaution may not be considering the risks associated with feeding a baby infant formula. Formula is not the nutritional equivalent of human milk. Babies who are formula-fed are at greater risk of illness and allergy. Also, abrupt weaning is traumatic for mother and baby. Mother may develop painfully engorged breasts, risking a breast infection and compounding the problems for which she was advised to take the medication in the first place. The mother/baby relationship is adversely affected by sudden weaning. Caring for the baby and keeping him contented becomes difficult or impossible; the baby is often utterly inconsolable.

In the 2002 edition of his book, *Medications and Mothers' Milk*, Thomas W. Hale, RPh, PhD, states:

> Although interrupting breastfeeding may seem safest to the physician, it is not really necessary in most cases as the amount of drug transferred to milk is normally quite small. It is well known that most medications have few side effects in breastfeeding infants because the dose transferred via milk is almost always too low to be clinically relevant or it is poorly bioavailable to the infant.

Most doctors have found that if a particular drug poses a potential risk for the baby, usually it is possible to substitute something else with less or no risk. When little is known about a drug's effect on a nursing baby, another medication about which there is more information can often be used instead. In some cases, the doctor may suggest monitoring the baby for side-effects of a medication taken by the mother. It may also be possible to alter or postpone treatment until the baby is older.

An increasing number of studies are being done on the subject of medications and their effects on breastfeeding. If there is any question about the safety of a drug for a nursing mother and her baby, it's a good idea to check with someone who is knowledgeable about medications as well as supportive of breastfeeding. Ask your doctor to talk with your baby's doctor. Pediatricians are often more familiar with the effects of medication on a breastfed baby than are physicians who treat only adults. Several reference books listed in the Appendix include information about the effects of medications on breastfeeding. The American Academy of Pediatrics publishes a listing of drugs that are safe to take while breastfeeding. Also check the articles listed in the References for this section. Information about drugs and breastfeeding is available to your doctor over the Internet. A La Leche League Leader may also be able to help you find more information, or she may be able to guide you to additional sources. Most questions about medications for the nursing mother can be resolved in a way that keeps baby at the breast.

Drugs that should be avoided while nursing

There are a small number of drugs that are contraindicated while you are breastfeeding. For example, the toxic drugs used in chemotherapy treatments for cancer are considered hazardous to the nursing baby. It is always necessary to wean if chemotherapy is required.

Some radioactive compounds used to diagnose and sometimes to treat certain conditions may appear in a mother's milk at levels high enough that there would be a risk to the baby. Depending on the type of compound used and the dosage, your baby may not be allowed to nurse at the breast for several hours, or even much longer. You can pump your milk during this time to keep up your supply, and discard it. Ask your doctor or the radiologist who will be supervising the test to investigate which substances are most compatible with breastfeeding.

Radioactive compounds used for treatment may require lengthy weaning, however, some mothers have pumped and discarded their milk, as necessary, for several months and then resumed nursing once their milk was free of radioactive material.

Immunizations

If your blood is Rh-negative and your baby's is Rh-positive, you will probably receive an injection of Rh antibodies (RhoGAM) very soon after you deliver. RhoGAM is used widely to prevent Rh complications, and it is not harmful to your nursing infant.

Along with RhoGAM, many other vaccines do not affect the breastfed baby through his mother's milk. According to the United States Centers for Disease Control (2002), "Neither killed nor live vaccines affect the safety of breastfeeding for mothers and infants. Acceptable vaccines include: chicken pox, smallpox, typhus, typhoid, yellow fever, oral and injected polio, tetanus, diphtheria, pertussis, rabies, measles, rubella, cholera, and influenza. Hepatitis B vaccine is also safe for nursing mothers."

With regard to immunizations for your baby, the same schedule is usually followed for the breastfed baby as for formula-fed infants.

Some doctors believe in delaying the immunization schedule for breastfed babies because of the protection they are receiving from their mother's milk.

In his book, *Listening to Your Baby*, pediatrician Jay Gordon, MD, expresses his opinion:

> My personal feeling is that your two-month-old baby's immune system is not yet ready to receive these shots and you should wait. This point of view is held by a very small minority of doctors, and I recommend discussing vaccines and their timing with your pediatrician.

There is no need to refrain from nursing the baby before or after administration of any vaccine, including the oral polio vaccine. Some studies indicate that breastfed babies respond better to immunizations, producing more immunities in their blood than babies who are formula-fed.

Other substances of concern

Smoking. Even if you are a smoker, you are probably acquainted with the disturbing statistics on the effects of smoking. The potential hazards of smoking during pregnancy may have been incentive enough for you to quit or cut down. However, despite your best intentions, you may find yourself still smoking when your baby is born, and you may be wondering how this will affect breastfeeding. Health professionals agree that the baby of a mother who smokes is better off breastfed than formula-fed. A breastfed baby in a smoking household will benefit greatly from the protection against respiratory disease that comes with mother's milk.

In general, if a mother smokes only a few cigarettes a day, the amount of nicotine in her milk is not usually enough to cause any problem for the baby. Though nicotine can be found in a mother's milk after she smokes, it is not readily absorbed by the baby's intestinal tract and is rather quickly metabolized. The fewer cigarettes smoked, the less chance there is that there will be any adverse effects on the baby. By keeping smoking to a minimum, a mother can decrease the potential risks to her baby.

When a nursing mother smokes heavily (more than twenty cigarettes a day), there may be reason for concern. Heavy smoking can reduce a mother's milk supply and on rare occasions has caused symptoms in the nursing baby such as nausea, vomiting, abdominal cramps, and diarrhea. One study found that smoking lowers prolactin levels in nursing mothers. In other studies, smoking was shown to interfere with the let-down reflex.

Many studies have shown that secondhand smoke is harmful for babies and young children. Through the years, numerous studies have found that babies and children exposed to smoke from adult cigarettes have significantly higher rates of respiratory disease, including pneumonia and bronchitis. The incidence of Sudden Infant Death Syndrome (SIDS) is also higher in babies exposed to secondhand smoke. If anyone in the household smokes, it should only be done away from the baby, in a separate room or outdoors.

Since there are legitimate concerns about the effects of smoking on a breastfeeding mother and her baby, the ideal solution is to avoid smoking. For those who can't quit, cutting down is an option that might seem more within reach. But don't stop breastfeeding.

Alcohol. Because of studies that show that alcohol can harm the unborn baby, many mothers do not drink alcohol at all while pregnant. These mothers may wonder if they must continue to abstain from alcohol during the time they are nursing.

The effects of alcohol on the breastfeeding baby are directly related to the amount the mother ingests. When the breastfeeding mother drinks occasionally or limits her consumption to one drink or less per day, the amount of alcohol her baby receives has not been proven to be harmful. If you enjoy an occasional glass of wine in the evening, or a cold beer on a hot summer day, there's no reason to deprive yourself of this because you are breastfeeding.

Alcohol does pass freely into a mother's milk and has been found to peak at 30 to 90 minutes after consumption of one alcoholic drink. Once the mother's body metabolizes the alcohol, a process that takes two to three hours, the alcohol is eliminated from her system and from her milk. However, the more alcohol that is consumed, the greater the amounts in her milk and the longer it takes to be eliminated. Large amounts of alcohol have been found to inhibit the let-down reflex. Other studies have shown that babies nursed more frequently but consumed less milk after their mothers had been given an alcoholic drink. Regular abuse of alcohol by a breastfeeding mother could result in slow weight gain or failure-to-thrive in her baby. Alcohol abuse will also interfere with a mother's ability to enjoy and care for her baby.

An anxious, overtired mother may sometimes find that a glass of wine or beer helps her to feel relaxed. But there are other ways to let go of stress. Many mothers find that tension drains away with a cup of hot or iced tea or another favorite beverage. Lying down can do wonders, and listening to music is soothing. Especially nice is having your husband's reassuring arms around you when you're feeling stressed by your new responsibilities.

Drugs of abuse. Marijuana, cocaine, amphetamines, heroin, and other illegal substances should be totally avoided by a breastfeeding mother. Research shows they can have harmful effects on the nursing baby and they can also be detrimental to a mother's ability to care for her baby. The use of marijuana, for example, has been found to cause significantly lower levels of prolactin, the "mothering" hormone that is important not only to an adequate milk supply but to the whole mother-baby relationship. THC, the active chemical in marijuana, is concentrated in human milk and appears in a baby's urine long after a breastfeeding mother has used it.

Cocaine and heroin pass into a mother's milk in significant amounts and can cause intoxication and addiction in the breastfed baby. Nursing mothers should avoid these substances.

Environmental contaminants

Contaminants in the environment have become an inescapable fact of modern life. We are all exposed to chemicals in the air we breathe and in our food and water. As a result, traces of environmental chemicals are found in human milk, as well as in cow's milk and in human urine, blood, and hair. Widespread publicity about the presence of certain chemicals found in mother's milk may raise questions about the overall safety of breastfeeding. In fact, testing human milk samples is used as a convenient way to monitor levels of a specific chemical in a human population group. The reports of chemicals found in human milk actually reflect their presence in the overall population. Environmental groups who report these results are not questioning the value of breastfeeding; they are trying to alert the public to the danger of these chemicals for everyone.

While the testing of milk samples from many mothers may provide valuable information for scientists seeking to clean up our environment, the situation can become intensely personal for a breastfeeding mother when reports in the media call attention to high levels of certain chemicals in human milk. What are the implications for her and her baby? Should she have her milk tested? Should she continue to breastfeed?

Our advice is to use common sense. Put the matter of contaminants in perspective. First of all, there is no evidence to date of any harm coming to a breastfed baby because of the presence of these substances in his mother's milk. In contrast, the risks of feeding babies artificial infant formula are well documented. Switching to infant formula may or may not lower the amount of that one chemical in the baby's diet, but it will definitely expose the baby to many other risks, including a greater likelihood of developing allergies and various illnesses.

One study in the US that examined a possible correlation between levels of certain chemicals in human milk and infant development found higher cognitive scores in the children who were breastfed, compared to those given formula—regardless of any chemicals in the milk. Another study published in 1996 in *Pediatrics* found that infants exposed to PCB and dioxin through human milk nevertheless scored significantly higher on mental and motor tests than artificially fed infants. The benefits of breastfeeding clearly outweighed any possible effects of exposure to environmental contaminants through human milk.

Contaminants are not to be taken lightly, of course. They pose a risk to all of us, and research must continue to determine the overall extent of this risk and what should be done about it. There will be times when human milk samples from many mothers are analyzed and the average levels of one or more chemicals will be reason for concern. But this does not mean that mothers should stop breastfeeding. While there is much that we don't know about the effects of contaminants in our environment, we know with certainty that artificial infant formula is inferior nourishment when compared to human milk. In addition, a baby being fed formula is exposed to chemicals beyond those in the formula itself, including lead and pollutants in the water used to prepare the formula. There is even concern about exposure to latex used in artificial nipples.

Analysis of human milk shows variability on a day-to-day and even a morning-to-evening basis, so testing a single milk sample cannot give a true picture of what the baby is actually getting. A study in Norway on insecticides in human milk showed a dramatic variance in the same mother's milk at different times. Repeated testing and careful analysis would be required to give meaningful results, and even then, safety levels have not been clearly defined. Testing milk samples may give scientists information about contaminants in the general population, but it does not provide useful information for individual mothers.

What can you do to lower the amount of environmental contaminants you, your baby, and the rest of your family receive? Give serious thought to what you eat and the products you use in your home. Discontinue the use of pesticides and other sprays in your home or on your lawn or garden. As much as possible, try to avoid eating foods that may contain residues of pesticides. Fruits and vegetables should be peeled or thoroughly washed under running water using a mild dish-washing soap. When you are pregnant and nursing, it's wise to avoid eating freshwater fish from waters that are known to be contaminated. Reduce your intake of red meat and dairy products and cut fat from meat and poultry, since most of the contaminants in animal-based foods are concentrated in the fat. If you minimize your exposure to chemicals in your home environment, you will be helping to keep your family healthy.

Mothers with Special Problems

A mother who is disabled in any way will find it convenient to breast-feed her baby. This is true of blind mothers, hearing-impaired moth-ers, mothers who are confined to wheelchairs, and mothers who are recovering from illness or injuries. Breastfeeding requires less effort than bottle-feeding, and nourishing her baby with her own milk may be especially satisfying to a mother with a disability. Many LLL publi-cations are available on cassette tape or in Braille for use by blind or handicapped parents.

Mothers with chronic illnesses also benefit from the ease and satis-faction of breastfeeding their babies. Illnesses such as diabetes, lupus, arthritis, epilepsy, or multiple sclerosis need not interfere with a mother's decision to breastfeed her baby. Most medications taken for these conditions are compatible with breast-feeding. Breastfeeding makes life eas-ier. One mother with diabetes says:

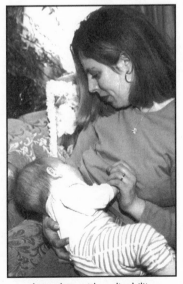

When a mother breastfeeds, she doesn't waste her time sterilizing bottles and preparing formula. The mother only has to bring the baby to bed, relax, and enjoy. Probably the biggest advantage is that the baby is healthier. Breastfeeding saves many trips to the doctor's office with ear infec-tions, digestive problems, and allergies.

A mother with a disability can take special pride in breastfeeding her baby.

Breastfed babies also tend to be less fussy because human milk is more easily digested than formula. If a breastfed baby is fussy, often just putting him to the breast is enough to calm him.

One physical advantage of breastfeeding is especially noteworthy. Many women with chronic illnesses find that the normal hormonal changes of pregnancy result in a temporary remission of their symptoms. When a woman breastfeeds, her hormonal levels do not revert back to their pre-pregnancy state right away; this happens gradually. If weaning occurs at a natural pace, her symptoms often return much later than if she were not breastfeeding, giving her better health when her tiny baby needs her most. Temporary remission during pregnancy and breastfeeding has been reported by mothers with rheumatoid arthritis, multiple sclerosis, lupus, and diabetes.

Breastfeeding can contribute to a woman's self-esteem and self-confidence as a mother. These kinds of positive feelings may also have a favorable effect on the course of her illness. One mother with epilepsy says:

> Breastfeeding has been a salvation for me, especially on days when I knew there was very little I could do for my child. At least I was giving the very best of myself in extremely important areas—food, warmth, affection, touching, and caring. I could never have gathered the strength or had the energy to give bottles.

There may be some things a mother can do, depending on her illness, to make nursing easier. For the mother with rheumatoid arthritis, it might help to set up a comfortable place to nurse with good support and extra pillows. An epileptic mother needs to have a safe place to lay the baby in the event of a seizure and to nurse in a chair that is well-padded or in a bed with guard rails or extra pillows.

Another benefit of breastfeeding for the chronically ill mother is the emotional closeness it adds to her relationship with her baby and the sense of normalcy that it brings to her situation.

Gail Stutler, who was recovering from brain surgery when her second child was born, recalls that she was helpless in many ways, but still, "I could scoop up a tiny bundle, put her to my breast, and nurse her close to my heart. I could satisfy at least one of the desperate needs I had when deprived of all my capabilities."

A mother with diabetes

Breastfeeding offers special advantages for diabetic mothers and their babies. Studies indicate that breastfeeding may reduce the baby's risk of developing both Type 1 and Type 2 diabetes later in life. Breastfeeding tends to make diabetes easier to manage after childbirth, since the mother's body makes a slower, more natural transition from the metabolic demands of pregnancy to the non-pregnant state. Stress, which is a normal part of adjusting to life with a new baby, can aggravate diabetes, but lactation hormones help mothers handle stress better.

Babies of diabetic mothers may routinely spend the first day or two after birth in the special-care nursery. This early separation can make it more difficult to get a good start at breastfeeding. Talk to your baby's doctor before the birth about your desire to breastfeed and room-in with your baby, if at all possible. The medical personnel will be checking to be sure your baby does not develop hypoglycemia. Frequent breastfeeding provides the baby with colostrum which will help to avoid hypoglycemia. You will be able to feed your baby more often if he is with you. A diabetic mother may find that her milk supply does not become more plentiful or "come in" until the fourth or fifth day after birth.

As breastfeeding continues, a diabetic mother may have to make adjustments in her diet based on how often her baby nurses from day to day. If she takes insulin, she will have to regulate the dosage as carefully as she did while she was pregnant in order to keep her diabetes under control while nursing. The insulin itself will not hurt the baby because its molecules are too large to pass into the milk. Mothers with diabetes may also be more likely to develop yeast infections. La Leche League's pamphlet, "The Diabetic Mother and Breastfeeding," provides further information. See the Appendix for details.

Epilepsy or seizure disorder

Mothers with epilepsy or seizure disorder benefit from the nursing hormones and the relaxation engendered by natural mothering. If the mother must take medication to control her seizures, she should check with her doctor about the drug's effects on breastfeeding. Most drugs prescribed for epilepsy won't harm the nursing baby. If your doctor is uncertain about the effects of a particular drug, perhaps one that is so new that little is known about it, he or she may be able to prescribe another drug instead. Another option is for the doctor to monitor the baby and watch for any signs that the drug is affecting his growth or development.

If you are a mother with a disability or chronic illness, it would be helpful for you to be in touch with your local LLL Leader. She will be able to offer you additional information and encouragement and may be able to put you in touch with another mother who has nursed her baby in circumstances similar to yours. Contacting someone who has "been there" can help give you the confidence you need to feel that you can do it, too.

Human immunodeficiency virus (HIV)

A mother who is HIV-positive faces a difficult situation when she considers whether or not to breastfeed her baby. Human immunodeficiency virus (HIV) is considered to be the virus that causes AIDS. HIV can be transmitted from mother to baby during pregnancy or at birth. Some evidence suggests that HIV can also be passed to the baby through breastfeeding. Whether or not a baby will become infected may be influenced by the stage of the mother's infection, what medical treatment she is receiving, the duration and exclusivity of breastfeeding, the mother's nutritional status, and other factors. A study published in 2001 showed that transmission rates of HIV were lower when mothers breastfed exclusively for three months or more than when infants were given both human milk and formula.

Whether or not an HIV-positive mother chooses to breastfeed will depend on her circumstances. In parts of the world where not breastfeeding puts a baby at serious risk of dying from infection or malnutrition, babies of HIV-positive mothers have a greater chance to survive if they are breastfed. In parts of the world where artificial feeding does not carry such grave risks, mothers with HIV may choose not to breastfeed. At this time, both the World Health Organization and the United States Centers for Disease Control advise against breastfeeding in HIV-infected women where safe alternatives are available.

More specific research on the relationship between HIV and breastfeeding is needed because many questions remain unanswered. A recent review article published in April 2003 lists twelve pivotal research questions about breastfeding and HIV that remain unanswered. A pregnant woman who is HIV-positive should seek out the most recent information before making a decision about breastfeeding.

AnotherLook is a nonprofit organization dedicated to gathering information, raising critical questions, and stimulating needed research about breastfeeding in the context of HIV/AIDS. Their Web site at www.anotherlook.org is updated regularly to reflect current research and recommendations.

Postpartum depression

Many mothers experience a day or so of "baby blues" in the first week postpartum. They suddenly find themselves crying for no apparent reason, wondering how they can feel so sad when they're supposed to feel so happy. The great changes and responsibilities that come with a new baby also bring worry and anxiety, and a mother's emotions may be magnified by shifting postpartum hormones and lack of sleep. For most women this period passes quickly, but for others, anxiety, sadness, mood swings, or other symptoms persist for weeks or even reappear months after giving birth. This is no longer "baby blues"; this is postpartum depression.

Depression is not something you can just "snap out of," though there may be people who suggest that a mother should do just that. Mild depression may lift with time, especially if a mother makes a disciplined effort to take care of herself. She should eat nutritious meals and snacks, take a daily walk or try some other form of exercise, get help with household tasks, and sleep when the baby sleeps. Most importantly, she should find other women with babies to talk with, friends who can reassure her that she is doing a good job and that she is not alone in her feelings. A La Leche League Group can be a valuable source of support for a mother struggling with postpartum adjustments.

When a mother is anxious about her ability to care for her baby, or is just plain feeling "down," breastfeeding may become the focus of her worries. She may find it hard to trust that her body will make enough milk for her baby, or she may begin to feel that breastfeeding itself is the cause of her unhappiness. While difficulties with nursing can certainly be upsetting, many mothers find that getting some assistance in order to resolve the breastfeeding problems is a more positive course of action than deciding to wean. Ultimately, both mother and baby benefit. It's also important to remember that the challenges often experienced by new mothers will still be there, even if the baby is switched to formula.

When a woman experiences persistent postpartum depression, she may need assistance from a counselor, a psychiatrist, or both, in getting herself back on track. A mother cannot care for her baby effectively if she is feeling sad or anxious much of the time, so it is important to seek help. It's a good idea to talk with several potential counselors or doctors before choosing one to work with. A mother will want to find a doctor or therapist who is supportive of breastfeeding and understands its importance to both mother and baby.

Depression can often be treated very effectively with medication, but there may be some concern about whether a particular drug is safe for the baby. This is a time to consider carefully the mother's need for the drug, the possible alternatives, and the latest information available about the medication. In many cases, it is possible to choose a medication that is compatible with breastfeeding. A mother may want to include her husband or a friend in these discussions with the doctor, to help make clear her desire to avoid weaning. Ending the breastfeeding relationship can be very difficult for a mother emotionally and sudden weaning may cause hormonal changes that intensify her depression. Any decisions about how to treat postpartum depression should take this into account. (See the Appendix and References for sources of information about medications and breastfeeding that can be shared with the mother's doctor.)

PART SEVEN

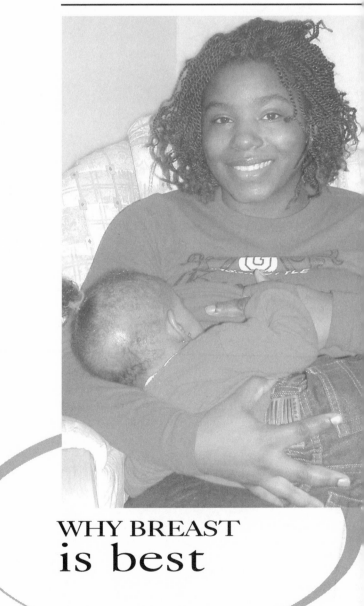

WHY BREAST
is best

CHAPTER EIGHTEEN

HUMAN MILK FOR
human babies

In the nearly half century since La Leche League was founded, science has learned a great deal about human milk and its role in babies' growth and development. Research has shown that human milk is far more than good food. It is a living fluid that protects babies from disease and actively contributes to the development of every system in baby's body. Human infants are relatively immature at birth, and feeding at mother's breast is nature's way of bridging the developmental gap between growing in the protective environment of the womb and being able to survive out in the world.

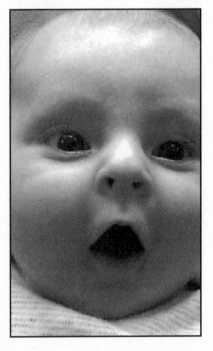

Breastfeeding plays a critical role in nature's plan for ensuring that human babies survive and grow. Feeding at mother's breast nourishes babies and provides the raw materials they need in order to develop in the way that nature intended. As science learns more about the complex ingredients in human milk and the ways in which mother's body is attuned to the needs of her breastfeeding infant, it becomes very clear that artificial feeding—formula feeding—is a substantial departure from nature's plan. While babies fed infant formula do grow and develop adequately,

339

manufactured infant formula does not promote optimal growth and development as does the milk designed by nature for human babies.

This chapter describes the many ways in which human milk and the whole process of breastfeeding play key roles in babies' development and well-being. Common sense has long dictated that milk made by mother herself is superior to manufactured substitutes, and a growing collection of scientific evidence fully supports this conclusion. Breastfeeding is not just an "extra" that you may or may not choose to give your baby. It is more than a few added vitamins or health-boosting antibodies. Human milk is the key to good health and development for human infants. Breastfeeding is every baby's birthright. After all, babies are born to breastfeed!

How Your Baby Grows

"My, how that baby has grown!" This admiring comment is music to a nursing mother's ears. Babies grow faster in the first months of life than at any other time. The human brain is one-third its adult size at birth and reaches the two-thirds mark by age one. Your baby's head grows about four-and-one-half inches (11.25 centimeters) during his first year to allow for the tremendous growth of his brain. Good muscle development and substantial increase in length are other significant signs of progress, along with baby's weight gain.

Babies also grow in ways that can't be measured with a tape measure or scale. During the first year of life, babies' nervous and endocrine systems mature, they develop better control of their muscles, and their immune systems become better able to protect their bodies from germs. In just twelve months, babies learn to sit up, to crawl, and to stand, and to focus on faces, objects, and tasks. At one year of age, babies still need a great deal of care, but they are well on their way to becoming independent.

Growing up is a complicated process for a baby, one that requires not just any food, but food that contains the right kinds of proteins, fats, and carbohydrates that babies need to build high-quality brains and muscles. Adult bodies can break down or transform one type of protein or fat into another, but babies cannot always do this efficiently. Human milk provides the specific nutrients that babies need to grow, both in size and maturity, for the first six months of life. Even after babies start to eat solid foods, sometime in the middle of the first year, human milk remains their nutritional mainstay for most of the first year. And along with the basic nutrients found in human milk, babies get a healthy dose of hormones, enzymes, and immunities that protect

them from disease and help every system in their bodies develop in the way
nature planned.

Your milk is uniquely suited to
meet your baby's nutritional needs.
No two mothers produce identical
milk (although all but the most malnourished mothers produce milk
whose high quality is remarkably consistent). The composition of your milk
varies from day to day and during different times of the day—just as other
fluids and systems in our bodies fluc-
tuate. The colostrum your baby
receives on the first day of his life is
different from the colostrum on day
two or three. Premature babies need
greater amounts of some nutrients
than full-term babies, and milk from

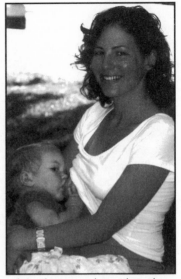

A mother can take pride in the
unique qualities of the milk she is
giving her baby.

mothers who deliver early contains higher levels of many of these
nutrients.

Even the taste of the milk changes with the diet of the mother.
One study showed that when mothers consumed garlic capsules, their
milk had the odor of garlic, and their babies sucked more vigorously
and took in more milk. You could say that your milk is programming
your baby's taste buds for the coming fare on the family dinner table.
During one feeding, your milk varies from skim to creamy, permitting
your breastfed baby to enjoy a change of tastes that could be compared
to a multi-course meal. Human milk will sustain, strengthen, protect,
and fill out your baby's precious body, and put a recognizable bloom on
his skin. Human milk is the food of choice for human infants; anything
else is a distant second.

Unique Milk for a Unique Species

All mammals produce milk but the composition of that milk differs
from one species of mammal to another. All milk consists mainly of
water, protein, fat, and lactose (a sugar), along with a generous dash of
vitamins and minerals and traces of enzymes and hormones. However,
the proportions of the various components of milk differ greatly from
one species to another to accommodate different growth rates, different behavior, and different needs.

Cow's milk, for example, contains larger amounts of protein than human milk since calves need to grow rapidly to keep up with mother in the meadow. Whale's milk is high in fat, because baby whales need a layer of blubber to keep them warm in cold seas. Human milk has higher levels of lactose and specific long chain fatty acids which are important to the development of humans' most important tool—the brain. The lower levels of protein in human milk mean that human babies need to feed often, so human mothers keep their babies close to them. This arrangement works out well, since human babies also need close human contact to be kept safe from danger and to develop the social skills that are important to their survival.

Artificial infant feeding products are only a rough imitation of human milk. Most infant formula is made from cow's milk that is diluted with water to decrease the protein content. Sugar must then be added to increase the level of carbohydrates and calories. Formula advertising may boast of fats that nurture brain development or of other modifications that promise that a specific brand is "best for baby." But tinkering with a few proteins or fatty acids will not transform artificial baby milk into anything close to the complex array of nutrients found in human milk. Completely missing in artificial infant feeding products are the live cells that help protect baby from disease and the enzymes and hormones that support baby's physiological development. Infant formula cannot duplicate all the subtle ways in which human milk supports infant growth and health. Human milk is uniquely suitable for human infants because of the complex balance of ingredients.

Proteins are the key to growth

Of all the substances that make up living things, proteins are the most distinctive, the most characteristic of the species. Proteins in your milk are as different from those in cow's milk (or other animal milks) as you are from a cow. The most notable distinction is the difference in relative amounts of casein and whey proteins. The large amount of casein protein in cow's milk forms large, tough, rubbery curds that are difficult for the human baby to digest. This explains why a formula-fed baby's tummy remains "full" longer than the breastfed baby's. Whey protein, which is more plentiful in mother's milk, is perfectly suited to the human baby's digestive system. It is higher in nutritive value than casein protein and makes for a softer, better-smelling stool. Many of the whey proteins in human milk also play important roles in protecting babies from infection.

Amino acids and taurine

Proteins break down into amino acids, the building blocks of body tissue. Your milk contains essential amino acids in the proper proportions that your baby needs.

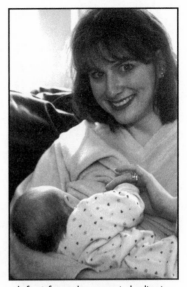

Infant formula cannot duplicate all the subtle ways that human milk supports a baby's health and growth.

Taurine, for example, is an important amino acid found in high concentrations in human milk. It is virtually absent in cow's milk. Research suggests that taurine has an important biologic role in the development of brain tissue and of the retina of the eye. The human infant is unable to make taurine out of other nutrients, so he is completely dependent on his food to supply this amino acid. This is only one example of how the nutrients in human milk match the specific needs of human infants. Because of its potential importance to brain development, some manufacturers add taurine to prepared infant formulas, but this does not begin to make these formulas the nutritional equivalent of human milk.

Fats provide energy and more

The fat in your milk provides energy for growth. And babies store some of this energy as a layer of fat under the skin. This fat tissue blankets a baby against heat loss and, along with his soft skin, it makes him especially nice to cuddle. A breastfed baby has firmer flesh and silkier skin than a formula-fed baby, probably because of the kind of fat in human milk.

The specific types of fat in human milk are important to the development of the brain and nervous system. For example, human milk contains large amounts of DHA and ARA (docosahexaenoic acid and arachidonic acid), which are long-chain polyunsaturated fatty acids. These fats are a prominent part of brain structures, and studies show that breastfed infants have higher concentrations of DHA in the blood and the brain than formula-fed infants. Other studies have found that higher blood levels of DHA and ARA are associated with better visual and cognitive development in infants. The availability of these particular fats in human milk is important, since infants have a limited capacity to manufacture these substances from other kinds of dietary fat. Formula manufacturers have begun to add DHA and ARA to artificial infant milks, though research has yet to demonstrate that adding this component to infant formula will ultimately make a difference in a baby's development. Science is only beginning to study the influence of nutrition on infant brain development, and DHA and ARA may be only one part of the story.

Anecdotal evidence seems to indicate that some babies develop gastrointestinal reactions when they are given formula fortified with DHA. Your breastfed baby will receive these important nutrients in human milk in just the right proportions with no unfortunate side effects.

Cholesterol is another type of fat used to build tissue in the brain and nervous system. Human milk contains generous amounts of cholesterol, which a baby needs in the first two years of life. Also, research suggests that exposure to cholesterol via human milk may enable a person to handle dietary cholesterol better as an adult. Infant formula contains far less cholesterol than human milk. Low-cholesterol formula might seem like a good thing, given that adults are encouraged to limit their intake of cholesterol, but the nutritional needs of growing babies are different from those of adults.

Human milk averages approximately two to three percent fat. Fat accounts for 30 to 55 percent of the total calories in human milk. Mothers who are severely undernourished and have no fat reserves of their own to draw on tend to produce milk that is somewhat lower in fat than that of well-nourished mothers, though the protein and lactose content of their milk is still within the normal range. Also, the types or proportions of the various fats in human milk vary according to the mother's diet.

The amount of fat in a mother's milk varies from feeding to feeding and changes during a feeding. The concentration of fat in the milk increases the longer baby nurses. As baby's sucking stimulates mother's let-down reflex, the milk-making cells in the breast release higher fat milk. This is why it's important to let a baby finish at the first breast before offering the second. He needs the high-fat milk that shows up late in the feeding as that first breast is emptied. The fat content of the milk is also related to the amount of time between feedings. Human milk's fat content decreases as the time between feedings increases. In other words, babies who go back to the breast for just a little bit more milk twenty or thirty minutes after a vigorous feeding will get a high-fat after-dinner snack.

The fat (or lipid) of human milk is absorbed and utilized by the baby with remarkable efficiency. Lipase, the enzyme needed to digest fat, is present in mother's milk and is active in the baby's intestine, aiding in the efficient digestion of milk lipids. This "self-digesting" feature of human milk is especially important to newborns and premature infants whose digestive systems are still maturing.

Lactose is essential

Sharing top nutritional billing with protein and fat is the sugar lactose. It is found only in milk and is frequently referred to as milk sugar. Among sugars, lactose has remarkable properties that benefit the newborn. In the familiar role of carbohydrate, it is a source of quick energy, but that is only one of its functions. Lactose contributes to the optimal development of your baby's brain and central nervous system. In general, the bigger the brain of a species, the higher the percentage of lactose in the milk. Human milk contains one and a half times as much lactose as is found in cow's milk—a fact that is readily verified by the sweet taste of human milk to the adult palate.

Infant formulas made from cow's milk contain lactose, but the sugar content of the milk must be increased by adding sucrose or other substitute sugars. These are not the equal of lactose. Lactose breaks down and releases its energy at a slow, steady pace, thus avoiding the highs and lows in blood sugar that follow the ingestion of sucrose.

Lactose has a beneficial effect on the environment in baby's intestines. It enhances the absorption of certain minerals, especially calcium, which is necessary for good bone and tooth development. It also promotes the growth of good bacteria in the infant gut. This thwarts the growth of undesirable bacteria that can cause diarrhea in the young. Evidence of the work of the good bacteria in baby's gut may be recognized by anyone who changes a breastfed baby's diaper. The bowel movements of the totally breastfed baby have a distinct, not unpleasant, buttermilk-like smell. This is proof that the small world within is populated by a preponderance of beneficial bacteria. The formula-fed baby's stools have a strong odor—very unbecoming to the baby.

Vitamins and minerals in perfect balance

Vitamins and minerals are essential to growth and health, and human milk is the best and most balanced source for infants. In fact, nutrition experts look to human milk when they are trying to determine how much infants need of a given nutrient. As a result, there is an ever-growing body of research on all these various nutrients, their presence in human milk, and the way they all work together to promote a baby's growth and keep him healthy. There is far more research than we can summarize in this chapter. This section concentrates on controversies over a few specific nutrients.

Even though human milk is recognized as the standard food for infants, there seems to be no end to the promotions aimed at persuading a mother that there is a danger that her milk is somehow inadequate or that her breastfed baby needs something in addition to human milk. The "something," it seems, can readily be supplied by a commercial product. Glossy advertisements will congratulate you on nursing your baby and then smoothly slip in a statement to the effect that some vitamin or other popular and important-sounding item is "borderline" in mother's milk. Or a chart in the ad will indicate that levels of a given nutrient in mother's milk fall within a range of values, from lower levels to higher ones. In contrast, the ads suggest that formula can be relied upon to provide a scientifically measured, predictable amount of that nutrient. Nursing mothers should be aware that what is really "borderline" is the scientific background of such ads. By telling only part of the story, ads mislead mothers and leave them unnecessarily worried about the nutritional content of their milk.

Iron

When it comes to vitamins and minerals for the baby, it is important to remember that more is not necessarily better. The workings of our bodies require a balance of nutrients. Dropping a supplemental dose of liquid vitamins or minerals into your baby's mouth "just in case" is not a good thing to do. Nor is it a good idea to rush the introduction of solids or supplement with formula. These unnecessary nutrients may interfere with the balanced nutrition in human milk. Supplementary doses of iron are a case in point.

The iron in human milk, while low in quantity, is extremely well absorbed. Manufacturers have to put lots of iron in formula precisely because so little of what's there can be used by the infant.

Studies have shown that breastfed infants do not become anemic in the first six months of life. One study found that infants exclusively breastfed (no formula, no solids) for seven months or longer were not anemic at their first birthday and had higher hemoglobin levels at one year and two years of age than breastfed babies given solids before seven months. Clearly, breastfed babies don't need routine iron supplements.

In fact, iron supplements may interfere with components in human milk that protect babies from disease and help them to grow. Infants who are more than six months old benefit from the iron in solid foods, however, introducing solids too early may lessen their ability to absorb the iron in human milk.

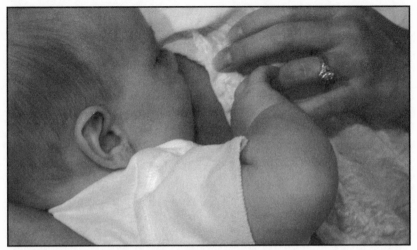

As baby peacefully nurses at his mother's breast, he receives a complex array of nutrients and protective substances.

Calcium and vitamin D

Calcium is well known for its role in the formation of strong bones and teeth. There is not as much calcium in human as in cow's milk, but the high level of lactose in human milk ensures that the calcium that is there is efficiently absorbed.

Vitamin D is needed to turn calcium into strong bones. Vitamin D is actually a hormone that is produced in the body when the skin is exposed to sunlight. Human milk contains only small amounts of vitamin D, since an infant stores vitamin D in his body before birth and can readily make more when his skin is exposed to sunlight. Infants and children who do not get enough calcium and/or vitamin D may develop rickets, a softening and bending of the bones. Rickets was rampant in the United States and other industrialized countries in the early 1900s, but vitamin D fortification of cow's milk eventually eliminated this problem. Rickets remains a serious public health problem in some developing countries at the beginning of the 21st century.

Rickets is not found in breastfed infants of well-nourished mothers who receive regular exposure to sunlight. A 1989 study in the *Journal of Pediatrics* reported that "unsupplemented human milk-fed infants had no evidence of vitamin D deficiency during the first six months." However, more recently, pediatricians have become concerned about cases of rickets in exclusively breastfed babies, an indication that some breastfed babies and their mothers may not be getting enough vitamin D from the sun. Darker-skinned individuals, who require longer exposure to the sun to produce sufficient amounts of vitamin D, may be at risk for vitamin D deficiency, as are mothers and babies who don't go outside much or whose skin is almost entirely covered by clothing or sunscreen when they are outside.

A few minutes a day of sun on your baby's cheeks is all that is needed to prevent vitamin D deficiency. Being sure that you get adequate amounts of vitamin D during pregnancy will ensure that your baby's body stores up vitamin D before he is born and that the levels in your milk are adequate. But physicians currently recommend that parents be cautious about exposing their babies to sunlight, because sun exposure has been linked to skin cancer later in life. In 2003, The American Academy of Pediatrics issued a statement recommending that all infants receive vitamin D supplements by two months of age. Not all experts agree with this recommendation. Supplements may be important for dark-skinned individuals, those who wear traditional clothing that leaves little skin exposed, and those who live in colder climates and northern latitudes where there is less exposure to sunlight. If you have concerns about how much vitamin D your baby is receiving from sunlight, discuss vitamin D supplements with your doctor.

Zinc

The zinc in human milk is better absorbed by your baby than the zinc in infant formula. In fact, human milk is a specific treatment for a rare, inherited metabolic disease called acrodermatitis enteropathica (AE). Infants with this condition suffer a zinc deficiency brought about by a reduced ability to absorb zinc. Babies who develop the disease improve dramatically when their feedings are switched from formula to human milk. Cow's milk formulas actually contain more zinc than human milk, but the zinc in human milk is absorbed more easily. The medical literature cites rare cases of mothers who themselves are deficient in zinc and whose milk is affected. However, this problem is easily resolved by giving a zinc supplement to the mother.

Other minerals besides zinc, such as copper and manganese, have been found to have a significantly better biological availability in human milk than in cow's milk or formula.

Fluoride

Over the years, fluoride supplements have received a great deal of attention, because studies have linked them to sound teeth and decreased dental caries. However, the use of fluoride supplements continues to be controversial among some experts. Mother's milk contains some fluoride, and while the amount is small, it seems to be perfectly suited to the baby's need. The American Academy of Pediatrics no longer recommends fluoride supplements for babies under six months. For children aged six months to three years, the AAP recommends fluoride supplements only for children living in areas where the drinking water has very low levels of fluoride. Too much fluoride can cause problems for some children. Some mothers who have used fluoride supplements have found they cause their babies to be fussy.

Enzymes and hormones

Human milk contains many substances whose precise role in infant physiology is yet to be determined. Enzymes present in human milk include the fat-digesting lipase, amylase, which helps break down carbohydrates, and protease which works on proteins; these help make the nutrients and immune factors in human milk more available to the baby. Hormones in human milk may influence how infant physiology responds to feedings as well and may guide other aspects of early development. Human milk contains high levels of a hormone called epidermal growth factor that may affect growth and development of the intestinal tract. Other growth factors in human milk may also help various infant tissues mature.

Human Milk—An Arsenal Against Illness

Mothers who breastfeed their babies have often noticed that when the rest of the family comes down with a cold or flu, the baby remains free of it or has only a mild case. On a larger scale, public health experts have long been aware that babies who are not breastfed are more vulnerable to infection. Infant mortality rates are higher among artificially fed infants, even in places where everyone has access to safe water and good medical care. Morbidity rates—how often babies get sick—are also higher among artificially fed infants in both the developed and the developing world. Breastfeeding is critical to infant survival in developing countries, and it plays a significant role in keeping babies healthy in families who enjoy a high standard of living.

Based on extensive research showing that breastfed babies are healthier than babies who are not breastfed, the United States government has initiated a Breastfeeding Awareness Campaign to promote the importance of breastfeeding as a public health issue in the United States.

A worldwide perspective

Study after study of mothers and babies living in poverty in developing countries confirms breastfeeding's importance to infant survival. In a 1996 survey of infants in the Philippines, deaths from respiratory infection and diarrhea were eight to ten times higher in babies who were artificially fed than in those who were even partially breastfed for six months. A study of infant deaths in metropolitan areas of Brazil found that the risk of death from diarrhea was 14.2 times higher in infants who were weaned from the breast than in fully breastfed babies; the risk of death from respiratory infection was 3.6 times greater. Infants who were partially breastfed were at greater risk than those who were fully breastfed, but were better off than those who were fully formula-fed. In Bangladesh, breastfeeding was found to reduce the mortality rate from diarrhea in the first six months of life by 24 to 27 percent; non-breastfed children were 4.2 times more likely to die from diarrhea before age five than were breastfed children.

These are only a few examples of the dramatic effect breastfeeding has on infant health in parts of the world where poor sanitation, unsafe water supplies, poverty, and lack of medical care add up to enormous public health problems. Mother's milk is the first line of defense for the community's smallest, most vulnerable members, but social change, urbanization, and the promotion of artificial infant feeding products have led to declines in breastfeeding rates in the developing world. As families move into cities hoping to improve their economic standing, mothers must work at jobs that separate them from their babies, making it difficult for them to breastfeed. Mothers who aspire to give their babies the best emulate Western formula-feeding practices, but with disastrous results, since they cannot afford to buy sufficient amounts of powdered formula, let alone the extra fuel required to boil water to prepare it safely. And as they attempt to bottle-feed their babies, their own milk supplies decline, so that even if they started out breastfeeding, eventually they don't have enough milk to satisfy their babies' hunger. As a result, babies are undernourished and sick, and many die. The World Health Organization, UNICEF, and other international public health organizations are committed to helping mothers around the world breastfeed their babies, whatever their life circumstances, but it is an uphill struggle.

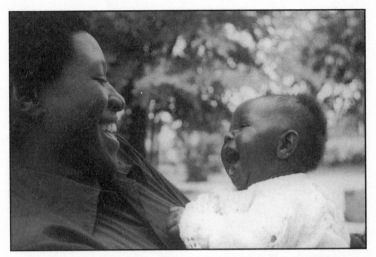

Human milk is critical to infant survival in developing countries.

Benefits of breastfeeding in developed countries

No one is surprised when research reveals that breastfed babies have a better chance at survival than formula-fed babies in places where there is no clean water and formula is too expensive for most families' budgets. But even in prosperous surroundings, where it's relatively rare for children to die of infectious diseases, breastfed babies are substantially better off than artificially fed infants. In affluent areas of the United States, Canada, New Zealand, Australia, and Western Europe, the contrast between breastfed and artificially fed infants is not as dramatic as in the developing world, but a growing body of research is demonstrating that even in affluent communities, breast-fed babies enjoy significant health advantages—and infants who are not breastfed may be at risk.

Before we describe the many good things associated with breast-feeding, we need to say something about changing perspectives on infant feeding. Breastfeeding supporters have long described the differences between breastfed infants and formula-fed infants as "advantages" of breastfeeding. But this understates the case. Breastfeeding is more than a nice "extra," like music lessons or summer camp, provided by conscientious parents who can manage to do so.

If you look at comparisons between breastfed and formula-fed infants from a different perspective the reasons to breastfeed become more than just "advantages." Anything that researchers describe as an advantage of breastfeeding can also be described as a risk associated with artificial feeding. For example, research shows that babies who are

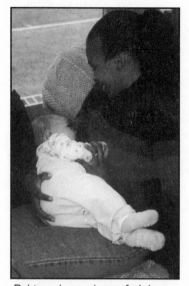

Babies who are breastfed do not get sick as often or as severely as those who are not breastfed.

breastfed are less likely to get ear infections; this means that formula-feeding places babies at greater risk for ear infections. We tend to think of runny noses and ear infections as being a matter of course in infants and small children, but these illnesses are actually a hazard of formula-feeding. Babies who are fed human milk do not get sick nearly as often.

As more and more scientific studies demonstrate significant differences between human milk and substitutes for human milk, mothers need to know that not only is breastfeeding better for their babies, artificial feeding carries health risks, both short-term and long-term.

Whether or not a mother breastfeeds her baby is obviously a very personal decision, and we know that there are situations in which human milk substitutes are truly needed. But holding back information and minimizing the differences between breastfeeding and formula-feeding keeps parents from being able to make informed decisions about their infant's care. As you read the rest of this chapter, keep in mind that breastfeeding is the norm for human infants—not just better or best, but the way that babies were meant to be fed. Babies are born to be breastfed.

Breastfeeding protects babies from infections

Research in industrialized nations has found that many kinds of infectious diseases occur at higher rates in formula-fed babies than in breastfed babies. These include respiratory infections, ear infections, urinary tract infections, haemophilus influenzae type B (HiB), pneumonia, and meningitis.

Breastfeeding's protective effect is especially significant in gastrointestinal illness. A study done in Israel reported that babies less than twelve months of age had a lower incidence of acute diarrhea during the months they were breastfed than formula-fed babies during those same months. A 1995 study in the United States found the incidence of diarrhea among formula-fed babies to be twice that of breastfed babies. In another study, babies breastfed for thirteen weeks or longer had lower rates of gastrointestinal illness throughout the first year of life than infants formula-fed from birth. Even in developed countries, diarrhea can be dangerous in infants; worldwide it's a leading killer of babies and small children.

The influence of feeding on respiratory infection is more difficult to study. Many factors besides breastfeeding can influence respiratory symptoms (parental smoking or allergies, for example). Nevertheless, studies have shown that breastfeeding protects babies against colds and other kinds of respiratory infections. Other studies have found that respiratory infections are less likely to be severe in babies who are breastfed.

Frequent ear infections can diminish babies' ability to hear, which can lead to problems with language development. This is why pediatric care professionals make diagnosing and treating ear infections a priority. In addition, mothers of babies who get ear infections often know all too well that they make babies miserable, especially at night. Many studies show that formula-fed babies are at a significantly greater risk for otitis media—infections of the middle ear—than breastfed babies. A 1998 study of infants attending regular medical clinics in Arizona found that breastfeeding for four months was associated with a lower risk of otitis media, and babies who were exclusively breastfed for six months had a lower incidence of recurrent ear infections. In another study, 80 percent fewer episodes of prolonged otitis media were reported in the breastfed group; this protection extended all the way into the second year of life.

Urinary tract infections are another example of a disease that is more likely to occur in formula-fed than in breastfed babies. The bacteria that cause urinary tract infections often originate in baby's stool, but since human milk encourages the growth of friendly bacteria in baby's intestines, the breastfed baby's stool contains lesser amounts of infection-causing germs. Immune factors present in human milk that eventually end up in the urine may also be involved in protecting the urinary tract from infection.

Breastfeeding and chronic illness

Breastfeeding has been associated with lower rates of juvenile (type 1) diabetes, adult onset (type 2) diabetes, celiac disease (sensitivity to gluten, a protein in wheat, rye, and barley), childhood cancer, rheumatoid arthritis, multiple sclerosis, dental caries, severe liver disease, and even acute appendicitis.

Scientists are particularly interested in the relationship between breastfeeding and autoimmune diseases such as type 1 diabetes. The immune system defends the body against foreign substances, but sometimes the immune system turns on the body and attacks and destroys normal tissues, causing an autoimmune disease. For example, in type 1 diabetes, the immune system attacks the insulin-producing cells in the pancreas, so that the body is unable to make enough insulin to handle dietary sugar. Immunologists have proposed two possible explanations for the lower incidence of type 1 diabetes in breastfed children. Since studies show a correlation between type 1 diabetes and the early introduction of cow's milk, breastfed babies may be protected simply because they are not exposed to foreign proteins as early as artificially fed children. Another explanation is that human milk helps build better immune systems in babies, and children who are not breastfed don't get the benefit of this. Breastfeeding's role in guarding against diabetes may involve both of these explanations; genetic predisposition and environmental influences also play a role in the development of diabetes and other autoimmune diseases such as celiac disease.

What is intriguing here is the idea that the immune components of human milk do more than just protect babies from infection during the months they are breastfed. Human milk also stimulates the development of the baby's own immune system. Several studies have noted that breastfed babies respond better to vaccines than formula-fed babies, another indication that breastfeeding is part of nature's design for the development of the infant's immune system. Depriving babies of the immunities in human milk can have consequences that last well beyond infancy.

Sudden Infant Death Syndrome

In recent years, researchers have found substantial evidence that breastfeeding lowers the risk of a baby dying of Sudden Infant Death Syndrome (SIDS). Large studies of SIDS in the United States, New Zealand, and England have shown that infants who were not breastfed had a two-to-three times greater risk than breastfed infants. This may be related to human milk's ability to protect babies from infection, or there may be other factors involved. SIDS rates have fallen dramatically since public information campaigns have instructed parents to place babies on their backs to sleep. Mothers who nurse in bed at night find that when babies let go of the nipple, they almost inevitably roll onto their backs to sleep!

Research continues

There is much more to be learned about the protective effects of breast-feeding, and physicians, epidemiologists, immunologists, and other scientists continue to study human milk's influence on infant health. Researchers interested in breastfeeding's benefits have learned that studies looking for relationships between infant feeding and the risk of disease must be designed carefully. It is important to know if the babies in the study group are exclusively breastfed or if they are receiving supplements. If babies are receiving milk or food other than human milk, it is important to know how much and when this food

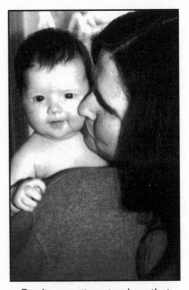

Studies continue to show that breastfed babies are healthier.

was introduced. Were the artificially fed infants in the study bottle-fed from birth, or did they receive human milk in the early weeks? Common sense suggests that infants who are exclusively breastfed—who get nothing but human milk—will probably benefit more from breastfeeding than those who are getting a combination of human milk and formula. (This is called a dose-response effect: the bigger the dose, the better the response.) But just a little bit of breastfeeding in the critical first days of life may also make a difference in some areas, and this could have an impact on research results.

Research on breastfeeding is complicated by these and many other factors. It is impossible for researchers to randomly assign one group of mothers to breastfeed and one group to formula-feed. This would be completely unethical. Yet there may be differences between mothers who choose to breastfeed and those who bottle-feed—differences that may affect how their babies grow and develop, independent of how they are fed.

Scientists, physicians, journalists, and ordinary people seeking information about breastfeeding must read research studies and reports on research in the popular media carefully. Some study results may not fit what we know about the overwhelming superiority of human milk over infant formula, and often limitations of the study design may help to explain the puzzling results. Keep in mind that scientific research is an ongoing process that zigs and zags on its way to the truth.

Epidemiology is the study of all the elements that contribute to the occurrence or non-occurrence of disease in a group of people. Epidemiologic research overwhelmingly shows that artificially fed infants are not as healthy as breastfed infants. Breastfeeding advocates have calculated that if every baby in the United States were breastfed, health care costs would decrease dramatically. The evidence comes down squarely on the side of human milk. But just what is it in human milk that makes this all happen?

Nature's Vaccine for the Newborn

What is it in human milk that makes the difference in babies' health? Babies' own immune systems are immature, unable yet to efficiently fight off the pathogens in the environment. Some kinds of protective antibodies are transferred from mother to baby via the placenta. The antibodies, which are also known as immunoglobulins, have been manufactured by your immune system in response to infections to which you have been exposed. These include some of the common contagious diseases of childhood and the everyday household germs found in your environment. While the immunity you have to these diseases is lifelong, the immunity that is passed on to your unborn baby in the form of immunoglobulins, known as IgG, gives him only temporary protection until his own immune system begins to develop.

Other kinds of immune protection are relayed from mother to baby via mother's milk. Many years ago, La Leche League's long time medical advisor Dr. Herbert Ratner coined a phrase that aptly describes human milk's unique anti-infective qualities—"nature's vaccine for the newborn." Since then, decades of increasingly sophisticated immunological research have discovered that human milk protects babies from disease in multiple ways:

- Babies who are exclusively breastfed have limited exposure to the germs that enter human bodies through water and food.

- Human milk destroys harmful bacteria and viruses, and it also enhances a baby's ability to fight these invaders.

- Human milk encourages the growth of healthier bacteria in the infant's digestive tract, which prevents harmful bacteria from proliferating.

- Substances in human milk help to regulate infants' immune responses to potential allergens, which puts breastfed babies at a lower risk for developing allergies.

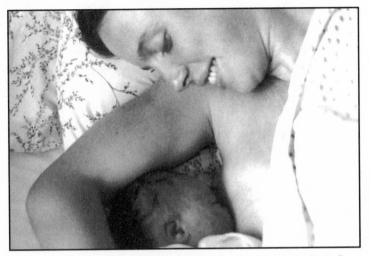

Colostrum has been called "nature's vaccine for the newborn."

- Human milk may "prime" a baby's immune system to operate better in later life.

Human milk accomplishes all these things through the complex interplay of many biologic substances. The immunological protection that comes with breastfeeding involves hormones, enzymes, growth factors, live cells, proteins, fats, immunoglobulins, and other specialized ingredients. As immunologists learn more about these processes, it becomes more and more apparent that manufactured substitutes for human milk cannot possibly compare with the real thing.

The germ-fighting properties of human milk

The most important antibody in human milk is called secretory immunoglobulin A, or sIgA. Its job is to protect the mucosal membranes in the body from germs, foreign proteins, and other harmful invaders. Mucous membranes line baby's stomach and intestines, as well as the respiratory tract and lungs. Germs and allergens can get through immature mucosal membranes and enter the blood. SIgA protects these tissues and captures the germs before they can do harm. SIgA stands as a sentry along the frontier that is the lining of the gastrointestinal tract and prevents germs or foreign proteins from penetrating the membranes and causing inflammation, infections, or allergic responses.

Colostrum has an abundance of sIgA. Although the concentration of sIgA decreases as milk volumes increase during the first week postpartum, baby still gets plenty of sIgA. An adult woman produces about 2.5

grams of sIgA daily for her own use; her baby, who is less than a tenth of her size, receives 0.5 to 1 gram of sIgA each day while breastfeeding. Even past your baby's first birthday, there are significant amounts of sIgA and other protective factors in your milk, and their concentration actually increases as your milk supply decreases during gradual weaning.

Early feedings of colostrum prepare the digestive system for future feedings. Researchers have found that the presence of sIgA in human milk stimulates the infant's own gastrointestinal production of sIgA. This is one of many reasons for insisting that your baby get nothing but your colostrum and milk in the first days of life. Those first doses of colostrum are designed to gently introduce baby's immune system to the world outside the womb. Breastfeeding-friendly neonatal intensive care units often save a mother's pumped colostrum for premature babies' very first feedings by mouth, even if these feedings don't take place until baby is several weeks old. All that sIgA in colostrum may be critically important to the early development of the baby's immune system.

The sIgA found in a mother's milk is produced locally in her breasts, but what kind of antibodies are produced in the breast is determined by immune responses in the mother's gut and her respiratory tract. When germs enter mother's body, her immune system responds by producing antibodies. Information about this response travels to the mucosal surfaces in the mammary gland, and the breast then makes sIgA antibodies that will fight the germs to which mother has been exposed. These antibodies end up in her baby and help him fight the bacteria and viruses in their shared environment. In other words, when baby comes into contact with a new germ, all he has to do is pass it on to his mother, perhaps by nursing at her breast, and her body will manufacture antibodies to that germ and give them back to baby in her milk. The antibodies in mother's milk will also reflect the germs with which she has come in contact in the past. These antibodies will protect her baby especially during the early months of life, until the time that he is better able to fight disease and infection on his own.

Colostrum is also full of many kinds of live cells. These cells, which are also found in blood, have the ability to destroy or thwart the bacteria and viruses that can cause serious disease. The live cells in human milk survive in baby's gastrointestinal tract and secrete hormones, growth factors, and other substances that regulate the body's immune response. They also manufacture IgA and travel through mucosal membranes and enter the blood where they can influence the development of other tissues in baby's body. The presence of live cells in milk means that milk is a living tissue, very much like blood. In fact, during the early weeks there are about as many live white cells in milk as there are in blood. Even before scientists knew about these live white cells, human milk was referred to by some doctors as "white blood," precisely because of its life-giving properties.

Lymphocytes are one type of live cell found in human milk. T lymphocytes ("T-cells") direct the immune response. Other types of lymphocytes produce antibodies and kill germ cells. Another type of live cell in human milk is the macrophage. Macrophages are capable of engulfing troublesome organisms. They swallow the germs, and with the help of the enzyme lysozyme, destroy them.

There are many, many other examples of ways in which specialized substances in human milk work together to destroy invaders. Some enzymes help other substances in milk survive the digestive process so that they can fight germs. In other cases, enzymes break down proteins or fats into components that can then go on to fulfill their immune functions. Some lymphocytes tell the body to attack germs; others tell the immune system to relax and tolerate substances, such as food proteins, that are foreign to the body but not dangerous. Lactoferrin, the main protein in human milk, kills certain kinds of bacteria, viruses, fungi, and tumor cells. It also has anti-inflammatory properties. Oligosaccharides, simple sugars found in human milk, prevent bacteria from binding itself to surfaces in the respiratory tract.

The direct, dynamic immune protection provided for infants in their mother's milk helps to explain how babies, as long as they are breastfed, can survive in a highly infected environment even before their own immune systems can protect them. The human immune system, viewed through the interaction of mother and baby in breastfeeding, is fascinating, and the details of how it all works add up to a very compelling reason to breastfeed your baby.

Avoiding Allergies

A greater risk of allergy is another of the many hazards of artificial feeding. Your baby will not be allergic to your milk; you can count on this with certainty. It is a law of nature that infants never become sensitized to their natural food. However, the ways in which human milk protects against allergies and asthma go beyond the early avoidance of allergy-causing foods such as cow's milk. The immune components in human milk help prevent babies from developing allergic reactions.

Allergies occur when an otherwise harmless substance, such as food, pollen, or mold, enters the body and the body recognizes it as foreign. The next time the immune system runs into this substance, it remembers that this substance, called an allergen, is foreign. The immune system attacks, producing chemicals that cause allergic symptoms, such as itchy eyes or a runny nose. It's not the food or the pollen that causes the misery of allergies, it's the body's reaction.

Besides learning how to recognize and destroy bacteria and viruses, baby's developing immune system also has to learn what foreign substances to tolerate. Human milk, with its various immune components, helps teach these lessons. It also helps prevent allergens from reaching the bloodstream at a time when baby's immune system is immature and more likely to overreact. This is part of sIgA's job of guarding the intestinal lining.

Many studies have found that babies who were exclusively breast-fed for several months or more had fewer allergic symptoms later in childhood. A 1995 study followed children from infancy through adolescence (seventeen years of age) and found that breastfeeding provided long-term protection from eczema and respiratory allergy as well as food allergy. Not every study of the relationship between infant feeding and allergy produces such dramatic results. Other factors, including heredity and the mother's diet during pregnancy, also factor into the development of allergies.

The proteins in cow's milk, in cow's milk formulas, and in soy formulas are well-known for causing allergies. Babies who are exposed to these foreign proteins at a young age may become sensitized. When they encounter them again, their immune systems react with a variety of symptoms: stomach upsets, vomiting, diarrhea, stuffy nose, rashes, general crankiness. Even one bottle of formula, fed during the night in the hospital nursery while mother "gets her rest," is enough to sensitize some babies to cow's milk or soy proteins and produce allergic symptoms months later.

The best way to avoid allergies, especially in babies with a family history of food allergies, is to breastfeed exclusively for the first six months of life, and then introduce solid foods very gradually. The immune components of human milk probably help babies tolerate new foods, so it is important to keep breastfeeding while baby learns to enjoy solids. A recent study found that children who continued to breastfeed for several months after wheat was introduced into their diet were less likely to develop celiac disease than those who weaned soon after beginning to eat wheat products.

A miracle cure

One of the most dramatic cases of an extremely allergic baby getting well because of mother's milk came early in La Leche League's history. Lorraine and Emil Bormet's two-and-one-half-month-old David, formula-fed since birth, had been suffering from almost continuous diarrhea, breathing difficulties, and eczema. Different formulas had been tried, including soy and meat-based varieties, with no improvement in David's condition. As a last resort, the doctor suggested that human milk was probably the only thing David could tolerate.

Lorraine located a nursing mother several miles from their Illinois farm home, and the mother agreed to help. Following David's first feeding of human milk late one evening, his astonished mother reported that "he fell asleep and slept through the night for the first time in his life."

Convinced of the value of human milk, the Bormets wondered if Lorraine could relactate and bring in her own milk supply, even though it had been almost three months since the baby's birth. They contacted La Leche League for information. Milk production, we could assure her, is stimulated by the baby's sucking, and so she began the painstaking work of encouraging David to take the breast. Lorraine stayed in close touch with Marian Tompson, one of La Leche League's Founders, and David continued to receive human milk from generous donor mothers. Eight days after Lorraine began her efforts to breastfeed, drops of milk appeared. Some weeks later, Lorraine Bormet was completely nursing her baby, who by then was symptom-free, healthy, and content.

In the years since the Bormet story unfolded, other mothers with similarly allergic babies have contacted La Leche League, and many have found that, despite a late start, they could provide their own milk for their babies.

Worth a try

Other enthusiastic accounts come from parents whose older children had problems with cow's milk allergies and who decided to try breastfeeding when expecting a new baby. They comprise a large group and are probably among the strongest advocates of breastfeeding. Kathy Driskell of Illinois tells the story of Michael, the Driskell's second child:

> **We had experienced a series of problems with our first child, Jennifer, who was formula-fed. She vomited after almost every feeding until she was nearly six months old. This was followed by chronic diarrhea until she was past two. Her**

pediatrician changed the formula numerous times, but to no avail. He finally concluded that it was an inherited allergy.

Needless to say, I was eager to avoid this nightmare with Michael. Some of my friends had tried to encourage me to breastfeed, but frankly, it scared me to death. Coming from a large, close-knit, strictly bottle-feeding family, I had visions of my relatives shaking their heads in pity at my poor starving baby. Finally, after much debate, my husband and I decided the best thing for Michael would be to give breastfeeding a try for a week or two. Now, fourteen months later, I have to look back and laugh, for Michael turned out to be the chubbiest, healthiest child I could have imagined. Needless to say digestive problems were nonexistent (he rarely even spit up). Nursing my son has been an experience I wouldn't have missed for anything.

A breastfed baby can still be allergic

Even with exclusive breastfeeding, some babies still develop allergies. A baby may react to foods other than cow's milk or soy formula—early solids, for instance, or even vitamins or medications. You'll do your baby a favor if you're careful to limit what goes into his tummy to what is compatible with his young system. Your milk alone is your best bet for about six months. While your baby remains on mother's milk, his intestinal tract is protected and given time to mature. Potentially allergenic foods, which might cause problems even at six months of age, may be better tolerated later on, especially if baby continues to nurse. Be careful about offering foods with a high potential for causing allergic reactions. These include: cow's milk, egg white, citrus fruits, corn, wheat, soy, fish, tomatoes, chocolate, cabbage, berries, and nuts, especially peanuts. If your baby shows signs of a reaction to a new food or if there is a history of allergy in your family, you may want to ask your doctor about postponing solids until eight or nine months. Be sure to read Chapter 13 on starting solids before introducing your baby to other foods.

Jani Howd of South Dakota did not think allergies would be a problem in her family, but she later found out her daughter Angie was highly allergic:

Avoiding allergies was not one of my primary reasons in deciding to breastfeed our first child. Now, two years later, I definitely know that it is an advantage that should not be taken lightly.

During her first year, Angie was a perfect example of a contented, healthy breastfed baby. Her only problem seemed to be a supersensitive skin. When I began introducing table food to her at about five-and-a-half months, she ate willingly with a good appetite. At twelve months any attempt to feed Angie cow's milk or eggs resulted in a reaction. By eighteen months, eggs were no longer a problem, and at twenty-one months she seemed to tolerate milk.

Shortly after this, Angie developed eczema. We immediately took cow's milk away, but the eczema did not disappear completely until I put Angie on a strict elimination diet to determine exactly which foods she was allergic to. Then the fading eczema wasn't the only change noticeable in Angie. Starting about the age of eighteen months, temper tantrums and sleepless nights had become a matter of course, along with a loss of appetite. John and I attributed it to her growing independence and tried to handle her with love and patience.

Now that she is eating foods that agree with her, it is a rare sight for her to have a temper tantrum. She is our happy, contented, breastfed toddler. Her appetite has returned and the change in her disposition is almost unbelievable. Breastfeeding does not entirely prevent allergies, especially with a very allergic individual like Angie, but it was reassuring to hear the dermatologist tell me that had she not been breastfed, her allergies would have been more severe, in greater number, and that she would have had food-related skin problems sooner, and would have kept them longer.

If there is a history of allergies in your family it is generally a good idea to avoid eating an excessive amount of any one food during pregnancy, particularly cow's milk and peanut products. There is evidence that a baby can become sensitized before birth to a food that his mother eats.

Can baby react to something mother eats?

In some instances, a food that a breastfeeding mother eats will cause a reaction in her baby. The protein from cow's milk, eggs, or some other food in the mother's diet may penetrate her gastrointestinal tract. These "stray" proteins in her blood find their way into her milk. The presence of foreign proteins in mother's milk may be nature's way of introducing these substances to baby in small amounts that will help his immune system learn to tolerate them. But some babies, especially those with a tendency toward developing allergies, may react to these foreign proteins. Eliminating the offending food from the mother's diet will clear the baby's symptoms. Keep in mind that the mother's milk itself is fine; the stray protein riding along is what's causing the problem. Switching the baby from human milk to an artificial infant food would overwhelm him with a large dose of potential allergens and more than likely make the problem worse. Plus this baby would then be exposed to all the other risks associated with infant formula.

Before you become too concerned about whether something in your milk is causing baby's fussiness, rash, diarrhea, or other symptoms, consider some other possibilities. The reason for the problem could be something quite simple. Did the baby receive any supplements of formula or juice? Vitamins or medication? He may be crying because he's coming down with an illness. A baby who is nursing very frequently may be going through a growth spurt. Consider your own situation. If you're continually tired or rushed, make life easier for yourself and your baby by slowing down. Are you taking any medication or food supplements? Are you consuming large amounts of caffeine or smoking cigarettes? One of these could be causing the problem. Something that the baby comes in contact with could be causing a rash. A few common possibilities include detergents, soaps, fabric softeners, dyes (colored sheets), wool, feathers, lotions, spray deodorants, and other hair and skin care products you use.

If the rash, fussiness, or whatever persists, your totally breastfed baby may indeed be reacting to something you are eating. Fortunately, there is a relatively simple and cost-free method of finding out if your diet is involved. Start by eliminating a particular food for a week or two and see if there's a difference in the baby. If you've been eating a lot of one particular food lately, perhaps something that's not a part of your regular diet, you might want to eliminate that first. Cow's milk is also a leading contender as a food in mother's diet that bothers babies. Besides eliminating milk, be sure you also exclude other dairy products such as cheese, yogurt, and ice cream, and all foods that are made with milk or dried milk solids. You'll have to read the labels of any prepared foods to be sure you are avoiding milk products completely. It may take ten days to two weeks to get the food out of your system, so don't expect your baby's reaction to clear up immediately.

If there's no change in your baby when you avoid dairy products, you might want to try eliminating other foods one at a time (or several at once) for a week or so to see if baby's symptoms disappear. Other

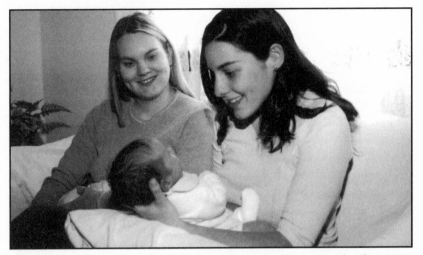

Interacting with your baby also enhances his social and cognitive development.

common allergens are eggs, wheat, citrus fruits, corn, onions, fish, peanuts, cabbage, chocolate, and other nuts. If baby seems to improve when you eliminate a group of foods, try reintroducing them one at a time in order to identify the source of the problem.

Occasionally, a mother can eat a small portion of a food as part of a meal with no reaction on the baby's part, but a large amount taken alone at one time will spell trouble. If you have a highly allergic child, a little experimentation may be necessary on your part, but you're already ahead of the situation by breastfeeding. If you find that your diet is greatly restricted by your baby's food allergies, you may want to get some help from a nutritionist in planning healthy and interesting meals for yourself. And remember, this won't last forever. Many mothers find that they can begin to introduce the troublesome food or foods back into their diet as baby gets older. Start with small amounts and don't eat the offending food at every meal or even every day.

If you have a baby who is sensitive to the foods you eat, you'll want to be especially careful to delay the introduction of solid foods and be cautious about which foods you offer.

More Reasons to Breastfeed
Cognitive development
Just as human milk plays an active role in the growth of baby's immunological system, it also contributes to the development of the brain and the nervous system. Studies comparing breastfed and formula-fed children at different ages and stages of development find that

those who receive human milk score higher on various measures of intellectual ability. Some studies have shown that these differences persist into later childhood and adolescence.

Many factors in a child's genetic make-up and social environment affect intellectual development. In places such as the US and Europe, the women most likely to breastfeed are well-educated mothers in middle to upper income groups, and the social and economic advantages enjoyed by their children are likely to boost their scores on IQ tests. The close, frequent interaction with mother that is an inevitable part of breastfeeding may also help to explain enhanced intellectual development in children who were breastfed. But even after these influences are accounted for or eliminated in the design of research studies, breastfed babies still come out ahead of those who do not receive human milk. Increasingly, researchers have come to believe that it is something in human milk itself that makes the difference.

One fascinating study compared premature infants who had received human milk in the hospital neonatal unit with those who had not. Children who were fed human milk had significantly higher IQs at 7 1/2 to 8 years of age when compared with those who had not received human milk. In the babies who were fed a combination of formula and banked human milk, their cognitive scores were directly related to the amount of mother's milk they received (a dose-response effect). When the children whose mothers had provided their own milk were compared to children of mothers who had intended to provide milk but were unsuccessful in doing so, the higher IQ scores were still apparent, suggesting that the enhanced intellectual development seen in the human milk-fed group could not be attributed to having the kind of mother who was willing to make the extra effort to pump. The researchers concluded that there is something in human milk that enhances brain development in premature babies.

Many other studies have used standardized tests to compare the intellectual development of children who were predominantly breast-fed with those who were predominantly formula-fed. The data from twenty such studies was examined in a meta-analysis, a study that combines and analyzes information from many research projects. The meta-analysis confirmed that children who were fed human milk consistently scored higher on various measures of cognitive ability. The longer the duration of breastfeeding the higher the scores. Making adjustments for the factors related to breastfeeding that also influence cognitive development (for example, socioeconomic status, maternal education, or birth weight), decreased the statistical differences between breastfed and formula-fed children, but even then, the human-milk-fed group came out ahead. The difference was small, but nevertheless significant. Breastfeeding appeared to be more crucial to cognitive development in low-birth-weight infants, where the differences between those who received human milk and those given formula were greater than in normal-weight babies. Babies who miss out on several weeks' worth of nutrients delivered in the womb via the placenta appear to be especially vulnerable to nutritional shortcomings of infant formula. Human milk gives them what they need to make up for the time missed in the womb.

Does this mean that your breastfed baby will be smarter than your neighbor's formula-fed baby? Of course not. Many factors in addition to breastfeeding influence when and how well your baby learns to walk, talk, read, and reason. The developmental differences researchers have found between artificially fed babies and breastfed babies are small, and it's important to remember that the numbers represent statistical differences between groups of children, not differences between individuals. But the fact that there are differences suggests that components of human milk play a part in how babies' brains develop. As science learns more about the way the brain works and how it develops its amazing capabilities, we will also learn more about the role of early infant nutrition in the growth and maturation of the brain and nervous system.

Jaw, teeth, and facial development

The fitness enthusiast working out in a gym and the little one at your breast—his fists tightly closed, drops of perspiration on his brow, and his jaws working vigorously—are both engaged in body shaping routines. The body-builder's exercise may result in developing big muscles; your baby's exercise in eating may affect the shape of his face, his teeth, and his smile.

Of course heredity lays the foundation for facial structure. A square jaw or a narrow chin, for example, may be a family trait. But whatever your child's potential, it is enhanced by the simple, repeated motions of sucking at mother's breast. Breastfeeding encourages proper facial development and may indeed spare your child dental or speech problems in future years.

A baby sucks differently on an artificial nipple than he does at his mother's breast. When your baby breastfeeds, he moves your nipple back into his mouth and up against the hard palate with his tongue, elongating the nipple and bringing his gums and lips around the areola (dark area). His cheek muscles are extremely active, enhancing facial development. The sucking techniques used in bottle-feeding do not involve as many muscles and may lead to underdeveloped facial structure. The faster flow from an artificial nipple may also encourage baby's tongue to thrust forward, causing the baby to develop an incorrect way of swallowing. If this habit persists beyond bottle-feeding days, there's the possibility that the alignment of permanent teeth will be affected. An artificial nipple, a pacifier, or baby's thumb may also press against the roof of his mouth, narrowing the upper dental arch and limiting the amount of room for teeth. Researchers from Johns Hopkins School of Public Health reported on a study of nearly 10,000 children in which they found that the longer the duration of breast-feeding, the lower the incidence of malocclusion. Children who were breastfed for a year or more required 40 percent less orthodontia than those who were bottle-fed.

Other aspects of development

There are many more ways in which breastfeeding affects how babies grow and develop. Studies have shown that infants who are breastfed are less likely to be obese in later childhood and adolescence. In the first days after birth, human milk contains high levels of endorphins, chemicals that reduce stress and thus may help babies adapt to living outside the womb. Nursing may affect how babies experience pain; in one study, babies who breastfed during a blood drawing procedure had lower pain scores than babies held in their mothers' arms without breastfeeding.

As science learns more about the development of infants' bodies and brains, they also learn more about the critical role of human milk in the process. Support for breastfeeding grows as it becomes apparent that mother's milk offers babies far more than calories. It is truly amazing to discover all the ways in which breastfeeding ensures that babies will survive and thrive. What is even more amazing is knowing that all the wonderful ingredients in human milk have been protecting babies from disease and helping them grow for thousands and thousands of years. Mothers who breastfed their babies centuries ago, or even just a few decades ago, may not have known the details about why their milk was so important for their babies. But the wonderful closeness of nursing and the joy of watching their little ones grow big and strong surely confirmed what they knew in their hearts—that what babies need most is mother's milk, mother's breast, and mother herself.

To learn more

Every year professional journals publish hundreds of articles reporting on research related to lactation. La Leche League International's

Center for Breastfeeding Information (CBI) maintains an extensive database along with a collection of more than 37,000 full length articles from professional journals. Check La Leche League's Web site at www.lalecheleague.org for access to selected bibliographies from the CBI. Also see the Appendix for details about other services available to health professionals and researchers.

CHAPTER NINETEEN

HOW BREASTFEEDING
affects a mother

Lactation is a natural and inevitable part of the human reproductive cycle. Pregnancy and childbirth are followed by breast-feeding. A mother's body makes milk for her newborn baby whether she chooses to breastfeed or not, and the lactation process affects more than just her breasts. Many of the changes in a mother's body that are associated with lactation benefit her directly. At the same time, however, she must remember that during breastfeeding, anything that affects her body may also affect her baby.

How the Breast Gives Milk

The way in which a mother's body makes and delivers milk is as remarkable as the milk itself. Mother's blood brings in the raw materials, and the breast transforms them into a secretion that perfectly nourishes the mother's offspring. It does this for months, even years, making subtle adjustments in the milk composition that correspond to baby's changing nutritional needs. The basic principles of lactation—that human milk is ideally suited to human babies and that the amount of milk mother makes matches baby's demand—are well known to breastfeeding mothers, but the details are topics of ongoing scientific investigation.

371

Breasts are secretory glands in which grape-like clusters of cells called alveoli make milk, which then travels through ducts to openings in the nipple. Each of these bunches of milk-producing cells and ducts is called a lobe, and most women have between seven and ten lobes of glandular tissue in each breast. Along with the glandular tissue that makes milk, breasts also contain fat, nerves, and blood vessels, with connective tissue holding everything else together. While breast size is determined mainly by the amount of fatty tissue present, the amount of fat in the breasts has no influence on the function of the breasts.

Breast changes are an early sign of pregnancy. As an expectant mother, you may have had trouble buttoning the buttons on a favorite shirt even before you found it difficult to zip your jeans. This increase in breast size comes as estrogen and progesterone stimulate the alveoli to grow and prepare to deliver milk to your infant. Already during pregnancy, the breasts make small amounts of colostrum, but it is the hormonal changes that follow birth that kick milk production into high gear.

Following the delivery of the placenta, estrogen and progesterone levels, which are high during pregnancy, fall rapidly, and prolactin, the hormone that tells the alveoli to make milk, takes over. The rate of milk production increases rapidly in the first days after birth, and a mother's breasts soon begin to feel full as her milk "comes in" to nourish her baby.

When the baby is put to the breast, his sucking stimulates nerves in the areola to send messages to the mother's brain. The brain responds by releasing another hormone, oxytocin, which causes cells around the alveoli to contract, forcing the milk in the alveoli down through the duct system to the nipple. This is the all-important letdown, or milk-ejection reflex, that makes a mother's milk readily available to her eagerly sucking baby.

Continued milk production depends on the baby regularly removing milk from the breasts. Breastfeeding mothers and the people who advise them have known for a long time that frequent, effective feedings, especially in the early weeks, are one of the keys to successful breastfeeding, but recent studies have looked more closely at how baby's breastfeeding behavior influences mother's milk production, even as her capacity to make and store milk may affect how often her baby feeds.

Supply responds to demand

Researchers have observed that milk production is not a steady, ongoing process. How much milk a mother makes varies from feeding to feeding. An empty breast makes milk faster than a breast that is relatively full. In other words, when a hungry baby takes a lot of milk from the breast, mother's body responds immediately by making more milk quickly. A baby who is growing quickly can thus depend on mother's breasts to supply the nutrients he needs when he needs them. When babies take only a small, "snack-size" feeding, milk is replaced at a slower rate.

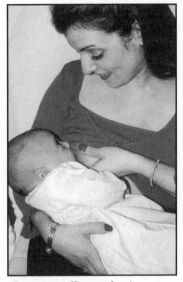

How much milk does a "full" breast hold? Researchers believe that this differs from one mother to another. Mothers whose breasts can store a lot of milk between feedings may have babies who nurse less often

Frequent, effective feedings are the key to a plentiful milk supply.

than mothers whose breasts store smaller amounts of milk. Differences in milk storage capacity may explain why some babies nurse at two-hour intervals and gain weight well, while others may be able to go longer between feedings and still get enough milk. Of course, there are many factors that influence how often a baby wants to nurse, including the baby's age, size, and personality. And since the amount of milk a baby takes at a feeding determines how much milk a mother produces, an individual baby's feeding preferences are an important influence on how much milk his mother produces and stores.

Scientists will continue to study how the breasts make milk, but breastfeeding mothers need not worry about making enough milk for their babies. Studies of the baby's side of the supply and demand equation of breastfeeding have shown that infants have a remarkable capacity to regulate their own food intake and thus, their mother's milk production. Different babies will follow different feeding patterns and an individual baby's breastfeeding pattern may change as he matures, but the elegant interplay between mother's milk production and baby's appetite makes it possible for every baby to get the nourishment he needs at his mother's breast. A mother who follows her baby's cues about when to breastfeed will find that her baby grows and thrives on just her milk.

There are times when the demand and supply equation can get out of balance. For example, a baby who is unable to suck effectively will not take much milk from his mother's breasts, causing milk production to slow down. Even if the baby is feeding frequently because he is hungry, mother's milk production will decrease, because much of the milk she is making is not being removed from the breast. Using a breast pump to remove milk from the breasts will help maintain her milk supply until her baby learns to breastfeed better. And the milk she pumps can be given to her baby.

Early feedings build the milk supply

Lactation researchers have found that frequent emptying of the breast in the first weeks after birth ensures that mother will have an ample milk supply when her baby is three or four months old. Researchers believe that more frequent feedings are associated with the development of an increased number of prolactin receptor cells in the breast. Receptor cells are there to capture prolactin molecules from the bloodstream so that they can do their job in the breast. More receptor cells may lead to better milk production.

Prolactin levels decline in the months after birth, even as a woman's body continues to produce milk. A lactating woman's prolactin levels are still higher than those of a non-lactating woman and levels go up after each feeding, but researchers believe that once lactation is fully established, milk production depends less on levels of prolactin in mother's circulation and more on what is happening within the breast itself.

Delivering high-fat hindmilk

The fat in human milk supplies calories for infant growth. The fat content of mother's milk changes during a feeding. As baby begins to suck, he receives low-fat foremilk, but after the mother's let-down reflex is triggered, the fat content of the milk increases as the alveoli release fat globules into the milk ducts. This high-fat hindmilk helps a baby feel full after a feeding, and it's important that a baby be allowed to nurse long enough at each breast to receive this high-calorie milk. An actively nursing baby is the best judge of when he is finished with the first breast offered at a feeding. (Sleepy newborn babies may need some encouragement from mother to keep nursing until their tummies are full of high-fat milk.)

Using ultrasound technology, researchers have been able 'o study what happens in the breast when the milk-ejection reflex is riggered by baby's sucking. They observed that the milk ducts dilate o accommodate the increased flow of milk. They also found that mc.t mothers in the study had more than one let-down per breast during feedings, and the more let-downs the mother experienced, the greater her baby's milk intake. (This supports the idea that babies should be allowed to "finish the first breast" before switching to the other side. If switched to the second breast too soon, they will miss out on the high-fat milk delivered by mother's second or third let-down.) Approximately one-third of the mothers did not feel their first let-down and most mothers did not feel any of the let-downs after the first one.

The ultrasound images actually came from the breast on which the baby was not feeding, so researchers were also able to watch what happens to milk that is released into the ducts but is not removed from the breast by the baby. They noted that the fatty milk globules that were pushed down toward the nipple by the milk-ejection reflex traveled back up the duct system and were stored in the alveoli and the smaller ducts deep in the breast. Other researchers have noted that the fat content of milk decreases as the amount of time between feedings increases. More frequent feedings may keep those fat globules in the milk rather than allowing them to be reabsorbed by breast tissue.

As with rates of milk production, the baby's feeding behavior influences the fat content of the milk he receives. A baby who nurses actively for a long time will trigger the release of more high-fat milk. A baby who goes back to the breast for just a little more milk twenty or thirty minutes after his last feeding will get milk with a high fat content, even if the amount of milk available to him is relatively small.

Breasts are not like bottles. Even though some lactation researchers talk about the importance of "emptying the breast," the breast is never really empty. You don't have to wait for your breasts to "fill up" with milk before you feed your baby. There is always some milk there. Your breast, after all, is not just a container for milk, it's the manufacturing site.

Breastfeeding hormones

Niles Newton, a psychologist who was a long-time friend and advisor to La Leche League, described oxytocin, the hormone that triggers the let-down reflex, as "the hormone of love." Oxytocin triggers nurturing behavior, which in Dr. Newton's words, is "an essential ingredient in the success of reproduction." Both prolactin and oxytocin may help to produce the feeling of relaxation that mothers come to associate with nursing sessions. Many women recognize that they feel calmer during the months they are nursing their babies and better able to cope with whatever comes along. A recent study showed that lactation suppresses the nervous system's hormonal response to stress. Nature intends for mothers to enjoy breastfeeding their babies, and

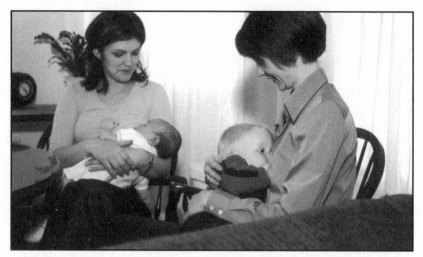

It helps when you know another mother who is also breastfeeding her baby.

the good feelings that come with breastfeeding help mothers become more attached to their babies.

Niles Newton's research years ago showed that the release of oxytocin is a conditioned response. A mother's body can produce oxytocin in response to familiar sights, sounds, and activities associated with breastfeeding (or with pumping), not just from the direct stimulation of the baby's suck. More recent research found that oxytocin levels increased in 30 percent of the mothers when their babies became restless and in 20 percent as they were preparing to nurse. Prolactin levels were found to increase only when the baby actually sucked at the breast.

Dr. Newton also showed that the let-down reflex could be inhibited by stress—in her research, the subject (herself) was made to do complex math problems in her head while breastfeeding. This resulted in less milk being available for the baby. Scientists believe that this interesting phenomenon developed in the early periods of the human race. When a wild creature or some danger threatened a mother and her baby it was time for mother and baby to flee, not sit and nurse.

There are no longer wild animals at our doors, but there are still plenty of times when mothers feel anxious and stressed. If your let-down reflex doesn't seem to be working, your baby may look up at you as if to say, "Where's the milk, Mom?" If this happens, you may need to make a deliberate effort to relax. Take a few really deep breaths, focus on your beautiful baby, and imagine your milk pouring out to him in all the profusion of a glorious Milky Way. A sixteenth century artist, Tintoretto, portrayed what has been identified as the milk let-down in a painting, appropriately titled, "The Origin of the Milky Way." It shows Hercules nursing at Juno's breast as her milk ejects in a spray of stars.

Guaranteed High-Quality Milk

Your body adapts to milk-making in many ways that are unseen. Just as with pregnancy, this is a time to marvel at how your body knows just what to do to nourish your baby. It is also a time to take special care of yourself—not because lactation is exhausting or a drain on your body, but because having a new baby is stressful. You will weather the challenges better if you are well-nourished, reasonably well-rested, and relaxed enough to concentrate on what's important.

One thing you don't have to worry about is your milk. How much milk you make is controlled by how much your baby nurses, and studies of breastfeeding babies show that they have a remarkable ability to regulate their own milk intake. Breastfed babies consume less milk than artificially fed infants. From four to twelve months they grow more slowly and are leaner than their formula-fed counterparts. But they are healthy and thriving—not hungry. Since human milk is the standard for human babies, it may be that formula-fed babies grow too quickly.

The quality of mothers' milk—the nutrients in it—is also something you can depend on. You would have to be severely malnourished before there would be reason to worry about whether your milk is meeting your baby's nutritional needs. The survival of the young of the species is so important that nature has made special provisions to ensure the quality of your milk.

One such arrangement is the extra fat you put on during pregnancy to fuel the milk-making process after baby's birth. Your body's metabolism becomes more efficient during lactation, another energy safeguard. Blood flow to the breasts increases, carrying needed nutrients. The calming effect of breastfeeding hormones is also in your baby's best interest.

Where do all the nutrients come from?

Does a mother's body rob itself of nutrients to make milk? There is no simple answer to the question of where all the good things in human milk come from, but concerns raised about nursing mothers being deficient in particular nutrients have proven to be unfounded.

Much of the dietary caution leveled at breastfeeding women is about calcium. Calcium, of course, is needed for strong bones, and cal-

cium deficiencies may contribute to osteoporosis, or bone degenera-
tion, as women age. The news that a lactating woman's body uses calcium from the reserves in her bones to make milk thus raises some
alarms. Do women who nurse their babies, especially for a long time,
place themselves at risk for bone problems later in life? The answer is
no, because here again, the body makes special allowances for lactation.

Calcium is absorbed more efficiently from the intestines during
lactation and for a time after weaning. Researchers have discovered
that while mothers' bones may lose a small amount of calcium during
the early stages of lactation, bones are built up again as baby begins to
take other foods and in the months immediately after weaning.

In studies of postmenopausal women, those who breastfed for
extended periods of time had comparable or higher bone mineral den-
sities than women who had never breastfed and actually had a lower
risk of hip fracture. Rather than being a cause for concern about osteoporosis, breastfeeding may actually offer some protection against it.

Mothers do, of course, need plenty of calcium in their diets. Milk
and dairy products, including cheese and yogurt, are good sources. If
you find you must avoid dairy products because of allergies or because
they bother your baby, you can get calcium from other foods. A cup of
cooked bok choy (a type of cabbage) provides almost as much calcium
as a cup of milk. Half a cup of ground sesame seeds has twice as much
calcium as a cup of milk. Other calcium-rich foods to include in your
diet are blackstrap molasses, calcium-enriched tofu, collards, broccoli,
turnip greens, kale, liver, almonds, Brazil nuts, and canned salmon and
sardines, which are normally eaten with the soft bones.

Breastfeeding and Your Reproductive Cycle

If your baby nurses often, day and night, you probably won't ovulate or
have menstrual periods for many months. The time when you can
again conceive is postponed. While eventually you may be able to
become pregnant while still nursing, it will not be as soon after your
baby's birth as it would be if you were not breastfeeding. Other than
milk production, this is the most noticeable effect of breastfeeding on
a mother's body.

Many mothers find that their periods do not return until the nursing baby is a year old or older. By this time, he is nursing less often and
eating a variety of foods. According to the late Dr. Herbert Ratner: "It
is the baby's sucking that controls the mother's ovulation. The more

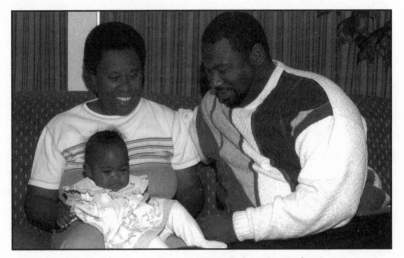

Mother, father, and baby all benefit from breastfeeding.

the baby has a need to suck, the less ready he is to be displaced by another. The less the baby has a need to suck, the more ready and able he is to cope with a new sister or brother."

Almost all mothers who are fully breastfeeding their babies are free of menstrual periods for the first six months. This is called lactational amenorrhea. Fully breastfeeding means the baby relies completely on mother for nourishment and for all of his sucking needs. Your baby's frequent nursing inhibits the release of hormones that cause your body to begin the monthly preparations for a new pregnancy. Ovulation does not take place, and you do not have menstrual periods.

Lactational amenorrhea is a normal, healthy part of the female reproductive cycle. Women who bear only two or three children during their reproductive years come to think of their monthly menstrual cycle as normal and the period of lactational amenorrhea as a departure from the norm. However, going for years without having a period is probably what women's bodies were meant to do. Mothers in traditional hunter-gathering cultures nursed each baby for two or three years and enjoyed long periods of lactational amenorrhea. When their periods returned, they would become pregnant again, and it might be another three years before they again had a menstrual period. As a result, these women experienced far fewer menstrual periods in their lifetime. Today, scientists believe that extended periods of lactational amenorrhea may help to explain the lower rates of ovarian, endometrial, and breast cancer found in women who breastfeed. The absence of the repeated hormonal ups and downs of regular menstrual cycles may leave the breasts and reproductive organs less vulnerable to cancer.

When your menstrual cycle is in the resting state, you are less likely to have problems with anemia and the fatigue that goes with it, since there is no monthly loss of blood. Also, you will not experience the mood swings and other premenstrual symptoms that bother many women. One husband listed this as an added advantage of breastfeeding because he found that "living was easy" during the months his wife was breastfeeding.

Breastfeeding's contraceptive effect

Numerous studies over many years have confirmed that breastfeeding reduces fertility. We learned this, too, from our own experience and the experience of the thousands of breastfeeding mothers who have been associated with La Leche League. John and Sheila Kippley, founders of the Couple to Couple League, gathered data on American women who practiced total breastfeeding for the first six months and then introduced solids gradually. They found there was an average of 14.6 months without periods following childbirth. LLL Leader Sheila Kippley writes in her book, *Breastfeeding and Natural Child Spacing*, "This is only average. Some, an exceptional few, will experience a return before 6.0 months postpartum. Others will go as long as 2.5 years without menses while nursing."

More recently, scientists specializing in the study of lactational infertility have developed the Lactational Amenorrhea Method of contraception (LAM), based on research done in a variety of cultures around the world. LAM has a 98 percent effectiveness rating in the first six months after birth, which compares well to other contraceptive methods.

Using LAM for contraception is safe, simple, inexpensive, and effective. Knowing exactly what conditions make it likely that you will remain infertile can help you use breastfeeding's effect on your reproductive cycle to your advantage. You are unlikely to become pregnant if you can answer "no" to all three of the following questions:

1. Have your menses returned?

2. Are you supplementing regularly or allowing long periods without breastfeeding, either during the day (more than four hours) or at night (more than six hours)?

3. Is your baby more than six months old?

If your answer to any of these questions is "yes," the chances of becoming pregnant increase. However, if you are separated from your baby regularly, frequent milk expression may provide enough breast stimulation to maintain infertility. A recent study of employed mothers in Chile suggests that hand-expressing milk at work at regular intervals was also effective in delaying a return of fertility.

When your periods do return

Fully breastfeeding will always delay ovulation for a time, but the resumption of regular periods is usually an indication that ovulation is occurring. For some women, especially those who are still exclusively breastfeeding, the first one or two menstrual periods may occur without previous ovulation. But a mother who has regular periods should consider herself able to conceive again. When menstruation does return, there is no reason to stop nursing the baby. Breastfeeding can and should continue.

When baby gets older, is nursing less, and eating a variety of other foods, a mother who has not been having periods is more likely to resume ovulation without a prior menstrual period and conception can take place before menstruation resumes. Ovulation may also resume if a mother returns to work and is separated from her baby for several hours each day and is not pumping her milk, or if a baby who was nursing often suddenly starts to sleep through the night.

Any time the amount of baby's sucking at the breast is reduced, a mother should realize that her hormone level could be affected and her menstrual cycle may resume. More importantly, if this change in nursing patterns has happened suddenly, ovulation is more likely to occur before the first menstrual period.

Early periods may be less regular than they were before you became pregnant, since it takes a while for the menstrual cycle to settle into a predictable schedule after childbirth, whether a mother is breastfeeding or not. You can find a more detailed and thorough explanation of the physical changes in your reproductive cycle while breastfeeding, and how you can become more aware of them, in Sheila Kippley's book, *Breastfeeding and Natural Child Spacing* and in *Your Fertility Signals: Using Them to Achieve or Avoid Pregnancy, Naturally* by Merryl Winstein. See the Appendix for details.

Since certain patterns of breastfeeding have been shown to significantly delay the return of fertility, you may not need to consider other methods of family planning in the early months. However, as your natural period of infertility is ending, you may want to think about family planning options. Your own values and preferences will certainly influence the choices you make, as will the fact that you are breastfeeding.

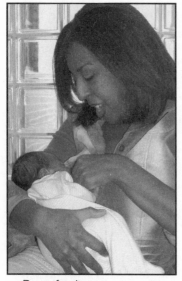

Breastfeeding saves money
for families, governments,
insurance companies, and
society as a whole.

If a breastfeeding mother chooses to use contraception, her safest choice would be one of the non-hormonal barrier methods. Health professionals agree that a mother's use of a spermicide does not present any problems for her nursing baby. The IUD (intrauterine device) is also thought to be safe for breastfeeding mothers.

Hormonal contraceptives that contain estrogen have been shown to decrease milk supply in some mothers as well as result in changes in milk composition. Health professionals knowledgeable about breastfeeding advise mothers to avoid hormonal contraceptives that contain estrogen during lactation. A woman who wants to use hormonal contraception while breastfeeding should use a progestin-only type. These are less likely to have a negative effect on her milk supply. Some mothers and health professionals, however, have found that even progestin-only contraception can reduce a mother's milk production, especially when introduced too early in the course of lactation. There are still no conclusive studies on long-term effects of hormonal contraceptives on mother or nursing baby. For this reason, some health professionals advise that hormonal contraceptives be avoided by nursing mothers, especially when their babies are under six months of age.

Protection against Breast Cancer

A steadily accumulating body of research shows that breastfeeding offers mothers protection against breast cancer. Protection against breast cancer is related to duration of breastfeeding, with the greatest risk reduction seen in women whose total amount of breastfeeding, for one or more children, totals several years.

A recent study of breastfeeding and breast cancer combined and reanalyzed data from 47 studies done in 30 countries. Combining data from many studies gave the researchers information on 50,000 women with breast cancer and 97,000 women in a control group without breast cancer. The results of the analysis showed that among women who had given birth to children, the risk of breast cancer decreased by 4.3 percent for every 12 months of breastfeeding. This was true regardless of the woman's age, whether she was pre- or postmenopausal, and whether she lived in a developed or a developing country. The researchers concluded that the higher incidence of breast cancer in developed countries (i.e., the United States, Western Europe) is largely due to the lack of breastfeeding or the short duration of breastfeeding. Apparently breasts that are used as nature intended are better protected against disease.

Another interesting finding about breast cancer rates was reported in a 1994 study that showed that women who were breastfed themselves had significantly less risk of developing breast cancer. Both premenopausal and postmenopausal breast cancer were decreased by 26 to 31 percent in women who had been breastfed. Interestingly, this study points out that women who had been breastfed were more likely to breastfeed their own children, but this was not part of the decreased risk shown in this research.

Even though reports show that breastfeeding decreases a woman's chances of breast cancer, a mother should not ignore a lump in her breast. In rare cases, a breastfeeding mother can develop breast cancer. Most lumps in the lactating breast are milk-filled cysts (galactoceles), inflammation (mastitis or plugged ducts), or benign tumors (fibromas). However, any lump that stays the same size or that gets bigger should be examined by your doctor. If further testing needs to be done, try to find a doctor who is familiar with breastfeeding and can evaluate the situation without insisting that you wean your baby.

Economy, Ecology, Convenience, and Enjoyment

"As a mother who has done both, I can tell you that nothing is more convenient than breastfeeding," states Katie Hartsell from Kansas. "When the baby begins to cry, the mother has a readily available supply of milk at the right temperature. There is no waiting for the bottle to be warmed. There is quite a savings to the family budget and no waste."

The savings with breastfeeding are considerable, especially compared to premixed formulas and disposable bottles. One young couple, trying to budget for their new baby and their first apartment, were shocked by the "substantial sum" that would be added to their weekly food bill with the regular purchase of formula. Recent estimates place the cost of buying infant formula for one child for one year to be somewhere between $1,160 and $3,915, depending on the brand and type of formula used.

Viola Lennon, one of La Leche League's co-Founders, suggests that the money you save by breastfeeding might be used to purchase a major appliance. A father from New Zealand, Harry Parke of Cambridge, told a group of fathers, "My wife and I figured that by nursing our first son, Christopher, we saved considerably in the first year by not using formula, sterilizers, early solids, electricity, birth control means, etc. Raewyn immediately decided that the money saved was to be a deposit on a freezer, and it now stands in the hall!"

At one point, in the United States, formula costs increased at such a rapid pace that the entire industry was investigated by the Federal Trade Commission. The price of infant formula increased six times faster than the price of cow's milk. Low income mothers in the United States can receive food supplements for themselves, their babies, and their young children through the WIC (Women, Infants, and Children) program developed by the federal government. Formula prices have escalated the cost of this program. In 1986, only 38 percent of WIC mothers were breastfeeding their babies at hospital discharge. In a 1987 Summary Report from the US Department of Agriculture, it was estimated that 29 million dollars could be saved annually if mothers in the WIC program breastfed their babies for just one month.

In 1996, the Colorado WIC program determined that they could save $74,000 per month if only 50 percent of the new mothers in their program breastfed for five to six months. They estimated that a nationwide savings of 9.3 million dollars a month could be realized if 50 percent of all the mothers in the WIC program across the country breastfed for five to six months.

Breastfeeding also saves health care dollars—for families, for insurance companies, for governments, and for society. A report from the US Department of Agriculture, published in 2001, calculated the savings that could result in the USA if more women breastfed. They say that a minimum of $3.6 billion would be saved if breastfeeding were increased from current levels (64 percent in hospital; 29 percent at 6 months) to those recommended by the US Surgeon General (75 percent in hospital; 50 percent at 6 months). This figure is likely an underestimation of the total savings because it represents cost savings from the treatment of only three childhood illnesses: otitis media, gastroenteritis, and necrotizing enterocolitis.

Worldwide implications

In Third World or developing countries, the impact on the economy is devastating when mothers choose to abandon breastfeeding. Gabrielle Palmer, a nutritionist and breastfeeding counselor from Great Britain, writes in *The Politics of Breastfeeding*:

Human milk is a commodity which is ignored in national inventories and disregarded in food consumption surveys, yet it does actually save a country millions of dollars in imports and health costs. The Mozambiquan Ministry of Health calculated in 1982 that if there were a mere twenty percent rise in bottle feeding, in just two years this would cost the country (the equivalent of) 10 million US dollars, and this did not include fuel, distribution, or health costs. They also calculated the fuel required for boiling the water would use the entire resources from one of the major forestry projects. Inventors of

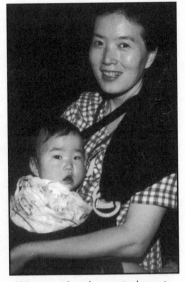

Women who choose to breastfeed are making a difference in the world.

fuel-saving cars are rewarded, why not energy-saving women? For every three million bottle-fed babies, 450 million tins of formula are used. The resulting 70,000 tons of metal in the form of discarded tins are not recycled in the developed countries.

Once you become an experienced nursing mother, you will probably spend two or three hours a day relaxing in your favorite chair, casually offering your baby the emotional, nutritional, and immunological benefits of breastfeeding. You will take this for granted as part of your daily routine. You may pause for a moment to reflect on the fact that you're giving your little one the very best start in life—but you may never stop to realize the global implications of what you are doing. You may not be aware that a mother's decision to breastfeed has economic, ecological, and political significance.

Worldwide trends toward artificial feeding have drastic consequences in terms of maternal and infant health. We can be proud of the involvement of La Leche League in efforts to reverse this trend. Forty-seven years ago, the seven Founders wanted to help their friends and neighbors experience the benefits of breastfeeding their babies. Now the organization's outreach extends to mothers in every part of the world who need that same kind of mother-to-mother support and encouragement. La Leche League also works with UNICEF, the World

Health Organization, and local governments to help provide mothers with breastfeeding information and support. Becoming a member of La Leche League and contributing to the organization are positive ways to convey a message of support to mothers all over the world who want to give their babies the best start in life.

Women who choose to breastfeed their babies are making a difference in the world. They are preserving the environment, improving infant health, and saving precious resources. And their loving, generous example models a caring way of life for their families and communities.

Your milk is always available

As a nursing mother, you can take off on short notice for a family excursion, a long trip, or a full-day picnic—situations in which formula can spoil. You can make your plans and pack your bags without worrying about having an adequate supply of formula for the baby—a formula that may not be available everywhere. You won't even have to be concerned that a strange water supply will make your baby sick, since a breastfed baby does not need extra water.

Wherever you and your baby are, so is your milk. It's a most reassuring thought, particularly in the rare, but always stressful time when the usual, normal supplies of food are cut off. This doesn't happen too often, but we do hear from mothers who have had such experiences and are most grateful that their little ones were spared the brunt of this disturbing situation.

In the Midwest, an unexpected and severe snowstorm stranded a family in their car. While the husband went for help, his wife snuggled the baby under her coat, keeping them both warm, and the baby nursed and slept. The young mother found the feeling of normalcy associated with feeding the baby helped to keep her own fears in check until a rescue crew came for them.

Emergency situations

Another family unexpectedly spent a night in the mountains. The four Walkers of Ohio—mom, dad, five-year-old Scott, and one-year-old Adam, in a backpack atop his father's shoulders—set out for an afternoon's hike and didn't make it back to their camper for twenty-one hours. "We had hiked these trails so often we thought we knew them all thoroughly," Judy Walker wrote. But when the Walkers started down the trail they thought led back to their car, they inadvertently went down another trail, which they learned later, "went right off the map." The night spent in the isolated area was cold, rainy, and so dark "we couldn't see each other." Judy concludes her story: "My husband kept scooping leaves over us trying to keep us dry, and all night, at least once an hour, Adam woke, hungry, wet, screaming. Each time I nursed him, as it was the only thing that calmed him. I thank God that throughout that cold, wet night I had warm milk to fill my baby's tummy and to comfort him."

Kay Troisi from Alabama tells of her family's experience:

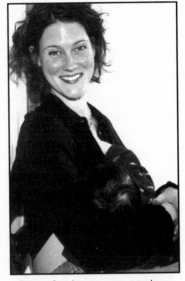

Breastfeeding is meant to be a pleasurable experience.

A hurricane came roaring through our community with little advance warning of its nearness or intensity. A lot of damage resulted, including many fallen wires, and snapped pine trees perilously perched on power lines. Consequently, we were without electricity for two-and-a-half days. During this time, I realized even more what an advantage breastfeeding is. Our daughter, Tamara, was only three weeks old and not having to worry about how to feed her was an immense relief. There was no concern over preparing formula, not to mention sterilizing, storing, or heating it without electricity. Not only did I have ready nutrition and reassurance for Tamara, but baby and mother were also consoled by our nursing session during the worst of the storm. We could be in our little world while nursing, oblivious to the external ragings. After the storm, continuous closeness ensured a peaceful baby, contented mother, and overall a happier family, during a time when other families might have been in chaos.

A pleasurable experience

Breastfeeding is intended to be a pleasurable experience for a mother. A woman who breastfeeds with pride and satisfaction is aware that breastfeeding is a sensual experience. She also knows that this is a perfectly healthy and normal aspect of her sexuality. Dorothy V. Whipple, MD, wrote in *The Journal of the American Medical Women's Association*:

Suckling a baby, for the woman who accepts and enjoys her femininity, is a particularly moving experience. The physical sensation is pleasant, the guzzling eager mouth against the sensitive erectile tissue of the nipple is enjoyable in itself. It also brings peace, contentment, fulfillment to the whole body and personality. The sensation is not orgasmic; it is more like the peaceful afterglow of orgasm. It brings to the woman a deep and personal understanding of her role as a woman. It brings to her also a bond with women in distant times and cultures. The mature woman who carries out the totality of her feminine functions knows she has a niche in the ultimate scheme of things.

And Selma Fraiberg, in describing how a baby learns to love, tells about the mutual satisfaction of breastfeeding:

In breastfeeding, the infant is cradled in the mother's arms. Pleasure in sucking, the satisfaction of hunger, intimacy with the mother's body, are united with his recognition of her face. The baby learns to associate this face, his mother's face, with an enjoyable and comforting experience. As we watch the nursing baby we see how gradually the skin surface of the body is suffused with pinkness—a sensual glow of pleasure and well-being.

When the baby is held at his mother's breast the entire ventral surface of his body is in contact with her body. And this sensual pleasure heightens his awareness of his own body. Nursing mothers also experience sensual pleasure through the baby's sucking. This should lead to no embarrassment. It is simply one of the rewards, one of the ways in which mutual sensual pleasure binds the mother to her baby and the baby to her.

To the list of breastfeeding's unique characteristics, we add yet one more—its universality. The baby at the breast represents the common language of mothering. Babies have basic needs that do not change, regardless of when or where they are born. And the beautifully natural act of nursing your little one has this same timeless quality. It is a link to other mothers and a sign, even, of womanly power. The ability of a mother's body to nurture her child is a source of strength to her. And through breastfeeding's gentling effect, an island of peace is secured. It is a small miracle, belonging rightfully to mothers, babies, and families the world over.

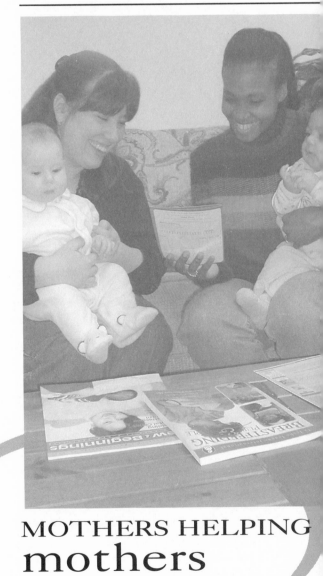

PART EIGHT

MOTHERS HELPING
mothers

CHAPTER TWENTY

ABOUT
la leche league

La Leche League began with a wish—a dream, really—that all mothers who want to breastfeed their babies would be able to do so. The seven of us who founded La Leche League had overcome a variety of difficulties before we were able to breastfeed with ease and confidence, and we knew of too many mothers who were unable to breastfeed at all simply because they had no one to turn to for information and advice.

How It All Began

It was at a church picnic that Mary White and Marian Tompson decided there had to be a way to help their friends who wanted to breastfeed their babies but found only frustration and failure when they tried. With their own nursing babies cradled in their arms on that summer afternoon in 1956, Mary and Marian talked about finding a way to help those women experience the joy and deep fulfillment of breastfeeding.

In the weeks that followed, Mary talked to Mary Ann Kerwin, her sister-in-law, and Mary Ann Cahill, who casually mentioned the idea to Betty Wagner. Marian contacted Edwina Froehlich, who got on the phone to call her good friend Viola Lennon. Each had nursed one or more babies. We had no grandiose plans about how to go about helping our friends, but we were willing to try. Two local physicians, Drs. Herbert Ratner and Gregory White, advised us on those aspects of breastfeeding that were commonly associated with the medical community, and gave us the benefit of their wisdom and insights into human nature.

Confident of our information, and enthusiastic about breastfeeding, we invited our pregnant friends to a meeting at Mary White's house one October evening in 1956. What we offered to interested neighborhood mothers then—and what the 40,000 La Leche League Leaders who have followed us continue to provide—was information, encouragement, and support. Personal mother-to-mother warmth and caring have been a cornerstone of our organization since its inception. Although La Leche League has grown into a worldwide organization with over 3,000 Groups in sixty-six countries (located in communities throughout the United States, Canada, New Zealand, Europe, Africa, Asia, Latin America, and South America), our focus still remains on the personal one-to-one sharing of information and encouragement that provides a new mother with the confidence she needs to breastfeed her baby.

Today La Leche League stands as the internationally recognized authority on breastfeeding. La Leche League has been contacted by mothers, fathers, doctors, nurses, lactation consultants, and other professionals throughout the world for expertise on breastfeeding. La Leche League International serves as a Non-Governmental Organization Consultant to UNICEF, an agency of the United Nations, and the World Health Organization (WHO), acts as a registered Private Voluntary Organization for the US Agency of International Development (USAID), is an accredited member of the US Healthy Mothers, Healthy Babies National Coalition, is a member of the Child Survival Collaborations and Resources Group (CORE), and is a founding member of the World Alliance for Breastfeeding Action (WABA).

La Leche League's Annual Seminars for Physicians, held in North America, attract doctors from all over the world. They are cosponsored by the American Academy of Pediatrics and the American College of Obstetricians and Gynecologists. The American Academy of Family Physicians participates as a Cooperating Organization. These seminars are also accredited by the American Medical Association—Category 1 of the Physician's Recognition Award, the American Osteopathic Association, The American Dietetic Association, and the International Board of Lactation Consultant Examiners.

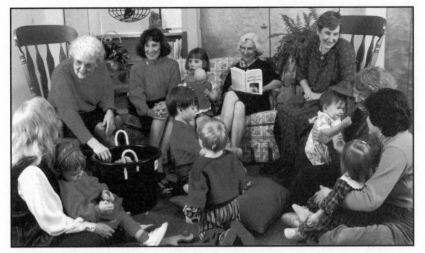

LLLI's Founders enjoy being involved with mothers and their children.

Workshops for Lactation Specialists are scheduled each year in the spring and fall in regional locations to meet the needs of health professionals who specialize in caring for the breastfeeding dyad. Continuing education credits are available to International Board Certified Lactation Consultants and to registered nurses.

How LLL Can Help You

Over the years it has been La Leche League's privilege to help hundreds of thousands of mothers breastfeed their babies. La Leche League, to us, is simply a mother with a baby in her arms and a smile on her face, proud of herself and eager to share all that she has learned and experienced. Mothers, like you, who find fulfillment and delight in nurturing an infant are the heart and soul of La Leche League.

La Leche League Leaders everywhere rejoice in the knowledge that by helping mothers to breastfeed their babies, they are playing a part in strengthening and deepening the love ties formed in infancy that will last a lifetime.

Our organization

Our name, La Leche, is Spanish and is pronounced la lay-chay. Simply translated, it means "the milk." The name of our organization was inspired by a shrine in St. Augustine, Florida, dedicated to the Mother of Christ under the title "Nuestra Senora de la Leche y Buen Parto," which translates freely, "Our Lady of Happy Delivery and Plentiful Milk."

Our international headquarters, located in Schaumburg, Illinois, USA, is staffed by 30 employees. Every year people throughout the world seeking breastfeeding help or information contact LLLI by phone, fax, email, and regular mail. There are LLLI Affiliate organizations in Canada, French Canada, Great Britain, Switzerland, Germany, and New Zealand. La Leche League is a not-for-profit, non-sectarian organization and is entirely supported by donations, memberships, and sales of materials.

Professional support

La Leche League International has a Health Advisory Council comprised of doctors and health professionals from all over the world. This council is consulted about medical situations and evaluation of new research. Members of the Health Advisory Council review La Leche League publications that include medical information. Complementing the Health Advisory Council are doctors throughout the world serving as Medical Associates of La Leche League.

A Legal Advisory Council and a Management Advisory Council complete the LLLI Professional Advisory Board.

Publications

La Leche League's basic manual, THE WOMANLY ART OF BREASTFEEDING, has sold more than 3 million copies and is available in nine languages, on audiotape, and in English Braille. Other LLLI publications are available in 23 languages.

La Leche League is the world's largest resource for breastfeeding information. Currently, we publish 35 books and more than 100 pamphlets and tear-off sheets. A selection of more than 200 books, information sheets, and pamphlets are listed in the LLLI Catalogue along with breast pumps, baby slings, CD-ROMs, videos, and other products of interest to breastfeeding families.

LLLI's award-winning Web site at www.lalecheleague.org offers many opportunities to learn more, including breastfeeding information in languages other than English. You can browse through the LLLI Catalogue and place orders securely online, learn more about the history of La Leche League, and read articles from NEW BEGINNINGS and other LLL publications. The Web site includes answers to frequently asked questions and Help Forms you can fill out to receive a personal response regarding a specific breastfeeding situation. You can also find links to Group pages in the USA and around the world to help you find an LLL Leader or LLL meetings near you. There are also opportunities to participate in online meetings.

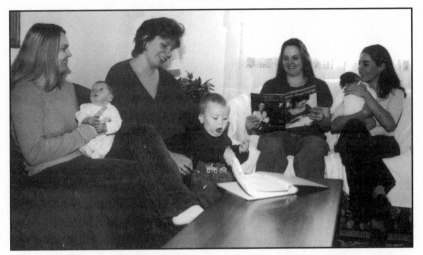

Mothers share information and support with one another at
LLL Group meetings.

Conferences

International and Area Conferences are held periodically for parents
and professionals. Speakers include experts in breastfeeding, parenting, childbirth, nutrition, childcare, and related topics. Doctors, educators, researchers, authors, and parents represent a wide range of
experiences and options as speakers and panelists.

Membership

Members of La Leche League care about giving their babies the best.
As an LLL member, you will have the satisfaction of being part of a
worldwide network of mothers with breastfeeding experience who
share information, support, and encouragement.

Membership in La Leche League offers you these benefits:

- one-year subscription (six bimonthly issues) to NEW BEGINNINGS
  a magazine filled with mothers' stories, inspiration, practical
  hints, photos, book reviews, and breastfeeding information.

- a 10 percent member's discount on most purchases from the
  LLLI Catalogue which features a wide variety of outstanding
  publications on breastfeeding, childbirth, nutrition, and parenting as well as products that have been found useful by breastfeeding mothers.

- the opportunity to share the companionship of other mothers of
  babies and young children at monthly meetings of your local LLL

Group and learn even more from the carefully selected books in the Group's library.

• participation in LLL special events, including local and international conferences, with a special member's discount on registration fees.

When you become a La Leche League member you support the efforts of your local Group Leaders who are volunteers, and you join an international mother-to-mother helping network with nearly fifty years of experience sharing practical mothering wisdom.

La Leche League Meetings

LLL meetings are informal discussion groups often held in the homes of members or at another easily accessible meeting location. Information is presented following a planned schedule of topics that cover practical, physical, and psychological aspects of breastfeeding.

La Leche League meetings offer a wonderful source of information and encouragement, and a ready source of new friendships among mothers who have many things in common. If you can attend LLL meetings while you are still pregnant, you will be well prepared for breastfeeding when your baby arrives.

At these La Leche League meetings, the LLL Group Leader shares her knowledge about breastfeeding and related topics and encourages mothers to ask questions and share their own experiences. For every question or difficulty that might be brought up, there are usually several mothers at the meeting who are able to offer various solutions or suggestions. It is both exciting and reassuring to watch other babies in the Group thrive and grow. It is fun to see how unique each baby is, and the wonderful, warm way in which each mother and baby relate to each other. Babies are always welcome at LLL meetings.

Our Leaders are primarily mothers who have breastfed their own babies and are willing to share their knowledge and enthusiasm about breastfeeding with mothers who look to them for help. The personal experience and special training of each Leader prepare her for this role. Every LLL Leader has completed a specific application process before she is considered qualified to act as an official representative of La Leche League.

How to find La Leche League

With more than 3,000 La Leche League Groups meeting every month all around the world, the chances are excellent that there are one or more Groups in your community. Group Leaders make every effort to publicize their meetings so that mothers will be able to find the local LLL Group quickly and easily.

Nearly all Groups place meeting notices in the local newspapers. Watch your paper, or simply call the newspaper office and ask if they know how to get in touch with the La Leche League Groups in the area.

In some of the larger cities, you will find La Leche League listed in the white pages of the telephone directory. If there is not a listing, try calling the maternity wards of the larger hospitals or some of the obstetricians and pediatricians in your area. Childbirth instructors or your local library may have information about La Leche League Groups in the community.

Be sure to ask around among your friends and neighbors who are pregnant or have young children. You will more than likely find one or more of them has been to La Leche League meetings and would be delighted to put you in touch with a local Leader.

In the USA and Canada, there are toll free numbers you can call for immediate answers to breastfeeding questions, a free copy of the LLLI or LLL Canada Catalogue, or the name of a La Leche League Leader near you. Just call 1-800-LA LECHE in the USA or 1-800-665-4324 in Canada. You can also visit La Leche League on the World Wide Web at http://www.lalecheleague.org where you will find an on-line catalogue, answers to frequently asked questions, listings of local LLL Groups, and other current information.

Or you can email us at llli@llli.org or write us at La Leche League International, 1400 N. Meacham Road, P.O. Box 4079, Schaumburg, Illinois, 60168-4079, USA. Our regular telephone number is 847-519-7730. By calling this number, you can locate a La Leche League Leader near you by using your zip code (in the USA). The fax number is 1-847-519-0035. Business hours are from 9:00 AM to 5:00 PM, Central Time.

Would you like to help?

Perhaps you are not able to locate a La Leche League Group in your community and this book has been your only source of guidance for your breastfeeding experience. As the months go by and your baby grows and thrives on your milk, you may notice other mothers asking you questions about breastfeeding. We know, because that's how we got started! If you find this is something you enjoy, why not write to us for information on starting a La Leche League Group?

La Leche League needs mothers just like you who have read this book, followed its recommendations, and happily breastfed their babies. If there is no La Leche League Group in your area and you think you'd be interested in becoming a La Leche League Leader, write to LLLI, c/o Leader Accreditation Department, and request a copy of our free brochure, "Becoming a La Leche League Leader."

If you are involved with an LLL Group, you can obtain more information about LLL leadership from the Leaders in your local LLL Group.

About This Book and Its Authors

When the seven of us wrote the first edition of THE WOMANLY ART OF BREASTFEEDING in the 1950s, we were all mothers at home full-time. Writing was done in between other chores, while the baby napped or played nearby, perhaps with a preschool brother or sister. More often than not, the desk was the family dining table, and manuscript pages had to be hastily gathered up at mealtime.

We had mutually agreed from the very beginning that our families were our first priority. This understanding freed us to set aside LLL work when our families needed us. As our children grew and circumstances changed, some of us took on salaried jobs at La Leche League International's office, but we are now all retired from those responsibilities. However, the interest that we shared nearly fifty years ago has not abated. All of us continue working on LLL projects when our help is needed and we serve as members of the Founders' Advisory Council.

When we started La Leche League, each of us knew one or more of the others, but some of us were getting acquainted for the first time. We were far from being carbon copies of each other. Some had bottle-fed older children; others had been fortunate enough to have breastfed their first babies. There is a span of sixteen years in our ages and great diversity among us. What solidly unites us is our belief in the importance of mothering and the value of breastfeeding.

Since our philosophy is based mainly on what we have found through experience to be the most valuable, we include some information about us as individuals.

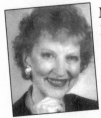 **Mary Ann Cahill,** McHenry, Illinois: In 1956, the year La Leche League was founded, the Cahills of Franklin Park, Illinois, were wholeheartedly into "people building." "The more common term would be parenting," Mary Ann explains, "But we were idealists and dreamers, as are all parents of young children to some extent. For Chuck and me, it was a wonderfully exciting time."

In the years to follow, the family grew from six to a total of nine children—Bob, Elizabeth, Tim, Teresa, Mary, Joe, Margaret, Charlene ("Charlie"), and Frannie, with room always at the table for Janet, a foster daughter who spent several of her grade-school years with her "Cahill family." The family moved to a bigger house in Libertyville in 1960, and more recently, Mary Ann moved to a smaller home in McHenry. Her husband, Chuck, died in 1978. "I will never forget the outpouring of love and sympathy from LLL people, their many kindnesses to me and my family at that time."

The days of intense parenting are now in the past, and the Cahill children have moved to different parts of Illinois and to Missouri, Wisconsin, and Colorado. They're mothers and fathers, and they work in maintenance, social work, designing, postal services, as a doctor, pharmacist, sign interpreter to the hearing impaired, librarian, and teacher. "When we're all together, we have a grand time," Mary Ann says. "The hopes and dreams, the prayers and hard work of 'people building' are well worth the effort. I can't imagine a more satisfying life." Mary Ann left the LLLI office staff in 1995 and worked part time at a local hospital. A favorite activity remains her work with the other Founders on the Founders' Advisory Council. In 2001, Mary Ann wrote a book reflecting the Founders' memories of the history of La Leche League. Introduced at the LLLI Conference that year, SEVEN VOICES, ONE DREAM was an immediate success.

Updating her family story for this edition of THE WOMANLY ART OF BREASTFEEDING, Mary Ann writes:

I'm still living in McHenry, now known as the "fastest growing community in Illinois." Soon, instead of open fields I'll be looking out over rooftops which, I've decided, have a beauty all their own.

I'm now working on the staff at the Church of Holy Apostles, five minutes up the road from where I live. It's a young, welcoming parish, full of life, and I enjoy being a part of it.

My children are my delight. Unfortunately, six of the ten live out of state. In June 2003, when Fran announced that her family was coming to McHenry from their home in Colorado for little David's baptism, word went out and the whole clan assembled—kids, grandkids, and great-grandkids—42 in all. The locals spiffed up Gram's house in anticipation and mowed an adjacent "volleyball field" for a big game. New arrivals hugged and greeted and helped cook up a storm. For three days, everybody celebrated. It was awesome, really awesome!

I am an optimist, if for no other reason than I see so many good, caring young mothers and fathers doing their best to bring up good, caring youngsters. Yes, there are tremendous pressures on today's families, which is all the more reason that we must be there for each other, to support, encourage, and offer the best possible guidance. Yes, to see that La Leche League remains strong, fresh, and accessible to ever more breastfeeding mothers, babies, and their families.

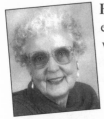

Edwina Froehlich, Inverness, Illinois. Although Edwina enjoyed the dozen or so years she spent doing secretarial work at various companies located in the heart of downtown Chicago, she always planned and expected to become a wife and mother. She and John met the year Edwina turned 33 and six months later they were married. She was 36 years old when she gave birth to her first child. Since most women in the 1940s and 1950s had their babies well before age 30, it was not surprising that Edwina was given dire warnings from all sides about the perils of having a first baby at such an "advanced" age. Moreover she was told that the breasts of a woman over thirty could never produce milk. Fortunately her "aged" mammary glands produced plenty of milk for her three sons. It is interesting that now, 50 years later, it has become quite common for women in their thirties to give birth to one or more babies and happily breastfeed.

The Froehlich family has grown to include Edwina's three daughters-in-law and the nine grandchildren they have given her. Paul and Marilyn, David and Sharon, and Peter and Paula each have three children. Edwina feels her sons outdid themselves in choosing their wives. All three are outstanding young women, devoted wives, and very nurturing mothers. Marilyn became a La Leche League Leader. After retiring from membership on the Board of Directors of LLLI, Edwina became active in the Founders' Advisory Council. As the designated facilitator, she sets up their meetings, takes notes, and distributes the minutes.

Her favorite role is that of Grandma to Leanne, Kristin, and Steven who are now in college, Katrina and Michael who will enter high school in the Fall of 2003, and Laura, Colleen, Jenna, and Christian who are still in grammar school. Their grandpa, John, died in 1997. In January 2003 Edwina finally left Franklin Park, her home for 40 years, and moved to a townhouse that is no more than 10 minutes away from her grandchildren and their parents.

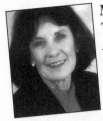

Mary Ann Kerwin, Denver, Colorado: When Mary Ann and Tom Kerwin became parents for the first time in 1955, Mary Ann was eager to breastfeed even though not one of her friends was breastfeeding. The combination of her inexperience and a sleepy baby made it difficult to get started. Helpful advice and support were forthcoming from Greg and Mary White (Mary is Tom Kerwin's sister). Soon, Mary Ann and her first baby were a contented nursing couple. Mary Ann's major regret regarding her first breastfeeding experience is that she weaned at nine months. It was a painful and upsetting time for both mother and baby, but Mary Ann learned from this experience. All of the other babies were allowed to wean at their own pace. The Kerwins have eight children: Tom, Ed, Greg, Mary, Anne, Katie, John, and Mike. Two are doctors, two are lawyers, one a bookseller, one a journalist, one a software engineer, and the youngest is a geology professor. They had one more child, Joseph, born in 1959, who died at six weeks of age—a victim of Sudden Infant Death Syndrome. They now have seven wonderful sons-in-law and daughters-in-law—and thirteen grandchildren.

After serving as Chairman of LLLI's Board of Directors from 1980-83, Mary Ann returned to school and earned a law degree in 1986. The education she received from her children gave her the necessary determination and self-discipline to achieve this goal. She practiced family law in Colorado until 2000 and continued as an active member of LLLI's Board of Directors until 2001. Currently Mary Ann is a member of the LLLI Founders' Advisory Council.

Mary Ann enjoys being closely involved with her children and their children. Six of the eight families live nearby. Often they celebrate holidays and special occasions together. Mary Ann tries to take her younger grandchildren on outings several times a week to give their busy mothers a bit of a break. She loves swimming, biking, reading, singing, hiking, tennis, and games, all of which she can enjoy with her grandchildren.

Mary Ann feels very fortunate that all of her grandchildren have been breastfed babies even though several mothers had to overcome challenges.

Mary Ann tells this story:

> Our first two grandchildren were born prematurely to our daughter, Mary. Although her first son, Michael, was two months premature, Mary was eventually able to breastfeed him completely. She received help and encouragement from LLL Leaders and LLL-trained lactation consultants.

The hospital staff was also very supportive. Dr. Marianne Neifert arranged for Mary to use an electric double breast pump to build up her milk supply so that Michael could be given her milk. Mary felt good about pumping her breasts because she was able to give her baby the best possible start in life. Providing her own milk for Michael also helped overcome the grief she felt because of his premature birth.

At first, Michael drank Mary's milk from a tube, then transitioned to a bottle, then to the breast with a nipple shield. Within a few weeks, he was strong enough to nurse fully on the breast. His brother, Ben, was born five weeks early, but he began breastfeeding in just a few days.

Both boys, now in their teens, are thriving and have no long-term effects from their premature births thanks in large part to successful breastfeeding.

Mary Ann's daughters-in-law have succeeded beautifully in breastfeeding and mothering eight more grandchildren. All breastfed immediately after birth.

Mary Ann's third daughter, Katie, however, experienced great difficulty nursing her first and third babies. It took Katie three weeks to get her first baby started because of latch-on problems. The second was a pro at breastfeeding from birth. But her third baby was not fully breastfeeding until she was two-and-a-half months old.

Mary Ann explains:

Katie would not have succeeded without extensive help from numerous LLL-trained lactation consultants. They helped her work through problems with a sleepy baby, poor latch-on, a high-arched palate, possible acid reflux, and ultimately an oversupply of milk that ironically caused poor weight gain. To overcome this, Katie had to pump before feeding the baby so that she would get enough of the rich hindmilk that breastfed babies need! After this last hurdle, her baby's weight increased significantly.

As Mary Ann ponders the legacy of La Leche League, her primary goal remains helping all mothers benefit from breastfeeding. As a member of the Colorado Breastfeeding Task Force, she is working to boost breastfeeding rates among low-income women in particular, focusing on helping mothers in the critical early weeks. Mary Ann knows that once a mother establishes a powerful bond with her baby, parenting will be enhanced for years to come. Mary Ann also is working to establish legislation in the US that would allow mothers to breast-feed their babies anyplace the mother has the right to be. She is disap-pointed that in this new millennium, mothers still face prejudice from people who try to prevent mothers from feeding their babies in places like airports, museums, restaurants, and stores.

Mary Ann believes her sons and daughters and their spouses are doing a better job with breastfeeding and parenting than she did. She knows that at times breastfeeding is not easy and that being a good parent presents daily challenges.

She believes, however, her children and their spouses have a head start thanks to the influence of La Leche League International. She says:

> **Whatever I might have done to help others during the past five decades has come back to me much, much more than a thousandfold. Undoubtedly La Leche League has enriched my life, the lives of my family, and the lives of innumerable families all over the world!**

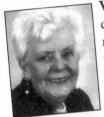

Viola Lennon, Park Ridge, Illinois: Vi's ten little Lennons came in all sizes, and just to prove that no challenge was too much for her, she even produced a set of twins in 1961. It was considered quite an accomplishment to nurse even one baby in those days, so Vi caused quite a stir in the neighbor-hood when she calmly proceeded to totally breastfeed both Catherine and Charlotte. Cathy was wakeful as an infant, nursing at least every two hours, while sleepy Charlotte nursed much less often, but gained more rapidly than her sister. She also weaned five months later than Cathy. The twins were sixth and seventh in the lineup, with Elizabeth, Mark, Mimi, Rebecca, and Matthew preceding them, and Martin, Maureen, and Gina following. Mimi was colicky as a baby, and Vi assumed that indicated a high-strung personality, but Mimi has grown into an easygoing, serene young lady.

Vi was the first official Board Chairman, and led Board meetings for several years. She also worked in the LLLI Funding Development Department for many years. She is currently acting as a consultant to La Leche League's Alumnae Association. She is also a member of the Founders' Advisory Council.

Viola was the last of the Founders to become a grandmother, but currently she has eighteen grandchildren. All of her children and grandchildren live nearby, so Lennon family gatherings are large and frequent.

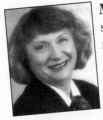

Marian Tompson, Evanston, Illinois: Even though she switched doctors with each of her first three babies, six months was the longest Marian was able to breastfeed them. Each doctor gave her advice that was standard for the time—nurse no more than every four hours, give an occasional supplementary bottle to ensure the baby was getting enough, and start solids by six weeks. With her third baby, it wasn't long before the doctor told Marian she had lost her milk; he explained that this was a common occurrence with mothers caring for several small children. Luckily, with the birth of their fourth baby in 1955, Marian and her husband, Tom, found the supportive help they needed from Dr. Gregory White and his wife, Mary. Baby Laurel, who was born at home, nursed past a year and weaned herself. This was also true for the three succeeding babies, each of whom nursed longer than the one before. Tom, "who was truly my partner and the main support of everything I was able to accomplish during my years as president of LLLI," died in 1981. The seven Tompson children— Melanie, Deborah, Allison, Laurel, Sheila, Brian, and Philip are grown now. Their own children were all breastfed. They live in Arizona, New Jersey, and Florida, with most of them still in Illinois. To Marian's great joy, most Christmases find the children and their spouses, 15 grandchildren, and now three breastfed great-grandchildren, gathered at her Evanston apartment for fun and games.

Marian served as LLLI's first and only president for twenty-four years. During seventeen of those years she also chaired meetings of the LLLI Board of Directors, served as the first editor of what is now NEW BEGINNINGS, and initiated the Breastfeeding Seminars for Physicians. Her enthusiasm for helping breastfeeding mothers is still evident today as she speaks at La Leche League conferences and other meetings around the world. In 1995 she was part of a group of breast-feeding supporters who attended the Fifth UN Conference on Women in Beijing, China to ensure that the value of breastfeeding was sup-ported as part of the solution to many of the issues being discussed. She serves on LLLI's Founders' Advisory Council and the International Advisory Council for WABA (World Alliance for Breastfeeding Action) and on the advisory boards of a number of other organizations concerned with childbirth and family life.

In 2000, Marian founded and currently serves as executive director of AnotherLook, a not-for-profit organization dedicated to gathering information, raising critical questions, and stimulating research about breastfeeding in the context of HIV/AIDS. "AnotherLook is really an outgrowth of my work in La Leche League," Marian explained.

"I want to make sure that all mothers, even those who have been diagnosed as HIV positive, get breastfeeding information that is based on scientific evidence that will ensure the best possible outcomes for their babies."

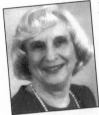

Betty Wagner Spandikow, Springfield, Tennessee: Betty breastfed all of her children, beginning back in 1943, thanks in large part to her mother, who was able to give her the practical help she needed. It was baby number six who presented Betty with new challenges. Dorothea cried a good deal and wasn't happy anywhere but in her mother's arms. Betty found it necessary to curtail all outside activities and rearrange her life around this little one who needed her so intensely. Dorothea was past her third birthday before she would venture very far from her mother, but about the time she was three and a half, she blossomed into a very self-confident, outgoing little girl. The Wagners had seven children—Gail, Robert, Wayne, Mary, Peggy, Dorothea, and Helen. Betty's daughter, Mary, was the first of the Founders' daughters to become a La Leche League Leader.

Betty Wagner was the Executive Director of LLLI for 19 years. She has retired from that position but continues to serve on the Founders' Advisory Council. Betty has twenty-four grandchildren and fourteen great-grandchildren; all have been happily breastfed.

Betty's husband died in 1979. In 1991 she married Paul Spandikow, the father of seven and grandfather of fifteen. They now reside most of the time in Springville, Tennessee with lots of travel to parts of the country where their children, grandchildren, and great-grandchildren live.

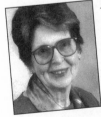

Mary White, River Forest, Illinois: Mary's first attempt at breastfeeding was just like that of most mothers in the 1940s—disastrous! In a short time, baby Joseph was a bottle-fed baby. When their second baby was born, her doctor husband, Greg, was home from the Army, and she had the support that a nursing mother needs. Bill, Peggy, Katie, Anne, Jeannie, Mike, Mary, Clare, Molly, and Liz were all happily breastfed with never a bottle in the house. Only the first three were hospital births; the others were born at home and arrived at intervals of two to five years due solely to the most natural family planning of all, breastfeeding. Liz was born when her mother was forty-seven, and Mary recalls, "It was the shortest pregnancy I ever had because for the first three months I thought I was in the menopause!"

Their eldest daughter Peggy died of cancer in 1968 at the age of 18. All three of their sons are doctors, in family practice as their father was.

Nine of their children are married and their 55th grandchild has just arrived. All of the grandchildren have been breastfed and almost all were born at home. Their youngest daughter, Liz, had an emergency cesarean birth with her first baby but after that had two natural births. There are now 16 great-grandchildren, including twins, Martin and Bridget, who each topped seven pounds at birth.

In 2001, Mary and Greg moved from their three-story family home into a condo in the same community. Greg retired from his practice in the summer of 2000 and sadly, he passed away in June 2003. The Whites had been married almost 60 years.

Mary still attends La Leche League Area Conferences and loves to talk on her favorite topic—moms and babies being together. Mary's devotion to the special kind of mothering that is so much a part of breastfeeding has always been a guiding influence in La Leche League. If you were to ask Mary, she would tell you that she believes her most important job as a mother is to instill in her children a love and trust in God for all of their lives.

Those who helped

A dedicated office staff and many professional consultants worked long hours to prepare the manuscript for the third edition of THE WOMANLY ART OF BREASTFEEDING in 1981. Mary Ann Cahill did most of the writing with lots of help from the other Founders.

The fourth revised edition, published in 1987, was compiled and edited by Judy Torgus, long-time La Leche League Leader and Executive Editor in LLLI's Publications Department. Judy has revised and edited all of the subsequent editions, with the help of Gwen Gotsch and others.

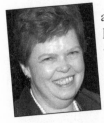 In this current 2004 edition, the information was once again updated by Judy Torgus, now LLLI's Director of Publications, and Gwen Gotsch, Senior Editor for LLLI, with computer assistance from Joyce Kashe. The Founders reviewed all of the revisions and added comments they thought were needed. Many of the new recommendations on latch-on, positioning, and milk supply in this edition are based on the information in the 2003 revised edition of LLLI's BREASTFEEDING ANSWER BOOK, which was written and researched by Nancy Mohrbacher, IBCLC, and Julie Stock, MA, IBCLC. Nancy Jo Bykowski, IBCLC, who works in the

LLLI Publications Department, helped provide background information on several topics, and solicited stories and comments from Leaders outside the USA. Carol Huotari, IBCLC, Manager of LLLI's Center for Breastfeeding Information, also provided research and reviewed the updated material.

Each time THE WOMANLY ART OF BREASTFEEDING is revised, the updated information is based on current research as well as the practical experiences of breastfeeding mothers. Although specific recommendations about breastfeeding have changed over the years, the basic questions and concerns that mothers have remain the same. And La Leche League's message has not changed in almost 50 years. We believe that breastfeeding is the ideal way for a mother to get to know her own baby and develop the skills she needs to make informed decisions that are right for her family.

Many of the personal stories that are included came from the pages of NEW BEGINNINGS, the LLLI bimonthly members' publication, and from *Aroha*, the New Zealand members' publication. We want to thank the parents who shared their experiences with us, as well as those who posed for the photographs that are used throughout the book.

We are deeply grateful to each of the above and to many others—too numerous to mention—who have helped to make THE WOMANLY ART OF BREASTFEEDING the classic that it is.

La Leche League's Influence

Many of the changes that have occurred in infant-care practices over the past 47 years can be attributed to La Leche League's influence. In 1956 babies were routinely introduced to solids between one and three months. Based on valid medical research as well as their success in keeping up their milk supply by delaying solids, the Founders of La Leche League recommended postponing the introduction of solids for four to six months. Today the American Academy of Pediatrics and the World Health Organization agree with delaying the start of solid foods for six months. Few mothers are told to give solid foods in the early months.

When La Leche League began, babies were routinely separated from their mothers following birth for as long as twenty-four hours. La Leche League spoke out—babies need their mothers, and mothers benefit, too, by early nursing and uninterrupted bonding. Today women expect to hold their newborn baby immediately after birth. What was unheard of forty-seven years ago is common practice now, and LLL helped mothers achieve this.

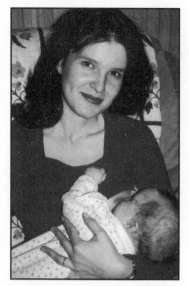

La Leche League began with the dream that all mothers who wanted to breastfeed their babies would be able to do so.

Dr. Ruth Lawrence, author of *Breastfeeding: A Guide for the Medical Profession,* collects historical data about breastfeeding. Quoting from magazines and advertisements dating from the 1940s and '50s, Dr. Lawrence points out that considerable doubt was posed in the mind of the average mother at that time. She was led to believe she should rear her child according to the advice of "experts."

Lynn Weiner, a historian and lecturer with the Women's Studies at Northwestern University, believes La Leche League's empowerment of women was the precursor of self-help groups and women's renewed control over family health-care issues. Seven women set out to give the baby back to the mother at a time when male experts dominated the child care field.

The women of the fifties came to La Leche League with very basic questions. How do I know if I have enough milk? How do I know when the baby is hungry? When will my child sleep through the night? Today's women still come to LLL in search of answers, encouragement, and the mother-to-mother support that we have become known for. More than 10,000 mothers a month call La Leche League's 800 number with questions about breastfeeding. The most common reason still given by mothers who stop nursing in the early weeks is that they didn't think they had enough milk.

From its small beginning, La Leche League has grown into an international organization, recognized worldwide as an authority on breastfeeding. La Leche League has matured into an experienced, well-seasoned, vital women's group making an impact on the world in which we live.

La Leche League remains in the forefront of placing the needs of the nursing baby on the world agenda. When heads of government met at the World Summit for Children in 1990, La Leche League was represented. In 1991, La Leche League participated in the formation of the World Alliance for Breastfeeding Action (WABA), a global network of organizations and individuals that is dedicated to protecting, promoting, and supporting breastfeeding.

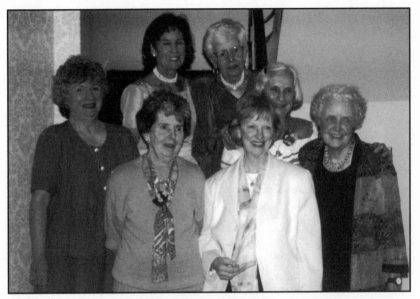

All seven of La Leche League's Founders attended the
LLLI Conference in 2001.

In the United States, a La Leche League program was developed
to encourage breastfeeding among low-income minority mothers which
has since spread to other countries. LLLI's Breastfeeding Peer
Counselor Program works in cooperation with local community health
care agencies, including WIC clinics in the USA, to offer accurate
breastfeeding information along with mother-to-mother support.

In 2003, La Leche League International was directly involved in
the planning and implementation of a three-year media campaign
sponsored by the US government to encourage more mothers to
breastfeed their babies. The US Department of Health and Human
Services recognizes breastfeeding as a public health issue and called on
La Leche League International's expertise and network of volunteers
to support this effort. This nationwide Breastfeeding Awareness
Campaign goes beyond anything the Founders could have imagined
when they met in Franklin Park, Illinois, 47 years ago to help their
friends and neighbors learn about breastfeeding.

A Final Word—From the Founders

In closing, we seven women wish to acknowledge and express heartfelt
thanks to those who have made important contributions to the development of La Leche League.

First we would like to recognize two physicians, Dr. Herbert
Ratner and Dr. Gregory White, both of whom recently passed away. As

the fathers of breastfed children, these two doctors were a rarity in 1956. Without their unfailing support and guidance, it is almost certain that we who began La Leche League would have found it extremely difficult to face the criticism and sometimes hostility of the medical community toward two basic womanly functions—natural childbirth and breastfeeding. Our own enthusiasm for and appreciation of these two functions survived because of the solid backing of those two physicians. We are eternally grateful to them, and we thank them also on behalf of the breastfeeding mothers to whom we have passed on what we learned. Over time, many other courageous physicians have also openly supported our efforts and generously shared their knowledge with us, and we are well aware of and grateful for their help. But it was Dr. Ratner and Dr. White who spoke out clearly and consistently at a time when their voices were most needed.

We also wish to recognize and gratefully acknowledge our volunteer La Leche League Leaders. It is the daily efforts of the thousands of generous volunteers who have become La Leche League Leaders who have built La Leche League. Without their continuing efforts over the years, we would not be the organization we are today.

A wide variety of books are available to help you learn more about breastfeeding, childbirth, parenting, and nutrition. We are proud of the books that are published by La Leche League International because they reflect the same philosophy you have found in the pages of this book. All of the books we publish can be ordered by mail and shipped directly to your home. Local La Leche League Groups also have these books available for purchase and/or loan, and some of them can be found in your local bookstore or public library.

We encourage you to read and learn as much as you can about your role as parents. Follow your instincts and natural inclinations in choosing the advice and information that seems right to you. The basic philosophy of La Leche League encourages you to learn about babies' and children's needs so you can understand and respond to those needs from earliest infancy and throughout the years as your child grows. And always remember, babies and children need lots and lots of love.

Books That We Publish

BREASTFEEDING ANSWER BOOK, Third Edition
by Nancy Mohrbacher & Julie Stock
This book is the definitive resource for those who are dedicated to helping mothers establish and enjoy a satisfying breastfeeding relationship with their babies. Also available on CD-ROM.
No. 1260-12 Hardcover, $68.00

BREASTFEEDING PURE & SIMPLE, REVISED EDITION
by Gwen Gotsch
Provides new mothers with a basic introduction that will guide them through the early months of their nursing relationship. Clear, straightforward text combined with lots of photos makes this book inviting and easy-to-read.
No. 803-12, $9.95

411

BREASTFEEDING YOUR PREMATURE BABY, Revised Edition
by Gwen Gotsch
Offers clear and concise information about how to breastfeed the premature baby and why breastfeeding is so important for these tiny infants. Also provides complete information on pumping, milk storage, and feeding your baby.
No. 150-12, $5.95

MOTHERWISE: 101 TIPS FOR A NEW MOTHER
by Alice Bolster
This concise book offers practical, nurturing wisdom in a format that is easily accessible to busy new mothers.
No. 148-12, $7.50

FATHERWISE: 101 TIPS FOR A NEW FATHER
by Alice Bolster
Offers practical, nurturing wisdom for new fathers. Written in an easy-to-read format, tips from new and experienced fathers are compiled to encourage a strong bond between father and child.
No. 933-12, $7.50

BECOMING A FATHER: HOW TO NURTURE AND ENJOY YOUR FAMILY, Revised Edition
by William Sears, MD
Dr. Sears shares his own story of maturing into fatherhood, discovering the joys of being an involved dad, and weathering the changes that children bring to a marriage.
No. 1377-12, $10.95

NIGHTTIME PARENTING: HOW TO GET YOUR BABY AND CHILD TO SLEEP, Revised Edition
by William Sears, MD
Explains how babies sleep differently than adults, how sharing sleep can help the whole family sleep better, and helps to reassure parents that meeting nighttime needs is important to their baby's well-being.
No. 160-12, $9.95

THE FUSSY BABY: HOW TO BRING OUT THE BEST IN YOUR HIGH-NEED CHILD, Revised Edition
by William Sears, MD
Suggestions include "back to the womb" security tips and a guide to interpreting a baby's cries. Chapters on coping with colic, feeding, fathering, soothing, and avoiding maternal burnout include plenty of support, reassurance, and day-to-day survival tips.
No. 1169-12, $9.95

GROWING TOGETHER: A PARENT'S GUIDE TO BABY'S FIRST YEAR
by William Sears, MD
Photos illustrate the growth of motor, language, social, and cognitive skills from birth to one year. Dr. Sears tells how parents can enhance their baby's development by their responsiveness. Includes tips on parenting, breastfeeding, and infant stimulation.
No. 158-12, $14.50

HOW WEANING HAPPENS
by Diane Bengson
Includes the personal experiences of mothers who have weaned in a variety of ways and covers the kinds of questions parents have about weaning.
No. 142-12, $10.95

MOTHERING MULTIPLES: BREASTFEEDING AND CARING FOR TWINS OR MORE!!! Revised Edition
by Karen Gromada
Full of practical tips from experienced mothers of twins. Everything mothers need to know to cope with the challenge of more than one baby.
No. 143-12, $14.95

MOTHERING YOUR NURSING TODDLER, Revised Edition
by Norma Jane Bumgarner
Warmth, wisdom, and wit illumine a lively discussion of breastfeeding past the age of one. Besides exploring the "why" of nursing a toddler, this book helps a mother cope with the challenges.
No. 157-12, $12.95

ADVENTURES IN TANDEM NURSING
by Hilary Flower
Combines the latest research with personal stories and humor to create an excellent reservoir of ideas for mothers who are defining breastfeeding boundaries while trying to prepare for the addition of a new baby to the family. Includes information to help mothers decide if being a "tandem mama" is right for them.
No. 1379-12, $14.95

DEFINING YOUR OWN SUCCESS: BREASTFEEDING AFTER BREAST REDUCTION SURGERY
by Diana West
Explores the many aspects of breastfeeding for a mother who has had breast reduction surgery; this book combines up-to-date research with experience and advice from breastfeeding mothers and addresses the questions and myths associated with breastfeeding after breast reduction surgery.
No. 1001-12 Softcover, $24.95

OF CRADLES AND CAREERS: A GUIDE TO RESHAPING YOUR JOB TO INCLUDE A BABY IN YOUR LIFE
by Kaye Lowman
Tips on breastfeeding and working, job-sharing, and maternity leave round out a book that encourages women to explore a variety of options and helps them choose what works best for themselves and their families.
No. 161-12, $7.95

PLAYFUL LEARNING: AN ALTERNATIVE APPROACH TO PRESCHOOL
by Anne Englehardt and Cheryl Sullivan
Designed to be a multi-purpose guide for adults who work with young children; includes a wide variety of craft projects, simple recipes, science experiments, plans for field trips, music activities, and much, much more.
No. 162-12, spiral-bound, $16.95

SAFE AND HEALTHY: A PARENT'S GUIDE TO CHILDREN'S
ILLNESSES AND ACCIDENTS
by William Sears, MD
Dr. Sears guides parents through some of the most stressful episodes of parenting
by answering the most frequently asked questions about childhood illnesses. Tells
when you should call the doctor and how to handle situations that don't require a
doctor's advice.
No. 164-12, $6.50

SEVEN VOICES, ONE DREAM
by Mary Ann Cahill
This colorful tapestry of memories explores the birth of La Leche League
International: the challenges, the joys, the ideas that were envisioned, and how
they came to fruition with the guidance of seven women.
No. 1000-12, $12.95

A SPECIAL KIND OF PARENTING: MEETING THE NEEDS OF HANDICAPPED
CHILDREN
by Julia Darnell Good and Joyce Good Reis
Children with disabilities challenge their parents' emotional and physical
resources. This book can guide parents through the problems and help them discover their disabled child as an individual.
No. 163-12, $6.50

Children's Books
THE CUDDLERS
by Stacy Towle-Morgan; illustrated by Marvin Jarboe
This children's book captures the warmth and love a family experiences when
children are drawn to the security of their parents' bed.
No. 155-12, $9.95

MAGGIE'S WEANING
by Mary Joan Deutschbein
A delightful, child's-eye view of the nursing experience. As Maggie reflects on the
time she once spent at her mother's breast, she offers her thoughts on the joys
and the challenges of slowly leaving breastfeeding behind.
No. 721-12, $6.95

MICHELE: THE NURSING TODDLER
by Jane M. Pinczuk; illustrated by Barbara Murray
This book talks about growing up in a family that loves to the fullest. From mother's milk to daddy's hugs and special visits from grandparents, Michele blooms
from an infant to a toddler, developing confidence and pride along the way.
No. 147-12, $14.95

Cookbooks

WHOLE FOODS FOR BABIES AND TODDLERS
by Margaret Kenda
This comprehensive introduction into the world of whole foods for little ones will give you the knowledge to help encourage healthy eating habits for all ages. With recipes that can be used for the whole family, this book will encourage a lifelong commitment to healthful eating.
No. 1002-12, $15.95

WHOLE FOODS FOR KIDS TO COOK
This children's cookbook includes recipes that are simple enough for preschoolers, with a little help from Mom and Dad. Others are meant for older children who have already developed simple cooking skills.
No. 149-12, spiral-bound, $9.95

WHOLE FOODS FOR THE WHOLE FAMILY Revised Edition
edited by Roberta Johnson
Filled with time-saving make-ahead meals, ideas for using leftovers, special diet and allergy recipes, suggestions for baby's first foods, and last-minute dinner menus. Uses only whole unprocessed foods and minimal amounts of salt and sweeteners. Complete with protein and calorie counts.
No. 151-12, spiral-bound, $18.95

WHOLE FOODS FROM THE WHOLE WORLD
edited by Virginia Sutton Halonen
This cookbook combines the goodness of whole foods with the variety of ethnic dishes from around the world.
No. 152-12, spiral-bound, $12.50

Other Helpful Books

In addition to the books we publish, La Leche League International distributes a selection of books that offer helpful information to parents and professionals. Some of these are listed here. For a complete, up-to-date listing plus ordering information, call 1-800-LA LECHE for a free copy of the LLLI Catalogue, or call the Order Department at 847-519-9585.

Breastfeeding

The American Academy of Pediatrics New Mother's Guide to Breastfeeding edited by American Academy of Pediatrics and Joan Younger Meek
No. 1248-7, $13.95

Bestfeeding: Getting Breastfeeding Right for You
by Mary Renfrew, Chloe Fisher, and Suzanne Arms.
No. 16-7, $14.95

Breastfeeding and Natural Child Spacing: How Ecological Breastfeeding Spaces Babies, Revised Edition
by Sheila Kippley
No. 50-7, $9.95

So That's What They're For! Breastfeeding Basics
by Janet Tamaro
No. 84-7, $10.95

Ultimate Breastfeeding Book of Answers
by Dr. Jack Newman and Teresa Pitman
No. 1057-7, $19.95

Pregnancy & Childbirth

The Birth Book: Everything You Need to Know to Have a Safe and
Satisfying Birth
by William and Martha Sears
No. 45-7, $13.95

The VBAC Companion: The Expectant Mother's Guide to Vaginal Birth
After Cesarean
by Diana Korte
No. 77-7, $12.95

Your Fertility Signals: Using Them to Achieve or Avoid Pregnancy
Naturally
by Merryl Winstein
No. 76-7, $14.95

Motherhood

Confessions of an Organized Homemaker: The Secrets of Uncluttering
Your Home and Taking Control of Your Life
by Deniece Schofield
No. 38-7, $11.99

The Hidden Feelings of Motherhood
by Kathleen Kendall-Tackett
No. 1211-7, $14.95

Child Rearing

The Discipline Book: Everything You Need to Know to Have a Better-
Behaved Child—From Birth to Age Ten
by William and Martha Sears
No. 2-7, $13.95

The Baby Book: Everything You Need to Know About Your Baby from
Birth to Age Two
by William and Martha Sears
No. 83-7, $21.45

The Family Bed: An Age Old Concept in Child Rearing
by Tine Thevenin
No. 91-7, $9.95

Good Nights, The Happy Parent's Guide to the Family Bed
by Jay Gordon
No. 1249-7, $13.95

How to Talk So Kids Will Listen and Listen So Kids Will Talk
by Adele Faber and Elaine Mazlish
No. 62-7, $12.50

The Successful Child, What Parents Can Do to Help Kids Turn out Well
By William and Martha Sears
No. 1229-7, $16.95

Sweet Dreams, A Pediatrician's Secrets for Your Child's Good
Night's Sleep
by Paul M. Fleiss
No. 1230-7, $14.95

Parenting Through Crisis: Helping Kids In Times of Loss, Grief, and Change
by Barbara Coloroso
No. 1105-7, $14.00

Professional Books
Breastfeeding: A Guide for the Medical Profession, 5th edition
by Ruth A. Lawrence, MD
No. 391-19, $61.95

Breastfeeding Conditions and Diseases
by Anne Merewood, MA, IBCLC, and Barbara L. Phillip, MD, IBLCE
No. 1122-19, $19.95

Impact of Birthing Practices on Breastfeeding: Protecting the Mother and
Baby Continuum
by Mary Kroeger, CNM, MPH and Linda J. Smith, BSE, FACCW, IBCLC
No. 1419-19, $39.95

Medications and Mothers' Milk
by Thomas Hale, PhD
No. 390-19, $24.95

Pamphlets and Information Sheets
Various booklets, pamphlets, and information sheets on specialized topics are
available from local La Leche League Groups and from La Leche League
International. For an up-to-date listing plus complete ordering information, send
for a copy of the LLLI Catalogue. Here is just a sampling of the items:

Approaches to Weaning, No. 307-17
Breastfeeding a Baby with Down Syndrome, No. 528-24
Breastfeeding after a Cesarean Birth, No. 327-17

418

Breastfeeding the Baby with Reflux, No. 524-24
Breastfeeding Twins, No. 301-17
The Diabetic Mother and Breastfeeding, No. 525-24
A Mother's Guide to Pumping Milk, No. 991-17
Nursing a Baby with a Cleft Lip or Cleft Palate, No. 523-24
Positioning Your Baby at the Breast, No. 1380-17
Working and Breastfeeding, The Balancing Act, No. 1165-17

Visually Impaired Resource List from LLLI
Provides current list of breastfeeding materials available in Braille and on cassette tapes. For more information send for free brochure.
No. 560

Center for Breastfeeding Information
A reliable source for health professionals, researchers, breastfeeding counselors, and medical students seeking breastfeeding literature, current references, bibliographic lists, and general information. For more information send for a free brochure or look into our LLLI Web site at www.lalecheleague.org/cbi/cbi.html
No. 419-20

Breastfeeding Products

Most breastfeeding mothers and their babies get along just fine without specialized equipment or products. However, in cases where some assistance is necessary to ensure continued breastfeeding success, La Leche League has certain products available that can be of help. Some of these items are available through local LLL Groups, or you can order directly from La Leche League International.

Whisper Wear Double Pump Kit
This pump, designed to mimic the feel and sucking pattern of a baby, is the first hands-free pump on the market.
No. 1428-21, $219.00

Medela Pump In Style® Breastpump
Original No. 457-21, $309.95
Traveler No. 1235-21, $329.95

Nurture III Double Electric Breast Pump
No. 436-21, (without accessories) $125.00
No. 437-21, (with accessories) $165.00

Ameda Purely Yours® Pump
Purely Yours Carry All. No. 1329-21, $249.00
Purely Yours Backpack. No. 1330-21, $299.00

Lact-Aid Nursing Trainer Systems
Ideal for short-term use, Lact-Aid Nursing Trainer System is a supplementation system for mothers who need to give a supplement of human milk or formula at the breast. A standard unit contains adjustable neck strap, bag hanger, strainer, funnel, cleaning syringe, and instructions. A supply of 50 bags is also included.
1066-21, $46.00

Medela Supplemental Nursing System (SNS)™

Two thin tubes, taped to each breast, deliver a supplement to the nursing baby from a plastic container that hangs around the mother's neck. The SNS is helpful for the baby who can latch on but has special needs. This device is used in relactation, for babies with a weak suck, and for adopted babies.
No. 451-21, $41.95

Medela Hazelbaker™ FingerFeeder

This device is a transitional tool that is used for a short time in order to teach non-latching babies how to latch on to the mother's breast. Soft, silicone bulb holds the mother's expressed breast milk or a supplement. Milk comes through a tube attached to the mother's finger and is fed to the baby.
No. 1069-21, $31.00

Ameda Breast Shells

Ameda's breast shells are designed to correct inverted nipples.
No. 1435-21, $11.95

Additional Items of Interest

Lansinoh® Brand Lanolin for Breastfeeding Mothers

Created especially for nursing mothers, using a patented process that removes allergens and impurities, Lansinoh® is the world's purest lanolin. 100% natural—with no water to dilute the effectiveness or additives to cause irritation, Lansinoh® does not have to be removed prior to nursing and can be used with complete confidence of safety for mother and baby. Lansinoh® for Breastfeeding Mothers is endorsed by LLLI.
No. 428-21, 2 oz., $11.50

Over the Shoulder Baby Holder

This sling has extra padding around the baby's head and legs. Fits newborns and toddlers and can be adjusted for both men and women to wear comfortably. Comes in a variety of prints. Includes free informational video. **$39.95**

SlingEzee

Made of 100% cotton fabric, SlingEzee is well-padded over the shoulder and around baby's torso and legs for maximum comfort. Can be worn from birth through 35 pounds to accommodate baby's growth. Video included with every sling. Comes in a variety of prints. **$39.95**

Home Phototherapy Treatment

These units can be rented for use at home to treat high levels of jaundice.

BiliBed from Medela
Medela, Inc.
P.O. Box 660, McHenry, IL 60051-0660
USA
800-435-8316, 888-633-3528
Fax: 815-363-1246
www.medela.com

Wallaby Phototherapy Unit
Fiberoptic Medical Products
Suite 300 Commerce Plaza
5100 Tilghman St.
Allentown, PA 18104 USA

Organizations that offer support

American College of Nurse-Midwives
818 Connecticut Ave., NW, Suite 900, Washington DC 20006 USA
202.728.9860 www.acnm.org
Health care providers who offer a natural approach to birth.

AnotherLook
P.O. Box 383, Evanston IL 60204-0383 USA
847.869.1278 www.anotherlook.org
Dedicated to gathering information, raising critical questions, and stimulating needed research about breastfeeding in the context of HIV/AIDS.

Association of Labor Assistants & Childbirth Educators (ALACE)
P.O. Box 390436, Cambridge MA 02139 USA
617.441.2500 www.alace.org
Provides referrals to expectant parents and trains birth attendants and educators.

The Bradley Method: American Academy of Husband-Coached Childbirth
Box 5224, Sherman Oaks CA 91413-5224 USA
800.423.2397 www.bradleybirth.com
Provides childbirth education through films, classes, lectures, and workshops.

Birth Works, Inc.
P.O. Box 2045, Medford NJ 08055 USA
888.862.4784 www.birthworks.org
Offers childbirth classes, childbirth educator certification programs, and doula certification programs.

Cesareans/Support, Education, and Concern, Inc. (C/SEC)
22 Forest Rd., Framingham MA 01701 USA
508.877.8266
Provides information on many aspects of cesarean childbirth.

The Compassionate Friends, Inc.
P.O. Box 3696, Oak Brook IL 60522-3696 USA
877.969.0010 630.990.0010 www.compassionatefriends.org
Self-help support organization that offers friendship and understanding to bereaved parents, grandparents, and siblings.

The Couple-to-Couple League
P.O. Box 111184, Cincinnati OH 45211-1184 USA
513.471.2000 www.ccli.org
An interfaith organization offering couples help with the practice of natural family planning; teaches ecological breastfeeding and the full sympto-thermal method of predicting ovulation.

Depression After Delivery, Inc.
91 East Somerset Street, Raritan NJ 08869 USA
1.800.944.4773 www.depressionafterdelivery.com
Provides support for women and families coping with mental health issues associated with childbearing.

Doulas of North America (DONA)
P.O. Box 626, Jasper IN 47547 USA
888.788.3662 www.dona.org
Locate a doula (labor and/or birth support person) in your area.

Family and Home Network (Formerly "Mothers at Home")
9493-C Silver King Court, Fairfax VA 22031 USA
800.783.4666 703.352.1072 www.familyandhome.org
Supports familes who care for their own children. Publishes a monthly newsletter, "Welcome Home."

Family Voices, Inc.
3411 Candelaria NE, Suite M, Albuquerque NM 87107
505.872.4774 888.835.5669 www.familyvoices.org
A national grassroots network of families and friends speaking on behalf of children with special needs.

The InterNational Association of Parents & Professionals for Safe Alternatives in Childbirth (NAPSAC)
Rt. 4 Box 646, Marble Hill MO 63764
573.238.2010 www.napsac.org
Parents, health care providers, and childbirth educators who promote education enabling parents to assume more responsibility for pregnancy and childbirth.

International Board of Lactation Consultant Examiners (IBLCE)
7309 Arlington Blvd., Suite 300, Falls Church VA 22042-3215 USA
703.560.7330 www.iblce.org
Develops and administers the certification examination for lactation consultants.

International Cesarean Awareness Network (ICAN)
1304 Kingsdale Avenue, Redondo Beach CA 90278 USA
800.686.4226 310.542.6400 www.ican-online.org
Seeks to prevent unnecessary cesareans and to promote vaginal birth after ceserean.

International Childbirth Education Association (ICEA)
P.O. Box 20048, Minneapolis MN 55420 USA
952.854.8660 www.icea.org
A volunteer organization which brings together persons interested in family-centered maternity and infant care.

International Chiropractic Pediatric Association
5295 Highway 78, Suite D362
Stone Mountain, GA 30087-3414 USA
770.982.9037 www.4icpa.org
Provides referrals to chiropractors with expertise in treating children.

International Lactation Consultant Association (ILCA)
1500 Sunday Dr., Suite 102, Raleigh NC 27607 USA
919.861.5577 www.ilca.org
Provides referrals to board-certified lactation consultants.

Lamaze International
2025 M Street, Suite 800, Washington DC 20036-3309 USA
800.368.4404 202.367.1128 www.lamaze.org
Provides training and certification in the Lamaze method of childbirth preparation.

National Association of Childbearing Centers (NACC)
3123 Gottschall Road, Perkiomenville PA 18074 USA
215.234.8068 www.birthcenters.org
An organization that can help you find a free-standing birth center near you.

Neuro-Developmental Treatment Association
1540 South Coast Highway, Suite 203
Laguna Beach, CA 92651 USA
800.869.9295 www.ndta.org
Provides referrals to therapists who use a neuro-developmental (whole child) approach.

Pediatric/Adolescent Gastroesophageal Reflux Association (PAGER)
P.O. Box 486, Buckeystown MD 21717-0486 USA
301.601.9541 www.reflux.org
Provides information and support to parents whose children have gastroesophogeal reflux.

World Alliance for Breastfeeding Action (WABA)
P.O. Box 1200, 10850, Penang, Malaysia
60.4.6584816 www.waba.org.my
Sponsors World Breastfeeding Week (August 1-7) and other projects that promote and support breastfeeding.

Web sites that offer helpful information

These Web sites include information that may be of interest to breastfeeding mothers. Some of them may stray from the focus of breastfeeding.

Dr. Thomas Hale
neonatal.ttuhsc.edu/lact/
By the author of the well-known book Medications and Mothers' Milk.

Kathleen Kendall-Tackett, Ph.D., IBCLC
www.GraniteScientific.com
LLL Leader, psychologist, and author of some LLLI publications. Frequent speaker on the subject of postpartum depression in breastfeeding mothers.

Dr. James McKenna
www.nd.edu/~jmckenn1/lab/
Sleep researcher who has studied sleep patterns of co-sleeping mothers and babies and how those patterns differ from non-co-sleeping mothers and babies.

Dr. Jack Newman
www.breastfeedingonline.com/newman.shtml
Well-known author and speaker on healthcare practices that support breastfeeding.

Dr. William Sears
www.askdrsears.com
Well-known author of many books available through the LLLI Catalogue.

Linda Smith, IBCLC
www.bflrc.com
Well-known author and speaker on technical lactation topics.

Breastfeeding After Reduction Information and Support Site
www.bfar.org
Provides information and support to mothers and health care providers; owned by Diana West, author of LLLI's book DEFINING YOUR OWN SUCCESS: BREASTFEEDING AFTER BREAST REDUCTION.

The Craniosacral Association of North America
www.craniosacraltherapy.org
Provides referrals to crainosacral therapists.

The Marmet Technique of manual expression and assisting the milk ejection reflex (MER) has worked for thousands of mothers—in a way that nothing has before. Even experienced breastfeeding mothers who have been able to hand express will find that this method produces more milk. Mothers who have previously been able to express only a small amount, or none at all, get excellent results with this technique.

Technique Is Important

When watching manual expression the correct milking motion is difficult to see. In this case the hand is quicker than the eye. Consequently, many mothers have found manual expression difficult—even after watching a demonstration or reading a brief description. Milk can be expressed when using less effective methods of hand expression. However, when used on a frequent and regular basis, other methods can easily lead to damaged breast tissue, bruised breasts, and even skin burns.

The Marmet Technique of Manual Expression was developed by a mother who needed to express her milk over an extended period of time for medical reasons. She found that her milk ejection reflex did not work as well as when her baby breastfed, so she also developed a method of massage and stimulation to assist this reflex. The key to the success of this technique is the combination of the method of expression and this massage.

This technique is effective and should not cause problems. It can easily be learned by following this step by step guide. As with any manual skill, practice is important.

Advantages

There are many advantages to manual expression over mechanical methods of milking the breasts:
- Some mechanical pumps cause discomfort and are ineffective.
- Many mothers are more comfortable with manual expression because it is more natural.
- Skin-to-skin contact is more stimulating than the feel of a plastic shield, so manual expression usually allows for an easier milk ejection reflex.
- It's convenient.
- It's ecologically superior.
- It's portable. How can a mother forget her hands?
- Best of all it's free.

425

How the Breast Works

The milk is produced in milk-producing cells (alveoli). When the milk-producing cells are stimulated, they expel milk into the duct system (milk ejection reflex).

A small portion of the milk may flow down the ducts and collect in the milk ducts under the areola known as terminal ducts (distal portion of lactiferous ducts).

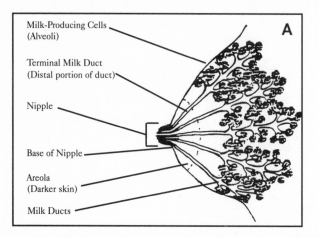

Milk-Producing Cells (Alveoli)

Terminal Milk Duct (Distal portion of duct)

Nipple

Base of Nipple

Areola (Darker skin)

Milk Ducts

A

Expressing the Milk

Draining the Terminal Milk Ducts

1. Position the thumb and first two fingers on the breast about 1" to 1 1/4" (2.5 to 3.125 cm) behind the base of the nipple.

   • Use this measurement, which is not neces-sarily the outer edge of the areola, as a guide. The areola varies in size from one woman to another.

   • Place the thumb pad above the nipple at the 12 o'clock position and the finger pads below the nipple at the 6 o'clock position forming the letter "C" with the hand, as shown. This is a resting position.

   • Note that the thumb and fingers are positioned so they are in line with the nipple.

   • Avoid cupping the breast.

2. Push straight into the chest wall.

   • Avoid spreading the fingers apart.

   • For large breasts, first lift and then push into the chest wall.

3. Roll thumb forward as if taking a thumbprint. Change finger pressure from mid-dle finger to index finger as the thumb rolls forward.

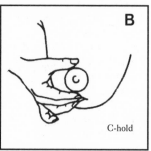

B

C-hold

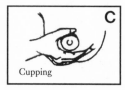

C

Cupping

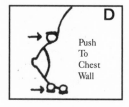

D

Push To Chest Wall

- **Finish Roll.** The rolling motion of the thumb simulates the wave-like motion of the baby's tongue and the counter pressure of the fingers simulates the baby's palate. The milking motion imitates the baby's suck by compressing and draining the terminal milk ducts without hurting sensitive breast tissue.

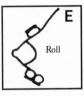

- Note the moving position of the thumbnail and fingernails in illustrations D, E, and F.

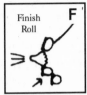

4. Repeat Rhythmically to drain the terminal milk ducts.

- Position, push, roll; position, push, roll...

5. Rotate the thumb and finger position to reach other terminal milk ducts. Use both hands on each breast. Illustration G shows hand positions on the right breast.

- Note clock positions of fingers in illustration G: 12:00 and 6:00, 11:00 and 5:00, 1:00 and 7:00, 3:00 and 9:00

Avoid These Motions
- Squeezing the breast. This can cause bruising.
- Pulling out the nipple and breast. This can cause tissue damage.
- Sliding on the breast. This can cause skin burns.

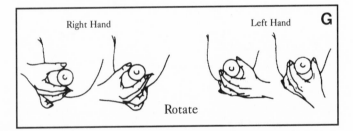

Assisting the Milk Ejection Reflex (MER)
Stimulating the flow of milk.

1. Massage the milk producing cells and ducts.

- Start at the top of the breast. Press firmly into the chest wall. Move fingers slowly, pressing firmly in a small circular motion on one spot on the skin.
- After a few seconds, pick fingers up and move to the next area on the breast. Do not slide on breast tissue.
- Spiral around the breast toward the areola using this massage.
- The pressure and motion are similar to that used in a breast examination.

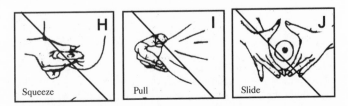

2. Stroke the breast from the chest wall to the nipple with a light tickle-like stroke.

- Continue this stroking motion from the chest wall to the nipple around the whole breast.
- This will help with relaxation and encourage the milk ejection reflex.

3. Shake the breast gently while leaning forward so that gravity will help the milk eject.

Procedure

This procedure should be followed by mothers who are expressing in place of a full feeding and those who need to establish, increase, or maintain their milk supply when the baby cannot breastfeed.

- Express each breast until the flow of milk slows down.
- Assist the milk ejection reflex (massage, stroke, shake) on both breasts. This can be done simultaneously, and only takes about a minute.
- Repeat the whole process of expressing each breast and assisting the milk ejection reflex twice more. The flow of milk usually slows down sooner the second and third time as the ducts are drained.

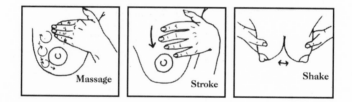

Massage   Stroke   Shake

Timing

The entire procedure should take approximately 20 to 30 minutes when manual expression is replacing a feeding.

- Express each breast 5 to 7 minutes.
- Massage, stroke, shake for about one minute.
- Express each breast 3 to 5 minutes.
- Massage, stroke, shake for about one minute.
- Express each breast 2 to 3 minutes.

Note: If the milk supply is established, use the times given only as a guide. Watch the flow of milk and change breasts when the flow gets small. If little or no milk is present yet, follow these suggested times closely. Any portion of the procedure or timing may be used or repeated as necessary.

Page 6   **Overall benefits of breastfeeding.**
American Academy of Pediatrics Work Group on Breastfeeding. "Breastfeeding and the use of human milk." *Pediatrics* 1997; 100(6):1035-37.

Heinig, M. J. and Dewey, K. G. "Health advantages of breastfeeding for infants: a critical review." *Nutr Res Rev* 1996; 9:89-110.

Cunningham, A. S., Jelliffe, D. B., and Jelliffe, E. F. P. "Breastfeeding and health in the 1980s: a global epidemiological review." *J Pediatr* 1991; 118(5):659-66.

Breastfeeding soon after birth causes uterus to contract.
Chua, S. et al. "Influence of breastfeeding and nipple stimulation on postpartum uterine activity." *Br J Ob Gyn* 1994; 101:804-05.

Breastfeeding promotes jaw and facial development.
Labbok, M. H. and Hendershot, G. E. "Does breastfeeding protect against malocclusion?" *Am J Prev Med* 1987; 3:227-32.

Protection from obesity.
Dewey, K. G. "Is breastfeeding protective against child obesity?" *J Hum Lact* 2003; 19(1):9-18.

Protection from allergies.
Oddy, W. H. et al. "Maternal asthma, infant feeding, and the risk of asthma in childhood." *J Allergy Clin Immunol* 2002; 110:65-67.

Saarinen, U. M. et al. "Breastfeeding as prophylaxis against atopic disease: prospective follow-up study until 17 years old." *Lancet* 1995; 346(8982):1065-69.

Wright, A. L. et al. "Relationship of infant feeding to recurrent wheezing at age 6 years." *Arch Ped Adolesc Med* 1995; 149:758-63.

Human milk protects infants from infection.
Goldman, A.S. "Modulation of the gastrointestinal tract of infants by human milk. Interfaces and interactions: An evolutionary perspective." *J Nutr* 2000; 130:426S-431S.

Goldman, A. S. et al. "Anti-inflammatory properties of human milk." *Acta Paediatr Scand* 1986; 75:689-95.

Dewey, K. G. et al. "Differences in morbidity between breastfed and formula-fed infants." *J Pediatr* 1995; 126(5) pt 1:696-702.

Enhanced development of baby's brain and nervous system.
Xiang, M. et al. "Long-chain polyunsaturated fatty acids in human milk and brain growth during early infancy." *Acta Pediatr* 2000; 89(2):142-47.

Anderson, J. W. et al. "Breastfeeding and cognitive development: a meta-analysis." *Am J Clin Nutr* 1999; 70:525-35.

Higher IQs are associated with components in human milk.
Lucas, A. et al. "Breast milk and subsequent intelligence quotient in children born preterm." *Lancet* 1992; 33:261-62.

Mortensen, E. L. et al. "The association between duration of breastfeeding and adult intelligence." *JAMA* 2002; 28(15): 2365-71.

Page 7   Breastfeeding delays menstruation and ovulation.
Lewis, P. et al. "The resumption of ovulation and menstruation in a well-nourished population of women breastfeeding for an extended period of time." *Fertil Steril* 1991; 55(3):529-36.

Breastfeeding mothers lose weight gradually without restricting calories.
Dewey, K. et al. "Maternal weight-loss patterns during prolonged lactation." *Am J Clin Nutr* 1993; 58:162-68.

Breastfeeding protects a mother from breast cancer.
Enger, S. M. et al. "Breastfeeding experience and breast cancer risk among post-menopausal women." *Cancer Epidemiol Biomarkers Prev* 1998; 7: 365-69.

Breastfeeding protects a mother from ovarian cancer, urinary tract infections, and osteoporosis.
Gwinn, M. L. et al. "Pregnancy, breastfeeding, and oral contraceptives and the risk of epithelial ovarian cancer." *J Clin Epidemiol* 1990; 43(6):559-68.

Coppa, G. V. et al. "Preliminary study of breastfeeding and bacterial adhesion to uroepithelial cells." *Lancet* 1990; 335:569-71.

Polatti, F. et al. "Bone mineral changes during and after lactation." *Obstet Gynecol* 1999; 94(1):52-56.

Page 13   Breastfeeding improves a mother's responsiveness to her baby.
Sears, W. BECOMING A FATHER. Schaumburg IL: La Leche League International, 2003.

Lavelli, M. and Poli, M. "Early mother-infant interaction during breast and bottle feeding." *Inf Behav Dev* 1998; 21(4): 667-84

Page 18   Feelings of self-esteem related to childbirth experience.
Korte, D. and Scaer, R. *A Good Birth, A Safe Birth,* 3rd ed. Boston: Harvard Common Press, 1992.

Page 20   Effects of medication used in labor and birth.
Rasjo-Arvidson, A. et al. "Maternal analgesia during labor disturbs newborn behavior: effects on breastfeeding, temperature, and crying." *Birth* 2001; 28(1):5-12.

Crowell, M. K. et al. "Relationship between obstetric analgesia and time of effective breastfeeding." *J Nurse Midwif* 1995; 39(3):150-56.

Sepkowski, C. et al. "The effects of maternal epidural anesthesia on neonatal behavior during the first month." *Dev Med Child Neurol* 1992; 34:1072-80.

Page 21   **Nursing soon after birth encourages milk to come in.**
Yamauchi, Y. and Yamanouchi, H. "Breastfeeding frequency during the first 24 hours after birth in full-term neonates." *Pediatrics* 1990; 86:171-75.

Separation of mother and baby may cause breastfeeding problems.
Righard, L. and Alade, M. "Effects of delivery room routines on success of first breast-feed." *Lancet* 1990; 336:1105-07.

Page 22   **Incidence of prematurity, respiratory distress, and other complications are higher with cesarean birth.**
Korte, D. and Scaer, R. *A Good Birth, A Safe Birth,* 3rd ed. Boston: Harvard Common Press, 1992.

Page 23   **Vaginal birth following a previous cesarean.**
Korte, D. *The VBAC Companion: The Expectant Mother's Guide to Vaginal Birth after Cesarean.* Boston: Harvard Common Press, 1997.

Page 24   **Choosing a health care professional.**
Wright, A. L. and Schanler, R. J. "The resurgence of breastfeeding at the end of the second millennium." *J Nutr* 2001-02; 13192): 421S-425S.

Freed, G. L. et al. "National assessment of physicians' breastfeeding knowledge, attitudes, training, and experience." *JAMA* 1995; 273(6):472-76

Page 26   **Effect of positioning on sore nipples.**
Frantz, K. "Baby's position at the breast and its relationship to sucking problems." LLLI Conference, 1983, 1985.

Page 27   **Montgomery glands cleanse and lubricate nipples.**
Williams, J. "Anatomy and physiology of breastfeeding." ILCA Conference, July 1992.

Page 29   **Treatment for inverted nipples.**
Main Trial Collaborative Group. "Preparing for breastfeeding: treatment of inverted and non-protactile nipples during pregnancy." *Midwifery* 1994; 10:200-14.

Page 36   **Effectiveness of mother-to-mother support.**
Grieve, V. and Howarth, T. "The counseling needs of women." *Breastfeeding Review* 2000; 8(2):9-15.

WABA. *Mother-to-Mother Support for Breastfeeding.* 1993.

Page 37   **Breastfeeding mothers need information and support.**
Lawrence, R. and Lawrence, R. *Breastfeeding: a Guide for the Medical Profession,* 5th ed. St Louis: Mosby, 1999.

Lawrence, R. A. "The management of lactation as a physiologic process." *Clin Perinatology* 1997; 14(1):1-10.

Page 45   **A newborn's capabilities.**
Klaus, M. and Klaus, P. *Your Amazing Newborn.* Cambridge, MA: Perseus Books, 1998.

Page 54   **The let-down or milk-ejection reflex.**
Newton, M. and Newton, N. "The let-down reflex in human lactation." *Pediatrics* 1948; 33:69-87.

Kent, J. "Physiology of the expression of breast milk, part 2." Presented at Medela Breast Pump Research Conference, Boca Raton FL, 2002.

Page 55   **Frequent nursing reduces engorgement.**
Moon, J. and Humenick, S. "Breast engorgement contribution variables and variables amenable to nursing intervention." *JOGNN* 1989; 18:309-15.

Hill, P. and Humenick, S. "The occurrence of breast engorgement." *J Hum Lact* 1994; 10:79-86.

Page 55   **Use of cabbage leaves to treat engorgement.**
Nikodem, V. et al. "Do cabbage leaves prevent breast engorgement? A randomized, controlled study." *Birth* 1993; 20:61-64.

Page 57   **Frequent, unrestricted breastfeeding does not cause sore nipples.**
de Carvalho, M. et al. "Does the duration and frequency of early breastfeeding affect nipple pain?" *Birth* 1984; 11:81-84.

Mohrbacher, N and Stock, J. THE BREASTFEEDING ANSWER BOOK, 3rd edition. Schaumburg, IL: La Leche League International, 2003.

Allow baby to decide when to end the feeding.
Woolridge, M. and Fisher, C. "Colic, 'overfeeding,' and symptoms of lactose malabsorption in the breastfed baby: a possible artifact of feed management?" *Lancet* 1988; 2(8605):382-84.

Using both breasts at each feeding.
Woolridge, M. et al. "Do changes in pattern of breast usage alter the baby's nutrient intake?" *Lancet* 1990; 336:395-97.

Page 61   **Breastfeed often and avoid artificial nipples.**
Nylander, G. et al. "Unsupplemented breastfeeding in the maternity ward." *Acta Obst Gyn Scand* 1991; 70:205-09.

Righard, L. "Are breastfeeding problems related to incorrect breastfeeding techniques and the use of pacifiers and bottles?" *Birth* 1998; 25(1): 40-44.

Page 64   **Use of silicone nipple shields.**
Wilson-Clay, B. "Clinical use of silicone nipple shields." *J Hum Lact* 1996; 12(4):279-85.

Page 65   **Avoid hospital gift packs that include formula samples.**
Snell, B.T. et al. "The association of formula samples given at hospital discharge with the early duration of breastfeeding." *J Hum Lact* 1991; 8:67-72.

Page 70   **New Guinea infants nurse frequently.**
Jelliffe, D. B. *Infant Nutrition in the Subtropics.* Geneva: World Health Organization, 1968.

Page 71   **No need to count feedings.**
Francis, B. "Successful lactation and a woman's sexuality." *J Trop Pediatr Env Health*1976; 22:4.

Page 72   **Pacifier use may lead to early weaning.**
Barros, F. C. et al. "Use of pacifiers is associated with decreased breastfeeding duration." *Pediatrics* 1995; 95(4): 497-99.

Howard, C. et al. "The effects of early pacifier use on breastfeeding duration." *Pediatrics* 1999; 103(3):e33(1-6).

Page 73   **Normal weight gain for a breastfed baby.**
Dewey, K. et al. "Growth of breastfed and formula-fed infants from 0 to 18 months. The DARLING study." *Pediatrics* 1992; 89(6):1035-41.

Page 78   Carrying baby reduces crying.
           Hunziker, U. and Barr, R. "Increased carrying reduces infant crying: a randomized
           controlled trial." *Pediatrics* 1986; 77-641.

Page 88   Even one bottle of formula can cause allergy.
           Host, A. et al. "A prospective study of cow's milk allergy in exclusively breastfed
           infants." *Acta Paediatr Scand* 1988; 77:663-70.

Page 92,   Effects of separation.
95   Sears, W. THE FUSSY BABY, Rev Edition. Schaumburg IL: La Leche League
           International, 2002.

Page 96   Mother's diet may cause colic.
           Clyne P. and Kluczycki, A. "Human breast milk contains bovine IgG.
           Relationship to infant colic?" *Pediatrics* 1991; 87(4):439-44.

Page 97   Chiropractic treatment for colic.
           Wiberg, J. et al. "Compared with Dimethicone, 2 weeks of spinal manipulation
           reduced infant colic behaviour at 4-11 days after initial treatment." *J Manip
           Physiol Ther* 1999; 22: 517-22.

Page 99   Nighttime needs.
           Sears, W. NIGHTTIME PARENTING, Rev Edition. Schaumburg IL: La Leche
           League International, 2000.

Page 99   Babies receive 25 percent of milk at night.
           Jelliffe, D. B. and Jelliffe, E.F.P. *Human Milk in the Modern World*, Oxford
           University Press, 1978.

Page 100   Sharing sleep decreases SIDS risk.
           Sears, W. *SIDS: A Parents' Guide to Understanding and Preventing Sudden Infant Death
           Syndrome.* Boston: Little, Brown and Company, 1995.

Page 110   Proper positioning prevents sore nipples.
           Mohrbacher, N and Stock, J. THE BREASTFEEDING ANSWER BOOK, 3rd edition.
           Schaumburg, IL: La Leche League International, 2003.

           Wilson-Clay, B. and Hoover, K. *The Breastfeeding Atlas*, 2nd edition. Austin, TX:
           LactNews Press, 2002.

Page 112   Moist wound healing is effective in treating sore nipples.
           Huml, S. "Cracked nipples in the breastfeeding mother." *Advance for Nurse
           Practitioners* 1995; 29-31.

Page 115   Treatment for thrush.
           Amir, L. et al. *Candidiasis and Breastfeeding.* Lactation Consultant Series II.
           Schaumburg, IL: La Leche League International, 2002.

Page 119   Selecting a breast pump.
           Frantz, K. *Breastfeeding Product Guide 1994.* Sunland, CA: Geddes Productions,
           1993.

           Mohrbacher, N and Stock, J. THE BREASTFEEDING ANSWER BOOK, 3rd edition.
           Schaumburg, IL: La Leche League International, 2003.

Page 122   Storage guidelines for human milk.
           Barger, J. and Bull, P. "A comparison of the bacterial composition of breast milk
           stored at room temperature and stored in the refrigerator." *IJCE* 1987; 2:29-30.

           Pardou, A. "Human milk banking: influence of storage processes and of bacterial
           contamination on some milk constituents." *Biol Neonate* 1994; 65:302-09.

Arnold, L. "Storage containers for human milk: an issue revisited." *J Hum Lact* 1995; 11(4):325-28.

Previously frozen milk can be kept refrigerated for 24 hours.
Arnold, L. *Recommendations for Collection, Storage, and Handling of a Mother's Milk for Her Own Infant in the Hospital Setting,* 3rd edition. Sandwich, MA, 1999.

Page 123 **Treatment of plugged ducts and mastitis.**
Lawrence, R. and Lawrence, R. *Breastfeeding: A Guide for the Medical Profession,* 5th ed. St Louis: Mosby, 1999.

Page 130 **No danger of breastfeeding with breast implants.**
Berlin, C. "Silicone breast implants and breastfeeding." *Pediatrics* 1994; 94(4):547-49.

FDA. "Breast implants: an information update." Rockville, MD: *US FDA,* March 1996.

Page 131 **Breastfeeding after breast surgery.**
West, D. DEFINING YOUR OWN SUCCESS: BREASTFEEDING AFTER BREAST REDUCTION SURGERY. Schaumburg, IL: La Leche League International, 2001.

Page 133 **Normal growth of breastfed babies.**
Dewey, K. et al. "Growth of breastfed babies deviates from a pooled analysis of US, Canadian, and European data sets." *Pediatrics* 1995; 96(3):495-503.

Page 142 **Breastfeeding protects against later obesity.**
Kramer, M. "Do breastfeeding and delayed introduction of solid foods protect against subsequent obesity?" *J Pediatr* 1981; 98:883-87.

Gillman, M. W. et al. "Risk of overweight among adolescents who were breastfed as infants." *JAMA* 2001; 285:2461-67.

Page 150 **How employed mothers feel about their breastfeeding experiences.**
Auerbach, K. and Guss, E. "Maternal employment and breastfeeding: a study of 567 women's experiences." *Am J Dis Child* 1984; 138:958-60.

Page 152 **Women who returned to work before their babies were two months old had more breastfeeding problems.**
Kearney, M. and Cronenwett, L. "Breastfeeding and employment." *JOGNN* 1991; 20(6):471-80.

Page 153 **Giving bottles too soon can cause nipple confusion.**
Neifert, M. et al. "Nipple confusion: toward a formal definition." *J Pediatr* 1995; 126(6):S125-S129.

Take full advantage of maternity leave.
Sears, W. and Sears, M. *The Baby Book,* revised ed. Boston: Little, Brown and Company, 2003.

Page 154 **Breastfeeding provides benefits to employers.**
Cohen, R. et al. "Comparison of maternal absenteeism and infant illness rates among breastfeeding and formula-feeding women in two corporations." *Am J Health Promo* 1995; 10(2):148-53

Storage guidelines for human milk.
Barger, J. and Bull, P. "A comparison of the bacterial composition of breast milk stored at room temperature and stored in the refrigerator." *IJCE* 1987; 2:29-30.

Pardou, A. "Human milk banking: influence of storage processes and of bacterial contamination on some milk constituents." *Biol Neonate* 1994; 65:302-09.

Arnold, L. "Storage containers for human milk: an issue revisited." *J Hum Lact* 1995; 11(4):325-28.

Page 158   **Previously frozen milk can be kept refrigerated for 24 hours.**
Arnold, L. *Recommendations for Collection, Storage, and Handling of a Mother's Milk for Her Own Infant in the Hospital Setting.* 3rd edition. Sandwich, MA, 1999.

Studies show human milk retards the growth of bacteria.
Pardou, A. "Human milk banking: influence of storage process and of bacterial contamination on some milk constituents." *Biol Neonate* 1994; 65:302-09.

Page 164   **Human milk provides protection for children in day care.**
Jones, E. et al. "Relationship between infant feeding and exclusion rate from child care because of illness." *J Am Diet Assoc* 1993; 93(7):809-11.

Page 169   **Baby's need for unchanging caregivers.**
Brazelton, T. B. and Greenspan, S. I. *The Irreducible Needs of Children: What Every Child Must Have to Grow, Learn, and Flourish.* Cambridge, MA: Perseus Publishing, 2000.

Pages 184   **Fathers get involved.**
Sears, W. Becoming a Father, Rev Ed. Schaumburg IL: La Leche League International, 2003.

Page 192   **Rewards of parenting.**
Stewart, D. *Fathering and Career: Keeping a Healthy Balance.* Marble Hill, MO: NAP-SAC, Int'l, 1987.

Page 216   **Nursing mothers' need for liquids.**
Dusdieker, L. et al. "Effect of supplemental fluids on human milk production." *J Pediatr* 1985; 106(2):207-11.

Page 217   **Sources of calcium for nursing mothers.**
Behan, E. *Eat Well, Lose Weight while Breastfeeding.* New York: Villard Books, 1994.

Page 218   **Effects of caffeine on breastfed babies.**
Berlin, C. and Daniel C. "Excretion of theobromine in human milk and saliva." *Pediatr Res* 1981; 15:492.

Nehlig, A. and Debry, G. "Consequences on the newborn of chronic maternal consumption of coffee during gestation and lactation: a review." *J Am Coll Nutr* 1994; 13(1):6-21.

Page 219   **Mothers on vegan diets may need to supplement.**
Kuhne, T. et al. "Maternal vegan diet causing a serious infantile neurological disorder due to Vitamin B12 deficiency." *Eur J Pediatr* 1991; 150:205-08.

Breastfeeding mothers tend to lose weight without restricting calories.
Dewey, K. et al. "Maternal weight-loss patterns during prolonged lactation." *Am J Clin Nutr* 1993; 58:162-66.

Heinig, M. et al. "Lactation and postpartum weight loss." *Mechanisms Regulating Lactation and Infant Nutrient Utilization* 1992; 30: 397-400.

Studies show that breastfeeding mothers can safely exercise.
Dewey, K. and McCrory, M. "Effects of dieting and physical activity on pregnancy and lactation." *Am J Clin Nutr* 1994; 59(Suppl):446S-59S.

Dewey, K. et al. "A randomized study of the effects of aerobic exercise by lactating women on breast milk volume and composition." *N Engl J Med* 1994; 330(7):449-53.

Exercise may increase a mother's milk supply.
Lovelady, C. et al. "Lactation performance of exercising women." *Am J Clin Nutr* 1990; 52:103-09.

Page 223   **Pediatricians recommend only human milk for 6 months.**
American Academy of Pediatrics Workgroup on Breastfeeding. "Breastfeeding and the use of human milk." *Pediatrics* 1997; 100(6): 1035-37.

Page 224   **Solid foods displace human milk in a baby's diet.**
Cohen, R. et al. "Effects of age of introduction of complementary foods on infant breast milk intake, total energy intake, and growth: a randomized intervention in Honduras." *Lancet* 1994; 344:288-93.

Starting solid foods early reduces protective antibodies for babies.
Duncan, B. et al. "Exclusive breastfeeding for at least 4 months protects against otitis media." *Pediatrics* 1993; 91(5):867-72.

Human milk protects against allergic reactions to other foods.
Taylor, B. et al. "Transient IgA deficiency and pathogenesis of infantile atopy." *Lancet* 1973; ii:111-13.

Vitamin supplements for breastfed babies.
American Academy of Pediatrics. "Fluoride supplementation for children: interim policy recommendations." *Pediatrics* 1995; 95:777.

Greer, F. R. and Marshall, S. "Bone mineral content, serum, vitamin D metabolic concentrations, and ultraviolet B light exposure in infants fed human milk with and without vitamin D2 supplements." *J Pediatr* 1989; 114(2):204-12.

Sunshine and vitamin D supplements.
American Academy of Pediatrics. "Prevention of rickets and vitamin D deficiency: new guidelines for vitamin D intake." *Pediatrics* 2003; 111(4):908-10.

Page 225   **Allow baby to decide which foods and how much he wants.**
Birch, L. et al. "The variability of young children's energy intake." *NEng J Med* 1991; 324(4):232-35.

Page 234   **Breastfeeding continues to offer immunity.**
Prentice, A. "Breastfeeding and the older infant." *Acta Paediatr Scand* 1991; 374: 78-88.

Goldman, A. "Immunologic components in human milk during the second year of lactation." *Acta Paediatr Scand* 1983; 72:461-62.

Van den Bogaard, C. et al. "The relationship between breastfeeding and early childhood morbidity in a general population." *Family Medicine* 1991; 23:510-15.

Page 241   **Weaning ages in other cultures.**
Mead, M. and Newton, N. "Cultural patterns of perinatal behavior," in *Childbearing: Its Social and Psychological Aspects*, ed. S. Richardson and Guttmacher, A. Baltimore MD: Williams and Wilkins Company, 1967.

Dettwyler, K. "A time to wean." Breastfeeding Abstracts 1994; 14:3-4.

Page 242   **Mothers report fewer illnesses when toddlers are still nursing.**
Gulick, E. "The effects of breastfeeding on toddler health." *Pediatric Nurs* 1986; 12:51-54.

Page 246   **Dental caries in breastfed children.**
Sinton, J. et al. "A systematic overview of the relationship between infant feeding caries and breast-feeding." *Ont Dent* 1998; 75(9): 23-27.

Oulis, C. et al. "Feeding practices of Greek children with and without nursing caries." *Pediatr Dent* 1999; 21(7): 409-16.

Roberts, G. et al. "Patterns of breast and bottle feeding and their association with dental caries in 1 to 4 year old South African children." *Comm Dent Hlth* 1993; 10:405-13.

Wendt, L. K. et al. "Analysis of caries-related factors in infants and toddlers living in Sweden." *Acta Odont Scand* 1996; 54(2):131-37.

Human milk may prevent cavities.
Erickson, P. R. and Mazhari, E. "Investigation of the role of human breast milk in caries development." *Pediatr Dent* 1999; 21(2): 86-90.

Erickson, P. et al. "Estimation of the caries related risk associated with infant formulas." *Pediatr Dent* 1998; 20(7): 385-403.

Rugg-Gunn. A. et al. "Effect of human milk on plaque pH in situ and enamel dissolution in vitro compared with bovine milk, lactose and sucrose." *Caries Res* 1985; 19(4): 327-34.

Page 250 Continuing to nurse when mother is pregnant.
Flower, H. ADVENTURES IN TANDEM NURSING: BREASTFEEDING DURING PREGNANCY AND BEYOND. Schaumburg, Il: La Leche League International, 2003.

Moscone, S. and Moore, J. "Breastfeeding during pregnancy." *J Hum Lact* 1993; 9(2):83-88.

Newton, N. and Theotokatos, M. "Breastfeeding during pregnancy in 503 women: does a psychobiological weaning mechanism exist in humans?" *Emotion and Reproduction* 1979; 20B:845-49.

Page 251 Nursing a toddler along with the new baby.
Gromada, K. "Breastfeeding more than one: multiples and tandem breastfeeding." *NAACOG* 1992; 3(4):656-66.

Page 253 Decisions about tandem nursing.
Flower, H. ADVENTURES IN TANDEM NURSING: BREASTFEEDING DURING PREGNANCY AND BEYOND. Schaumburg, Il: La Leche League International, 2003.

Page 257 Discipline and punishment.
Sears, W. and Sears, M. *The Discipline Book.* Boston: Little, Brown, and Company, 1995.

Page 259 What does spanking teach?
Brazelton, T. B. and Greenspan, S. I. *The Irreducible Needs of Children: What Every Child Must Have to Grow, Learn, and Flourish.* Cambridge, MA: Perseus Publishing, 2000.

LeShan, E. *When Your Child Drives You Crazy.* New York: St. Martin's Press, 1985.

Page 260 The need for self-esteem.
Samalin, N. *Loving Your Child Is Not Enough.* New York: Penguin Books, 1987.

Page 263 Influence of television on children's behavior.
American Academy of Pediatrics Committee on Communications. "Children, adolescents, and television." *Pediatrics* 1995; 96(4):786-87.

Sears, W. and Sears, M. *The Successful Child.* Boston: Little, Brown and Company, 2002.

Page 272 **Effects of anesthetics used for cesarean birth.**
Spigset, O. "Anaesthetic agents and excretion in breast milk." *Acta Anaesthesiol Scand* 1994; 38:94-103.

Righard, L. and Alade, M. "Effects of delivery room routines on success of first breast-feed." *Lancet* 1999; 336:1105-07.

Sepkowski, C. et al. "The effects of maternal epidural anesthesia on neonatal behavior during the first month." *Dev Med Child Neurol* 1992; 34:1072-80.

Effects of cesarean birth on breastfeeding.
Kearney, M. et al. "Cesarean delivery and breastfeeding outcomes." *Birth* 1990; 17(2):97-103.

Page 275 **Full-term babies who are jaundiced suffer no long term adverse effects.**
Newman, T. and Maisels, M. "Evaluation and treatment of jaundice in the term newborn: a kinder, gentler approach." *Pediatrics* 1992; 89(5):809-18.

Frequent breastfeeding keeps bilirubin levels within the normal range.
Gartner, L. and Herschel, M. "Jaundice and breastfeeding." *Ped Clinics in N Amer* 2001; 48(2):389-99.

Page 277 **Higher bilirubin levels may be beneficial.**
Hegyi, T. et al. "The protective role of bilirubin in oxygen-radical diseases of the preterm infant." *J Perinatol* 1994; 14(4):296-300.

Page 278 **Breastfeeding duration is affected by treatment for jaundice.**
Kemper, K. "Neonatal jaundice in the development of the vulnerable child syndrome." BREASTFEEDING ABSTRACTS 1990; 10:7.

American Academy of Pediatrics (AAP) Subcommittee on Neonatal Hyberbilirubinemia. "Neonatal jaundice and kernicterus." *Pediatrics* 2001; 108(3):763-65.

Using phototherapy to lower bilirubin levels while continuing to breast-feed.
Martinez, J. et al. "Hyperbilirubinemia in the breastfed newborn: a controlled trial of four interventions." *Pediatrics* 1993; 91(2):470-73.

Page 279 **Water supplements do not reduce jaundice.**
Gartner, L. and Lee, K. "Jaundice in the breastfed infant." *Clin Perinatol* 1999; 26(2);431-35.

Kuhr, M. and Paneth, N. "Feeding practices and early neonatal jaundice." *J Pediatr Gastroenterol Nutr* 1982; 1:485-88.

Nicoll, A. et al. "Supplementary feeding and jaundice in newborns." *Acta Paediatr Scand* 1982; 71:759-61.

Page 280 **Early and frequent breastfeeding stabilizes blood glucose levels.**
Eidelman, A. "Part 2: The management of breastfeeding: hypoglycemia and the breastfed neonate." *Pediatr Clin N Am* 2001; 48(2):1-10.

Hawdon, J. et al. "Prevention and treatment of neonatal hypoglycemia." *Arch Dis Child* 1994; 70:F60-F65.

Wang, Y. S. et al. "Preliminary study on the blood glucose level in the exclusively breastfed newborn." *J Trop Pediatr* 1994; 40:187-88.

Page 281   **Human milk is more easily digested by preterm infants.**
Schanler, R. et al. "Feeding strategies for premature infants: randomized trial of gastrointestinal priming and tube-feeding method." *Pediatrics* 1999; 103(2):434-39.

Schanler, R. et al. "Feeding strategies for premature infants: beneficial outcomes of feeding fortified human milk versus preterm formula." *Pediatrics* 1999; 103(6):1150-57.

Schanler, R. and Hurst, N. "Human milk for the hospitalized preterm infant." *Sem Perinatol* 1994; 18(6):476-84.

Improved IQ scores for preterm infants fed human milk.
Lucas, A. et al. "Breast milk and subsequent intelligence quotient in children born preterm." *Lancet* 1992; 339:261-64.

Golding, J. et al. "Association between breastfeeding, child development, and behaviour." *Early Human Dev* 1997; 49 Suppl:S175-84.

Fewer infections in preterm infants fed human milk.
Caplan, M. et al. "Necrotizing enterocolitis: a review of pathogenic mechanisms and implications for prevention." *Pediatric Pathology* 1993; 13:357-69.

Hylander, M. et al. "Human milk feedings and infection among very low birth weight infants." *Pediatrics* 1998; 102(3):1-6.

Differences in milk of mothers who deliver prematurely.
Luukkainen, P. et al. "Changes in fatty acid composition of preterm and term human milk from 1 week to 6 months of lactation." *J Pediatr Gastroenterol Nutr* 1994; 18:355-60.

Lemons, J. et al. "Differences in the composition of preterm and term human milk during early lactation." *Pediatr Res* 1982; 16:113-16.

Page 282   **Supplements or fortifiers may be added to human milk for preterm infants.**
Robertson, A. and Bhatia, J. "Feeding premature infants." *Clin Pediatr* 1993; n:36-44.

Valentine, C. et al. "Hindmilk improves weight gain in low birthweight infants fed human milk." *J Ped Gastro Nutr* 1994; 18:474-77.

Page 284   **The effects of kangaroo care on infant physiology.**
Acolet, D. et al. "Oxygenation, heart rate, and temperature in very low birth-weight infants during skin-to-skin contact with their mothers." *Acta Paediatr Scand* 1989; 78:189-93.

Anderson, G. "Kangaroo care and breastfeeding for preterm infants." BREASTFEEDING ABSTRACTS 1989; 9:7-8.

Ludington-Hoe, S. with Golant, S. *Kangaroo Care: The Best You Can Do to Help Your Preterm Infant.* New York: Bantam Books, 1993.

Mothers are more confident after kangaroo care.
Affonso, D. et al. "Reconciliation and healing for mothers through skin-to-skin contact provided in an American tertiary level intensive care nursery." *Neonat Network* 1993; 7(6):43-51.

Mothers produce more milk after kangaroo care.
Hurst, N. et al. "Skin-to-skin holding in the neonatal intensive care unit influences maternal milk volume." *J Perinatol* 1997; 17(3):213-17.

Page 285   Cup feedings used for premature babies.
Dowling, D. et al. "Cup-feeding for preterm infants: mechanics and safety." *J Hum Lact* 2002; 18(1):13-20.

Lang, S. et al. "Cup feeding: an alternative method of infant feeding." *Arch Dis Child* 1994; 71:365-69.

Marinelli, K. et al. "A comparison of the safety of cup feedings and bottle feedings in premature infants whose mothers intend to breastfeed." *J Perinatol* 2001; 21(5):350-55.

Breastfeeding less stressful for preterm infants than bottle-feeding.
Meier, P. "Bottle and breastfeeding: effects on transcutaneous oxygen pressure and temperature in small preterm infants." *Nurs Res* 1988; 37:36-41.

Page 286   A nipple shield makes latch-on easier for some preterm infants.
Meier, P. "Nipple shields for preterm infants: effect on milk transfer and duration of breastfeeding." *J Hum Lact* 2000; 16(2):106-14.

Page 287   Use of an electronic scale to monitor baby's intake.
Meier, P. et al. "The accuracy of test-weighing for preterm infants." *J Ped Gastro Nutr* 1990; 5:50-52.

Page 288   Breastfeeding a baby with Down Syndrome.
Aumonier, M. and Cunningham, C. "Breastfeeding in infants with Down's Syndrome." *Child Care Health Development* 1983; 9:247-55.

Mizuno, K. and Ueda, A. "Development of sucking behavior in infants with Down's Syndrome." *Acta Paediatr* 2001; 90:1384-88.

Page 289   Surgery for cleft lip or palate.
American Society of Anesthesiologists (ASA). "Practice guidelines for preoperative fasting and the use of pharmacologic agents to reduce the risk of pulmonary aspiration: application to healthy patients undergoing elective procedures." *Anesthesiology* 1999; 90(3):896-905.

Cohen, M. et al. "Immediate unrestricted feeding of infants following cleft lip and palate repair." *J Craniofac Surg* 1992; 3(1):30-32.

Weatherly-White, R. et al. "Early repair and breastfeeding for infants with cleft lip." *Plas Reconstruc Surg* 1987; 79:886-87.

Page 290   Babies with cleft palate may feed more effectively with a palatal obturator.
Turner, L. et al. "The effects of lactation education and a prosthetic obturator appliance on feeding efficiency in infants with cleft lip and palate." *Cleft Palate-Craniofac J* 2001; 38(5):519-24.

Immunological benefits of breastfeeding for a baby with a cleft palate.
Paradise, J. et al. "Evidence in infants with cleft palate that breast milk protects against otitis media." *Pediatrics* 1994; 94(6):853-60.

Symptoms of cystic fibrosis may be delayed if infant is breastfed.
Holliday, K. et al. "Growth of human milk-fed and formula-fed infants with cystic fibrosis." *J Pediatr* 1991; 118:77-79.

Page 291   Infants with PKU can be partially breastfed.
Greve, L. et al. "Breastfeeding in the management of the newborn with phenylketonuria: a practical approach to dietary therapy." *J Am Diet Assoc* 1994; 94:305-09.

Babies who had been breastfed prior to PKU testing scored higher on IQ tests at school age.
Riva, E. et al. "Early breastfeeding is linked to higher intelligence quotient scores in dietary treated phenylketonuric children." *Acta Paediatr* 1996; 85:56-58.

Page 295 **Breastfeeding is less stressful than bottle-feeding for a sick baby.**
Marino, B. et al. "Oxygen saturations during breast and bottle feedings in infants with congenital heart disease." *J Pediatr News* 1995; 10(6):360-64.

Page 296 **Breastfeeding more than one baby.**
Gromada, K. K. MOTHERING MULTIPLES: BREASTFEEDING AND CARING FOR TWINS OR MORE!!! Schaumburg, IL: La Leche League International, 1999.

Page 301 **Breastfeeding triplets or quadruplets.**
Mead, L. et al. "Breastfeeding success with preterm quadruplets." *JOGNN* 1992; 21(3):221-27.

Duggin, J. "Breastfeeding triplets—it can be done!" *Breastfeed Rev* 1994; II(10):469-70.

Page 302 **Relactation.**
Auerbach, K. and Avery, J. "Relactation: a study of 366 cases." *Pediatrics* 1980; 65:236-48.

Phillips, V. "Relactation in mothers of children over 12 months." *J Trop Pediatr* 1993; 39:45-48.

Page 305 **Herbs and medications may be used to stimulate lactation.**
DaSilva, O. et al. "Effect of domperidone on milk production in mothers of premature newborns: a randomized, double-blind, placebo-controlled trial." *Can Med Assoc J* 2001; 164(1):17-21.

Ehrenkranz, R. and Ackerman, B. "Metoclopramide effect on faltering milk production by mothers of premature infants." *Pediatrics* 1986; 78(4):614-20.

West, D. DEFINING YOUR OWN SUCCESS: BREASTFEEDING AFTER BREAST REDUCTION SURGERY. Schaumburg, IL: La Leche League International, 2001.

Page 307 **Continuing to breastfeed if baby has diarrhea.**
Vonlanthen, M. "Management of diarrhea: to continue to breastfeed or not?" BREASTFEEDING ABSTRACTS 1995; 14:26-27.

No need to avoid breastfeeding when baby has diarrhea or is vomiting.
Brown, K. and Lake, A. "Appropriate use of human and non-human milk for the dietary management of children with diarrhoea." *J Diarrhoeal Dis Res* 1991; 9(3):168-85.

Page 308 **If baby can take anything by mouth it should be his mother's milk.**
Ruuska, T. "Occurrence of acute diarrhea in atopic and nonatopic infants: the role of prolonged breastfeeding." *J Pediatr Gastroenterol Nutr* 1992; 14L27-33.

Page 310 **Secondary lactose intolerance.**
Sears, W. SAFE AND HEALTHY. Schaumburg, IL: La Leche League International, 1989.

Breastfed babies have fewer episodes of reflux.
Heacock, H. et al. "Influence of breast versus formula milk on physiological gastroesophageal reflux in healthy, newborn infants." *J Pediatr Gastroenterol Nutr* 1992; 121:913-15.

Newman, J. and Pitman, T. *The Ultimate Breastfeeding Book of Answers.* Roseville, California: Prima Publishing, 2000.

Page 311   **Length of fasting time before surgery for a breastfeeding baby.**
American Society of Anesthesiologists (ASA). "Practice guidelines for preoperative fasting and the use of pharmacologic agents to reduce the risk of pulmonary aspiration: application to healthy patients undergoing elective procedures." *Anesthesiology* 1999; 90(3):896-905.

Initial weight loss and regaining birth weight in breastfed babies.
DeMaijo, S. et al. "Initial weight loss and return to birth weight criteria for breastfed infants: challenging the 'rules of thumb.'" *Am J Dis Child* 1991; 145:402.

Page 315   **Use of breast compression.**
Newman, J. and Pitman, T. *The Ultimate Breastfeeding Book of Answers.* Roseville, California: Prima Publishing, 2000.

Use of silicone nipple shields.
Wilson-Clay, B. and Hoover, K. *The Breastfeeding Atlas,* 2nd edition. Austin, TX: LactNews Press, 2002.

Page 318   **Cup feeding as an alternative to bottles.**
Lang, S. et al. "Cup feeding: an alternative method of infant feeding." Arch Dis Child 1994; 71:365-69.

Supplementing with the mother's own milk.
Valentine, C. et al. "Hindmilk improves weight gain in low birth weight infants fed human milk." *J Ped Gastro Nutr* 1994; 18:474-77.

Page 319   **Possible causes of slow weight gain: caffeine, nicotine, hormonal contraceptives, mother's health.**
Nehlig, A. and Debry, G. "Consequences on the newborn of chronic maternal consumption of coffee during gestation and lactation: a review." *J Am Coll Nutr* 1994; 13(1):6-21.

Dahlstrom, A., et al. "Nicotine and cotinine concentrations in the nursing mother and her infant." *Acta Paediatr Scand* 1990; 79:142-47.

Erwing, P. "To use or not to use combined hormonal oral contraceptives during lactation." *Fam Plan Perspect* 1994; 26(1)26-33.

Lawrence, R. and Lawrence, R. *Breastfeeding: a Guide for the Medical Profession,* 5th edition. St. Louis: Mosby, 1999.

Page 320   **A baby with a short frenulum may have difficulty sucking correctly.**
Ballard, J. L. et al. "Ankyloglossia: assessment, incidence, and effect of frenuloplasty on the breastfeeding dyad." *Pediatrics* 2002; 110(5):e63.

Using herbs and medication to increase milk supply.
DaSilva, O. et al. "Effect of domperidone on milk production in mothers of premature newborns: a randomized, double-blind, placebo-controlled trial." *Can Med Assoc J* 2001; 164(1):17-21.

Ehrenkranz, R. and Ackerman, B. "Metoclopramide effect on faltering milk production by mothers of premature infants." *Pediatrics* 1986; 78(4):614-20.

Huggins, K. "Fenugreek: one remedy for low milk production." *Medela Rental Roundup* 1998; 15(1):16-17.

West, D. DEFINING YOUR OWN SUCCESS: BREASTFEEDING AFTER BREAST REDUCTION SURGERY. Schaumburg, IL: La Leche League International, 2001.

Rarely, a mother may not be able to produce enough milk for her baby.
Neifert, M. and Seacat, J. "Lactation insufficiency: a rational approach." *Birth* 1987; 14:182-88.

Willis, C. and Livingstone, V. "Infant insufficient milk syndrome associated with maternal postpartum hemorrhage." *J Hum Lact* 1995; 11(2):123-26.

Widdice, L. "The effects of breast reduction and breast augmentation surgery on lactation: an annotated bibliography." *J Hum Lact* 1993; 9(3):161-67.

Page 321 **Breastfed babies gain more slowly after three months of age.**
Dewey, K. et al. "Breastfed infants are leaner than formula-fed infants at one year of age: the Darling study." *Am J Clin Nutr* 1993; 57:140-45.

Page 322 **Breastfeeding is safe for a mother with hepatitis.**
American Academy of Pediatrics (AAP) Committee on Infectious Diseases. *Red Book.* 25th ed. Elk Grove Village, IL: AAP, 2000.

Breastfeeding is safe for a mother with tuberculosis.
Lawrence, R. and Lawrence, R. *Breastfeeding: a Guide for the Medical Profession,* 5th edition. St. Louis: Mosby, 1999.

Page 324 **Medications used for general anesthesia are not harmful to the nursing baby.**
Spigset, O. "Anaesthetic agents and excretion in breast milk." *Acta Anaesthesiol Scand* 1994; 38:94-103.

Sources of information about breastfeeding and medications.
American Academy of Pediatrics Committee on Drugs. "The transfer of drugs and other chemicals into human milk." *Pediatrics* 2001; 108(3):776-89.

Anderson, P. "Drug use during breastfeeding." *Clin Pharmacy* 1991; 10:594-623.

Briggs, B., Freeman, R., and Yaffe, S. *Drugs in Pregnancy and Lactation,* 6th ed. Philadelphia/London: Williams and Wilkins, 2002.

Hale, T. *Medications and Mothers' Milk,* 10th ed. Amarillo, TX: Pharmasoft, 2002.

Mohrbacher, N. and Stock, J. THE BREASTFEEDING ANSWER BOOK, 3d rev. ed. Schaumburg, IL: La Leche League International, 2003.

Rose, M. et al. "Excretion of iodine-123-hippuran, technetium-99m-red blood cells, and technetium-99m-macroaggregated albumin into breast milk." *J Nucl Med* 1990; 31:978-84.

Page 326 **Vaccines safe for nursing mothers.**
Centers for Disease Control. "General recommendations on immunization." *MMWR* 2002; 51(RR02); 1-36.

Page 327 **Immunization schedule for breastfed babies.**
Gordon, Jay. *Listening to Your Baby: A New Approach to Parenting Your Newborn.* New York: Perigee, 2002.

Breastfed babies respond better to immunizations.
Pabst, H. et al. "Differential modulation of the immune response by breast- or formula-feeding of infants." *Acta Paediatr* 1997; 86(12):1291-97.

Breastfeeding protects a baby in a smoking household from respiratory disease.
Nafstad, P. "Breastfeeding, maternal smoking and lower respiratory tract infections." *Eur Respir J* 1996; 9:2623-29.

Woodward, A. et al. "Acute respiratory illness in Adelaide children; breastfeeding modifies the effect of passive smoking." *J Epid Commun Health* 1990; 44:224-30.

Page 328   **Smoking may decrease milk production, lower prolactin levels, and interfere with the let-down reflex.**
Hopkinson, J. et al. "Milk production by mothers of premature infants: influence of cigarette smoking." *Pediatrics* 1992; 90(6):934-38.

Andersen, A. et al. "Suppressed prolactin but normal neurophysin levels in cigarette smoking breastfeeding women." *Clin Endocrinol* 1982; 17:363.

Lawrence, R. and Lawrence, R. *Breastfeeding: a Guide for the Medical Profession*, 5th edition. St. Louis: Mosby, 1999, p. 534.

Alcohol passes into mother's milk.
Lawton, M. "Alcohol in breast milk." *Aust NZ Obstet Gynecol* 1985; 25(1):71-73.

Babies sucked more but got less milk after mothers had an alcoholic drink.
Mennella, J. and Beauchamp, G. "The transfer of alcohol to human milk: effects on flavor and the infant's behavior." *N Engl J Med* 1991; 325(14):981-85.

Mennella, J. "Regulation of milk intake after exposure to alcohol in mothers' milk." *Alcohol Clin Exp Res* 2001; 25(4):590-93.

Page 329   **Substances of abuse should be avoided.**
Wilton, J. "Breastfeeding and the chemically dependent woman." *NAACOG Clin Issues Perinat Women Health Nurs* 1992; 3(4):667-82.

THC appears in human milk and baby's urine.
Perez-Reyes, M. and Wall, M. "Presence of delta-9-tetrahydrocannabinol in human milk." *N Engl J Med* 1982; 307:819-20.

Cocaine appears in mother's milk.
Chasnoff, I. et al. "Cocaine intoxication in a breastfed infant." *Pediatrics* 1987; 80:836-38.

Page 330   **Higher cognitive scores in breastfed children.**
Koopman-Esseboom, C. et al. "Effects of polychlorinated biphenyl/dixoin exposure and feeding type on infants' mental and psychomotor development." *Pediatrics* 1996; 97(5):700-6.

Rogan, W. J. and Gladen, B. C. "Breastfeeding and cognitive development." *Early Hum Dev* 1993; 31:181-93.

Levels of insecticides in human milk vary at different times.
Johansen, H.R. et al. "Congener-specific determination of polychlorinted biphenyls and organochlorine pesticides in human milk from Norwegian mothers living in Oslo." *J Tox Envir Hlth* 1994; 42:157-71.

Page 331   **Mothers with chronic illness or disabilities can breastfeed.**
Lawrence, R. and Lawrence, R. *Breastfeeding: a Guide for the Medical Profession*, 5th edition. St. Louis: Mosby, 1999.

Page 332   **Mothers may experience temporary remission of symptoms while breastfeeding.**
Butte, N. et al. "Milk composition of insulin-dependent diabetic women." *J Pediatr Gastroenterol Nutr* 1987; 6:939.

Nelson, L. "Risk of multiple sclerosis exacerbation during pregnancy and breastfeeding." *JAMA* 1988; 259:3441-43.

Page 333   **Mothers with diabetes can breastfeed.**
Gagne, M. et al. "The breastfeeding experience of women with type 1 diabetes." *Health Care Women Int* 1992; 13:249-60.

Webster, J. et al. "Breastfeeding outcomes for women with insulin-dependent diabetes." *J Hum Lact* 1995; 11(3):195-200.

Page 334   **HIV transmission rates are lower with exclusive breastfeeding than with combined feeding.**
Coutsoudis, A. et al. "Method of feeding and transmission of HIV-1 from mothers to children by 15 months of age: prospective cohort study from Durban, South Africa." *AIDS* 2001; 15(3):379-87.

Coutsoudis, A. "Morbidity in children born to women infected with human immunodeficiency virus in South Africa: Does mode of feeding matter?" *Acta Paediatr* 2003; 92:890-95.

Unanswered questions on HIV and breastfeeding.
Coutsoudis, A. and Rollins, N. "Breast-feeding and HIV transmission: the jury is still out." *J Pediatr Gastroenterol Nutr* 2003; 36:434-442.

Page 335   **Choosing an antidepressant compatible with breastfeeding.**
Birnbaum, C. et al. "Serum concentrations of antidepressants and benzodiazepines in nursing infants: a case series." *Pediatrics* 1999; 104(3):e11(1-6).

Hale, T. and Berens, P. *Clinical Therapy in Breastfeeding Patients,* 2nd ed. Amarillo, TX: Pharmasoft, 2002.

Lamberg, L. "Safety of antidepressant use in pregnant and nursing women." *JAMA* 1999; 282(3):222-23.

Newport, D. et al. "Antidepressants during pregnancy and lactation: defining exposure and treatment issues." *Sem Perinatol* 2001; 25(3):177-90.

Page 336   **Abrupt weaning may intensify depression.**
Nicholas, L. et al. "Psychoneuroendocrinology of depression: prolactin." *Psychoneuroendocrinology* 1998; 21(2):341-57.

Susman, V. and Katz, J. "Weaning and depression: another postpartum complication." *Am J Psychiatry* 1988; 145(4):498-501.

Page 341   **Mother's milk changes throughout the day.**
Harzer, G. "Changing patterns of human milk lipids in the course of lactation and during the day." *Am J Clin Nutr* 1983; 37:612-21.

Milk of mothers who give birth to preterm babies is more suited to the nutritional needs of the premie.
Lemons, J. et al. "Differences in the composition of preterm and term human milk during early lactation." *Pediatr Res* 1982; 16:113-16.

Infants sucked more vigorously after mothers consumed garlic capsules.
Menella, J. and Beauchamp, G. "Maternal diet alters sensory qualities of human milk and the nursling's behavior." *Pediatrics* 1991; 88(4):737-44.

Page 343   **Taurine's role in infant development.**
Gaull, G. E. "Taurine in the nutrition of the human infant." *Acta Paediatr Scand* 1982; 269(Suppl):38-40.

Importance of long-chain polyunsaturated fatty acids in human milk.
Birch, E. E., et al. "Breastfeeding and optimal visual development." *J Pediatr Ophthal Strab* 1993; 30:33-38.

Bjerve, K. N. et al. "Omega-3 fatty acids: essential fatty acids with important biological effects, and serum phospholipid fatty acids as markers of dietary W-3 fatty acid intake." *Am J Clin Nutr* 1993; 57(Suppl):801-95S.

Page 344   **Breastfed babies have lower cholesterol later in life.**
Bergstrom, E. et al. "Serum lipid values in adolescents are related to family history, infant feeding, and physical growth." *Atherosclerosis* 1995; 117:1-3.

Severely undernourished mothers may have milk that is lower in fat than well-nourished mothers.
Smith, C. "Effects of maternal undernutrition upon newborn infants in Holland (1944-1945)." *J Pediatr* 1947; 30:229-43.

Fat content of milk decreases as the time between feedings increases.
Woolridge, M. "Baby-controlled breastfeeding: biocultural implications," in *Breastfeeding: Biocultural Perspectives*, ed. P. Stuart Macadam and K. A. Dettwyler. New York: De Gruyter, 1995.

Page 346   **Iron absorption from human milk.**
Griffin, I. and Abrams, S. "Part 2: The management of breastfeeding: iron and breastfeeding." *Pediatr Clin N America* 2001; 48(2):1-12.

Exclusively breastfed infants were not anemic at one year of age.
Pisacane, A. et al. "Iron status in breastfed infants." *J Pediatr* 1995; 127(3):429-31.

Iron supplements may interfere with immune components in human milk.
Bullen, J. J. et al. "Iron-binding proteins in milk and resistance to escherichia coli infection in infants." *Br Med J* 1972; 1:69-75.

Page 347   **Rickets not found in breastfed infants.**
Greer, F. R. and Marshall, S. "Bone mineral content, serum vitamin D metabolite concentrations, and ultraviolet B light exposure in infants fed human milk with and without vitamin D2 supplements." *J Pediatr* 1989; 114(2):204-12.

Page 348   **A few minutes of sunshine daily prevents vitamin D deficiency.**
Specker, B. "Do North American women need supplemental vitamin D during pregnancy or lactation?" *Am J Clin Nutr* 1994; 59(Suppl):4845-915.

Specker, B. et al. "Sunshine exposure and serum 25-hydroxyvitamin D concentrations in exclusively breastfed infants." *J Pediatr* 1985; 107:372-76.

Current guidelines on vitamin D.
American Academy of Pediatrics. "Prevention of rickets and vitamin D deficiency: new guidelines for vitamin D intake." *Pediatrics* 2003; 111(4):908-10.

Zinc absorption from human milk.
Sandstrom, B. et al. "Zinc absorption from human milk, cow's milk, and infant formulas." *Am J Dis Child* 1983; 137:726-29.

American Academy of Pediatrics. "Fluoride supplementation of children: interim policy recommendations." *Pediatrics* 1995; 95(5):777.

Page 350   **Reduced morbidity and mortality in breastfed infants.**
Yoon, P. W. et al. "Effect of not breastfeeding on the risk of diarrheal and respiratory mortality in children under 2 years of age in Metro Cebu, the Philippines." *Am J Epidemiol* 1996; 143(11):1142-48.

Victora, C.G. et al. "Evidence for protection by breastfeeding against infant deaths from infectious diseases in Brazil." *Lancet* 1987; 2:319-22.

Clemens, J. D. et al. "Breastfeding and the risk of severe cholera in rural Bangladeshi children." *Am J Epidemiol* 1990; 131(3):400-11.

Page 352 **A study done in Israel on acute diarrhea.**
Lerman, Y. et al. "Epidemiology of acute diarrheal diseases in children in a high standard of living in a rural settlement in Israel." *Pediatr Infect Dis J* 1994; 13(2):116-22.

Incidence of diarrhea in breastfed and formula-fed children.
Dewey, K. G. et al. "Differences in morbidity between breastfed and formula-fed infants." *J Pediatr* 1995; 126:696-702.

Less gastrointestinal illness in infants breastfed for at least 13 weeks.
Howie, P. W. et al. "Protective effect of breastfeeding against infection." *BMJ* 300:11-16, 1990.

Page 353 **Breastfeeding protects against colds and other respiratory infections.**
Wright, A. L. et al. "Breastfeeding and lower respiratory tract illness in the first year of life." *Br Med J* 1989; 299:945-49.

Howie, P. W. et al. "Protective effect of breastfeeding against infection." *Br Med J* 1990; 300:11-16.

Respiratory infections are less severe in breastfed babies.
Cushing, A. H. et al. "Breastfeeding reduces risk of respiratory illness in infants." *Am J Epidemiol* 1998; 147:863-70.

Bachrach, V. R. G., et al. "Breastfeeding and the risk of hospitalization for respiratory disease in infancy: A meta-analysis." *Arch Pediatr Adolesc Med* 2003; 157:237-43.

Formula-fed babies are at greater risk for otitis media.
Owen, M. J. et al. "Relation of infant feeding practices, cigarette smoke exposure, and group child care to the onset and duration of otitis media with effusion in the first two years of life." *J Pediatr* 1993; 123:702-11.

Duffy, L. C. et al. "Exclusive breastfeeding protects against bacterial colonization and day care exposure to otitis media." *Pediatrics* 1997; 100:e7.

A 1998 study in Arizona found a lower risk of otitis media in breastfed babies.
Duncan, B. et al. "Exclusive breastfeeding for at least 4 months protects against otitis media." *Pediatrics* 1993; 91:867-72.

Eighty percent fewer episodes of prolonged otitis in breastfed group.
Dewey, K. G. et al. "Differences in morbidity between breastfed and formula-fed infants." *J Pediatr* 1995; 126:696-702.

Urinary tract infections more likely in formula-fed infants.
Marild, S., U. Jodal, L. and A. Hanson. "Breastfeeding and urinary tract infection [letter]." *Lancet* 1990; 336:942.

Pisacane, A. et al. "Breastfeeding and urinary tract infection." *J Pediatr* 1992; 120:87-89.

Immune factors in human milk protect urinary tract.
Hanson, L. A. "Breastfeeding stimulates the infant immune system." *Science and Medicine* 1007; 4(6):12-21.

Lower rates of chronic illness in breastfed children.
Davis, M. K. "Breastfeeding and chronic disease in childhood and adolescence." *Pediatr Clin N Am* 2001; 48(1):125-41.

Page 354 SIDS incidence higher in babies not breastfed.
Hoffman, H. J. et al. "Risk factors for SIDS: results of the National Institute of Child Health and Human Development SIDS Cooperative epidemiological study." *Ann N Y Acad Sci* 1988; 533:13-30.

Page 356 Breastfed baby receives 0.5 to 1.0 gram of IgA each day.
Hanson, L. A. "Breastfeeding stimulates the infant immune system." *Science and Medicine* 1007; 4(6):12-21.

Page 358 Human milk stimulates the development of the immune system.
Oddy, W. H. "The impact of breastmilk on infant and child health." *Breastfeeding Review* 2002; 10(3):5-18.

Mother produces antibodies for her baby.
Hanson, L. A. "Breastfeeding stimulates the infant immune system." *Science and Medicine* 1997; 4(6):12-21.

Live cells from human milk survive in the infant's gastrointestinal tract.
Oddy, W. H. "The impact of breastmilk on infant and child health." *Breastfeeding Review* 2002; 10(3):5-18.

Page 359 Exclusively breastfed babies have fewer allergies.
Merrett, T. G. et al. "Infant feeding and allergy: 12-month prospective study of 500 babies born into allergic families." *Ann Allergy* 1988; 61:13-20.

Lucas, A. et al. "Early diet of preterm infants and development of allergic atopic disease: randomized prospective study." *Br Med J* 1990; 300:837-40.

Halken, S., A. Host, L. Hansen, et al. "Effect of an allergy prevention programme on incidence of atopic symptoms in infancy." *Ann Allergy* 1992; 47:545-33.

Saarinen, U. M. et al. "Breastfeeding as prophylaxis against atopic disease: propsective follow-up study until 17 years old." *Lancet* 1995; 346(8982):1065-69.

Wright, A. L. et al. "Epidemiology of physician-diagnosed allergic rhinitis in childhood." *Pediatrics* 1994; 94(6):895-901.

Page 360 Continued breastfeeding protects against celiac disease.
Ivarsson, A. et al. "Breastfeeding protects against celiac disease." *Am J Clin Nutr* 2002; 75:914-21.

Page 363 Can baby react to something mother eats?
Gerrard, J. W. "Allergies in breastfed babies to foods ingested by the mother." *Clin Rev Allergy* 1985; 2-143-49.

Jakobsson, I. and Lindberg, T. "Cows' milk proteins cause colic in breastfed babies: a double-blind crossover study." *Pediatrics* 1983; 71:268-71.

Lust, K. et al. "Maternal intake of cruciferous vegetables and other foods and colic symptoms in exclusively breastfed infants." *J Am Diet Assoc* 1996; 96(1):46-48.

Clyne, P. and Kulczycki, A. "Human breast milk contains bovine IgG: relationship to infant colic?" *Pediatrics* 1991; 87(4):439-44.

Page 366 Higher IQ in premature infants fed human milk.
Lucas, A. et al. "A randomised multicentre study of human milk versus formula and later development in preterm infants." *Arch Dis Child* 1994; 70:F141.46.

Studies on intellectual development.
Anderson, J. W. et al. "Breastfeeding and cognitive development: a meta-analysis." *Am J Clin Nutr* 1999; 70:525-35.

Mortensen, E. L. et al. "The association between duration of breastfeeding and adult intelligence." *JAMA* 2002; 28(15): 2365-71.

Page 367   Breastfeeding protects against malocclusion.
Labbok, M. H. and Hendershot, G. E. "Does breastfeeding protect against malocclusion? An analysis of the 1981 Child Health Supplement to the National Health Interview Survey." *Am J Prev Med* 1987; 3:227-32.

Davis, D. et al. "Infant feeding practices and occlusal outcomes: a longitudinal study." *J Can Dent Assoc* 1991; 57(7):593-94.

Page 368   Breastfed babies less likely to be obese in adolescence.
Gillman, M. W. et al. "Risk of overweight among adolescents who were breastfed as infants." *JAMA* 2001; 285:2461-67.

Endorphins in human milk.
Zanardo, V. et al. "Beta endorphin concentrations in human milk." *J Pediatr Gastroenterol Nutr* 2001; 23(2):160-64.

Lower pain scores in babies who were breastfeeding.
Carbajal, R. et al. "Analgesic effect of breastfeeding in term neonates: randomised controlled trial." *BMJ* 2003; 326:13-15.

Page 372   An empty breast makes milk faster.
Daly, S. E. et al. "The determination of short-term breast volume changes and the rate of synthesis of human milk using computerized breast measurement." *Exp Physiol* 1992; 77:79-87.

Wilde, C. J. "Autocrine regulation of milk secretion by a protein in milk." *Biochem J* 1995; 305:51.

Milk storage capacity.
Cregan, M. and Hartmann, P. "Computerized breast measurement from conception to weaning: clinical implications." *J Hum Lact* 1999; 15(2):89-96.

Daly, S. et al. "The short-term synthesis and infant-regulated removal of milk in lactating women." *Exp Physiology* 1993; 78:209-20.

Infants can regulate their own food intake.
Marasco, L. and Barger, J. "Cue feeding: wisdom and science." BREASTFEEDING ABSTRACTS 1999;18(4):27-28.

Page 374   Increased number of prolactin receptor cells.
De Coopman, J. "Breastfeeding after pituitary resection: Support for a theory of autocrine control of milk supply?" *J Hum Lact* 1993; 9(1):35-40.

Perry, H. M. and Jacobs, L. S. "Rabbit mammary prolactin receptors." *J Biologic Chem* 1978; 253:1560.

Ultrasound study of the milk-ejection reflex.
Kent, J. "Physiology of the expression of breast milk, part 2." Presented at the Medela Innovations in Breast Pump Research Conference, Boca Raton, Florida, July 2002.

Page 375   Fat content decreases as the amount of time between feedings increases.
Woolridge, M. "Baby-controlled breastfeeding: biocultural implications," in *Breastfeeding: Biocultural Perspectives*, ed. P. Stuart Macadam and K. A. Dettwyler. New York: De Gruyter, 1995.

Breastfeeding helps a mother deal with stress.
Altremus, M. et al. "Suppression of hypothalmic-pituitary-adrenal axis responses to stress in lactating women." *J Clin Endocrinol Metab* 1995; 80(9):2954-59.

Page 376   **The milk ejection reflex.**
Newton, M. and Newton, N. R. "The let-down reflex in human lactation." *J Pediatr* 1948; 33:698-704.

Oxytocin levels increased when babies became restless.
McNeilly, A. S. et al. "Release of oxytocin and prolactin in response to suckling." *BMJ* 1980; 281:834.

Page 377   **Breastfed babies consume less milk and grow more slowly.**
Butte, N. et al. "Human milk intake and growth in exclusively breastfed infants." *J Pediatr* 1984; 104:187-95.

Dewey, K. et al. "Growth of breastfed and formula-fed infants from 0 to 18 months." The DARLING study. *Pediatrics* 1992; 89(6):1035-41.

Page 378   **Calcium metabolism during lactation.**
Kalkwarf, H. J. et al. "Intestinal calcium absorption of women during lactation and after weaning." *Am J Clin Nutr* 1996; 63(4):526-31.

Sinigaglia, L. et al. "Effect of lactation on postmenopausal bone mineral density of lumbar spine." *J Reprod Med* 1996; 41(6):439-43.

Henderson, P. et al. "Bone mineral density in grand multiparous women with extended lactation." *Am J Obstet Gynecol* 2000; 182(6):1371-77.

Lower risk of hip fracture in women who breastfed.
Cumming, R. and Klineberg, R. "Breastfeeding and other reproductive factors and the risk of hip fractures in elderly women." *Int J Epidemiol* 1993; 22(4):684-91.

Page 380   **Breastfeeding delays fertility.**
Kippley, Sheila. *Breastfeeding and Natural Child Spacing.* Cincinnati, OH: Couple-to-Couple League International, Inc., 1999.

Lactational amenorrhea method of contraception.
Labbok, M. "The lactational amenorrhea method (LAM): another choice for breastfeeding mothers." BREASTFEEDING ABSTRACTS 1993; 13:3-4.

Page 381   **LAM for employed mothers.**
Valdes, V. et al. "The efficacy of the lactational amenorrhea method (LAM) among working women." *Contraception* 2000; 62:217-19.

Page 382   **Estrogen decreases milk supply.**
Tankeyoon, M. et al. "Effects of hormonal contraceptives on milk volumes and infant growth: WHO Special Programme of Research, Development, and Research Training in Human Reproduction Task Force on Oral Contraceptives." *Contraception* 1984; 30(6): 505-22.

Progestin-only contraception may affect milk production.
Nichols-Johnson, V. "The breastfeeding dyad and contraception." BREASTFEEDING ABSTRACTS 2001; 21(2):11.

Long-term effects of hormonal contraceptives on breastfed babies.
Harlap, S. "Exposure to contraceptive hormones through breast milk: are there long-term health and behavioral consequences?" *Int J Gynecol Obstet* 1987; 25(Suppl):47-55.

Study combines and reanalyzes data on breastfeeding and breast cancer.
Collaborative Group on Hormonal Factors in Breast Cancer. "Breast cancer and breastfeeding: collaborative reanalysis of individual data from 47 epidemiological studies in 30 countries, including 50,302 women with breast cancer and 96,973 women without the disease." *Lancet* 2002; 360:187-95.

Page 383   **Women who were breastfed have a lower risk of breast cancer.**
Freudenheim, J. et al. "Exposure to breast milk in infancy and the risk of breast cancer." *Epidemiology* 1994; 5(3):324-31.

Recent estimates of the cost of buying infant formula.
Breastfeeding Support Consultants. *Information on Infant Feeding Costs.* April 1998 (based on Illinois and North Carolina suburban supermarket prices).

Page 384   **Calculations of savings in the USA if more women breastfed.**
Weimer, D. *The Economic Benefits of Breastfeeding: A Review and Analysis. Economic Research Service.* US Department of Agriculture, Food Assistance and Nutrition Research Report No. 13. March 2001.

Worldwide savings
Palmer, G. *The Politics of Breastfeeding.* London: Pandora Press, 1999.

Page 387   **Pleasure of breastfeeding.**
Whipple, D. V. "Breastfeeding in today's world." *J Am Med Women Assoc* 1965; 10:936-37.

Page 389   **Baby's responses.**
Fraiberg, S. "How a baby learns to love." *Redbook* 1971.

Photos on the following pages are by David Arendt:
3, 7, 33, 35, 43, 45, 48, 49, 52, 53, 59, 69, 71, 77, 79, 85, 91, 93, 95, 100, 106, 119, 130, 137, 147, 149, 151, 153, 156, 164, 167, 169, 172, 175, 179, 187, 189, 191, 193, 197, 199, 203, 205, 207, 213, 233, 235, 239, 243, 250, 253, 255, 257, 262, 264, 267, 269, 292, 295, 297, 307, 331, 337, 341, 343, 365, 371, 373, 376, 379, 382, 385, 387, 406, 410.

Other photos by:

Page 5, Eric Walsworth

Pages 10, 17, 223, 231, 355, Subhadra Tidball

Pages 13, 21, 39, Mimi de Maza

Pages 15, 31, 183, 260, 313, 319, Judy Torgus

Page 18, Choice Photography by Edie Simon

Pages 63, 65, 67, 109, 111, 217, 281, 309, 391, 408, Kim Cavaliero

Pages 97, 393, 398, 400, 401, 403, 404, 405, Rae Cassin

Page 102, William Sears

Page 123, 181, 322, 347, John T. Franklin III

Page 140, Daria Amato

Page 195, Josh Smith

Page 210, Darrell Rideout

Page 221, 225, Erik Haskins

Page 228, Bill Finnerty

Page 273, Katy Lebbing

Page 276, Peggy Eaton

Page 283, Gene Cranston Anderson

Would You Like to Know More?

As you read this book, you find that La Leche League is mentioned over and over again as a source of information, support, and encouragement. La Leche League Groups meet monthly in communities all over the world to share breastfeeding and mothering experiences. Call 1-800-LA LECHE for a referral to a local LLL Group. Or visit the LLL Web Site at www.lalecheleague.org.

Perhaps you'd like to be a part of this mother-to-mother network. It is easy to become an LLL Member. Just return the coupon below along with your annual membership fee. You will receive six bimonthly issues of NEW BEGINNINGS, a magazine filled with personal stories, helpful hints, and up-to-date parenting information. Members automatically receive our LLLI Catalogues by mail and they are entitled to a 10% discount on most purchases. You don't need to attend Group meetings in order to join—though most members enjoy the interaction with other mothers that meetings provide.

Why should you join La Leche League? Because you care—about your own family and about mothers and babies all over the world.

Return this form to:

La Leche League International,
Post Office Box 4079, Schaumburg, IL 60168-4079 USA
* In Canada, write to LLLC National Office,
   18C Industrial Drive, Box 29, Chesterville, Ontario K0C 1H0

☐ I'd like to join La Leche League International. Enclosed is my annual membership of $36.

☐ In addition, I am enclosing a tax-deductible donation of
   $_____ to support the work of La Leche League.

☐ Please send me a copy of THE WOMANLY ART OF BREASTFEEDING, softcover $16.95 plus $4.25 for shipping and handling. (In California and Illinois, please add sales tax.)

☐ Please send me the La Leche League FREE Catalogue.

Name _____

Address _____

State/Province _____   Zip/Postal Code _____

Country _____

Prices may vary outside the USA.   1-04